D1036056

Autism
Spectrum
Disorder

Autism
Spectrum
Disorder

Edited by

Martin J. Lubetsky, MD
Western Psychiatric Institute and Clinic of UPMC
University of Pittsburgh School of Medicine
Pittsburgh, PA

Benjamin L. Handen, PhD, BCBA-D
Western Psychiatric Institute and Clinic of UPMC
University of Pittsburgh School of Medicine
Pittsburgh, PA

John J. McGonigle, PhD
Western Psychiatric Institute and Clinic of UPMC
University of Pittsburgh School of Medicine
Pittsburgh, PA

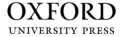

OXFORD
UNIVERSITY PRESS

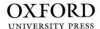

OXFORD
UNIVERSITY PRESS

Oxford University Press, Inc., publishes works that further
Oxford University's objective of excellence
in research, scholarship, and education.

Oxford New York
Auckland Cape Town Dar es Salaam Hong Kong Karachi
Kuala Lumpur Madrid Melbourne Mexico City Nairobi
New Delhi Shanghai Taipei Toronto

With offices in

Argentina Austria Brazil Chile Czech Republic France Greece
Guatemala Hungary Italy Japan Poland Portugal Singapore
South Korea Switzerland Thailand Turkey Ukraine Vietnam

Copyright © 2011 by Oxford University Press, Inc.

Published by Oxford University Press, Inc.
198 Madison Avenue, New York, New York 10016

www.oup.com

Oxford is a registered trademark of Oxford University Press

Library of Congress Cataloging-in-Publication Data

Autism spectrum disorder / edited by Martin J. Lubetsky, Benjamin L. Handen, John J. McGonigle.
    p. ; cm. — (Pittsburgh pocket psychiatry series)
  Includes bibliographical references and index.
  ISBN 978-0-19-975385-7 (alk. paper)
  1. Autism in children—Diagnosis. 2. Autism in children—Treatment. I. Lubetsky, Martin J.
II. Handen, Benjamin L. III. McGonigle, John J. IV. Series: Pittsburgh pocket psychiatry series.
  [DNLM: 1. Autistic Disorder—diagnosis. 2. Adolescent. 3. Autistic Disorder—therapy.
4. Child. WS 350.6]
  RJ506.A9A92374 2011
  618.92'85882—dc22   2010054146

9 8 7 6 5 4 3 2 1

Printed in the United States of America
on acid-free paper

To the children, adolescents and adults with autism and their families with whom we have worked and who teach us so much.

Series Introduction

We stand on the threshold of a new Golden Age of clinical and behavioral neuroscience with psychiatry at its fore. With the Pittsburgh Pocket Psychiatry series, we intend to encompass the breadth and depth of our current understanding of human behavior in health and disease. Using the structure of resident didactic teaching, we will be able to ensure that each subject area relevant for both current and future practicing psychiatrists is detailed and described. New innovations in diagnosis and treatment will be reviewed and discussed in the context of existing knowledge, and each book in the series will propose new directions for scientific inquiry and discovery. The aim of the series as a whole is to integrate findings from all areas of medicine and neuroscience previously segregated as "mind" or "body," "psychological" or "biological." Thus, each book from the Pittsburgh Pocket Psychiatry series will stand alone as a standard text for anyone wishing to learn about a specific subject area. The series will be the most coherent and flexible learning resource available.

David J. Kupfer, MD
Michael J. Travis, MD
Michelle S. Horner, DO

About Autism Spectrum Disorder

It has been our experience that many professionals are seeking additional training in working with individuals who have autism spectrum disorder (ASD). With a prevalence rate of one in 110 people having a diagnosis of ASD, more medical, behavioral health, and allied health care professionals are needed to serve this growing population. Consequently, there is a need for increased training in ASD, especially for psychiatry residents and child and adolescent psychiatry fellows, as well as residents in pediatrics, neurology, family medicine, internal medicine, and other fields in medicine. Medical schools are increasingly recognizing the importance of training physicians in how to screen, diagnose, and treat individuals with ASD. Primary care physicians are more frequently being expected to provide early identification and ongoing care for individuals with ASD. In addition, allied health care professionals, such as psychologists, dentists, speech and language specialists, occupational therapists, and physical therapists, as well as educators and teachers, are more involved in providing services to this population. In the future, adult health care professionals will provide clinical care to an increasing number of adults with ASD.

It is our goal in writing and editing *Autism Spectrum Disorder–Pittsburgh Pocket Psychiatry Series* to compile relevant and useful instruction from educators, clinicians, and researchers at Western Psychiatric Institute and Clinic (WPIC), University of Pittsburgh Medical Center (UPMC), the University of Pittsburgh, and the School of Medicine. Throughout the text we will refer to autism spectrum disorder as ASD (the term "autism" will be used in the chapter on historical perspective). With the upcoming changes in DSM-5 (Diagnostic and Statistical Manual of Mental Disorders–5, American Psychiatric Association), the separate diagnostic classifications under "pervasive developmental disorder" (PDD) may be subsumed under one category of ASD (DSM-5 Workgroup, APA). ASD will now include autistic disorder (autism), Asperger's disorder, childhood disintegrative disorder, and pervasive developmental disorder—not otherwise specified. Also, we will refer to "intellectual disability" rather than the old terminology of "mental retardation," which is also likely to be changed in DSM-5.

The reader will find a standard format for each chapter. Key Fact boxes summarize pertinent points to remember. Tables and diagrams are used to organize selected important information. Questions are located at the end of each chapter to test the reader's knowledge, and each chapter has further readings to help enhance understanding.

We hope that the reader will gain clinically useful knowledge from *Autism Spectrum Disorder—Pittsburgh Pocket Psychiatry Series* and will share it with other professionals, and that families will find it useful as well.

Martin J. Lubetsky, Benjamin L. Handen, and John J. McGonigle
Pittsburgh, Pennsylvania, 2011

Contents

1 Autism—Historical Perspective, Theories,
  and DSM Diagnostic Criteria   **3**
    Tiberiu Bodea and Martin J. Lubetsky

2 Recognition of Autism Spectrum
  Disorder—Early Identification and Diagnosis   **19**
    *John J. McGonigle, Virginia Martin, and
    Martin J. Lubetsky*

3 Medical Evaluation and Comorbid
  Psychiatric Disorders   **41**
    *Carla A. Mazefsky, Robyn Filipink,
    Jodi Lindsey, and Martin J. Lubetsky*

4 Neurobiology of Autism Spectrum Disorder   **85**
    *Kathryn McFadden, Nancy J. Minshew, and
    K. Suzanne Scherf*

5 Functional Behavioral Assessment (FBA)   **115**
    *Jennifer B. Alfieri, Rebecca Burkley, and
    John J. McGonigle*

6 Introduction to Treatment Chapters:
  Treatment Overview   **135**
    *Benjamin L. Handen, Johanna Taylor,
    Kylan Turner, and Martin J. Lubetsky*

7 Early Childhood Interventions   **147**
    *Louise A. Kaczmarek, Kylan Turner, and
    Jennifer B. Alfieri*

8 Language Interventions   **173**
    Diane L. Williams and Lori J. Marra

9 Feeding, Sleep, and Toileting Interventions 193
  Kristine Kielar, Cynthia R. Johnson, and
  Benjamin L. Handen

10 Educational Issues: School-Age 215
  Michelle Lubetsky, Virginia Martin, and
  Benjamin L. Handen

11 Transition-Age and Adult Interventions 231
  John J. McGonigle, Allen Meade Gregory, and
  Martin J. Lubetsky

12 Addressing Behavioral and
  Emotional Challenges in School-Age
  Children and Adolescents with ASD 253
  Carla A. Mazefsky and Benjamin L. Handen

13 Social Challenges and Social Skills Interventions 271
  Michelle Lubetsky, Melissa Smiley Jacobson, and
  Benjamin L. Handen

14 Pharmacological Interventions 295
  Benjamin L. Handen, Tiberiu Bodea,
  Rameshwari V. Tumuluru, and Martin J. Lubetsky

Future Directions 325
  Martin J. Lubetsky, Benjamin L. Handen,
  John J. McGonigle, and co-authors

Index *329*

Contributors

Jennifer B. Alfieri, MS, BCBA
Western Psychiatric Institute and
Clinic of UPMC
Pittsburgh, PA

Tiberiu Bodea, MD
Western Psychiatric Institute and
Clinic of UPMC
University of Pittsburgh School of
Medicine
Pittsburgh, PA

Rebecca Burkley, MS
Western Psychiatric Institute and
Clinic of UPMC
Pittsburgh, PA

Robyn Filipink, MD
Division of Child Neurology
Children's Hospital of Pittsburgh
of UPMC
University of Pittsburgh School of
Medicine
Pittsburgh, PA

Allen Meade Gregory, MA
Western Psychiatric Institute and
Clinic of UPMC
Pittsburgh, PA

**Benjamin L. Handen, PhD,
BCBA-D**
Western Psychiatric Institute and
Clinic of UPMC
University of Pittsburgh School of
Medicine
Pittsburgh, PA

**Melissa Smiley Jacobson,
MSW, LCSW**
Western Psychiatric Institute and
Clinic of UPMC
Pittsburgh, PA

**Cynthia R. Johnson, PhD,
BCBA-D**
Departments of Pediatrics and
Psychiatry
Children's Hospital
of UPMC
University of Pittsburgh School of
Medicine
Pittsburgh, PA

Louise A. Kaczmarek, PhD
Department of Instruction &
Learning
School of Education
University of Pittsburgh
Pittsburgh, PA

Kristine Kielar, MS, BCBA
Western Psychiatric
Institute and Clinic
of UPMC
Pittsburgh, PA

Jodi Lindsey, MD
Department of Pediatrics
Children's Hospital of Pittsburgh
of UPMC
University of Pittsburgh School of
Medicine
Pittsburgh, PA

Martin J. Lubetsky, MD
Western Psychiatric Institute and
Clinic of UPMC
University of Pittsburgh
School of Medicine
Pittsburgh, PA

**Michelle Lubetsky, MEd,
BCBA**
Allegheny Intermediate
Unit
Homestead, PA

Lori J. Marra, MA, CCC-SLP
Department of Speech-Language
  Pathology
Duquesne University
Pittsburgh, PA

Virginia Martin, PsyD
Western Psychiatric Institute and
  Clinic of UPMC
Pittsburgh, PA

Carla A. Mazefsky, PhD
Western Psychiatric Institute and
  Clinic of UPMC
University of Pittsburgh
  School of Medicine
Pittsburgh, PA

Kathryn McFadden, MD
Department of Pathology
University of Pittsburgh
  School of Medicine
Pittsburgh, PA

John J. McGonigle, PhD
Western Psychiatric Institute and
  Clinic of UPMC
University of Pittsburgh
  School of Medicine
Pittsburgh, PA

Nancy J. Minshew, MD
Departments of Psychiatry and
  Neurology
Western Psychiatric Institute and
  Clinic of UPMC
University of Pittsburgh
  School of Medicine
Pittsburgh, PA

K. Suzanne Scherf, PhD
Center for the Neural
  Basis of Cognition
Department of
  Psychology
Carnegie Mellon
  University
Pittsburgh, PA

Johanna Taylor, MEd, BCBA
Department of Instruction &
  Learning
University of Pittsburgh
  School of Education
Pittsburgh, PA

**Rameshwari V. Tumuluru,
MD**
Western Psychiatric
  Institute and Clinic
  of UPMC
University of Pittsburgh
  School of Medicine
Pittsburgh, PA

Kylan Turner, MEd, BCBA
Department of Instruction &
  Learning
University of Pittsburgh
  School of Education
Pittsburgh, PA

**Diane L. Williams, PhD,
CCC-SLP**
Department of Speech-Language
  Pathology
Duquesne University
Pittsburgh, PA

Autism
Spectrum
Disorder

Autism—Historical Perspective, Theories, and DSM Diagnostic Criteria

Tiberiu Bodea and Martin J. Lubetsky

Early Observations of Autistic-like Behaviors 5

Leo Kanner (1894–1981): The Introduction of the Concept of "Autism" 6

Hans Asperger (1906–1980): Identification of Asperger's Disorder 7

Kanner and Asperger: Similarities and Differences 8

Refuting the "Psychogenic Theory" of Autism 10

History of "Autism" and "Pervasive Developmental Disorder" as Diagnostic Categories in the Diagnostic and Statistical Manual of Mental Disorders 12

Future Directions—DSM-5 14

Further Reading 15

Questions 16

Answers 17

Autism is a developmental neurobiological disorder characterized by severe and pervasive impairments in reciprocal social interaction skills and communication skills (verbal and nonverbal), and by restricted, repetitive, and stereotyped behavior, interests, and activities. The current DSM-IV-TR (Diagnostic and Statistical Manual of Mental Disorders–IV, American Psychiatric Association) applies "pervasive developmental disorder" (PDD) as the diagnostic umbrella, with five subtypes. With the upcoming proposed changes in DSM-5, the separate diagnostic classifications under PDD may be subsumed under one category, "autism spectrum disorder" (ASD—www.dsm5.org). ASD would include autistic disorder (autism), Asperger's disorder, childhood disintegrative disorder, and pervasive developmental disorder—not otherwise specified. Rett's disorder is proposed to be removed, as it is now recognized as a genetic disorder.

Throughout this book, the diagnostic label of autism spectrum disorder (ASD) will be used, except the term "autism" makes historical sense in this chapter. Also, "intellectual disability" will be used rather than the old terminology of "mental retardation," which is also likely to be changed in DSM-5. This chapter will describe the early pioneering advances in the field, a retrospective review of the theoretical systems that have been proposed, and the rationale that leads to current knowledge of this condition. Understanding the evolution of autism as a concept, and reviewing the efforts that have been made over the last seven decades to describe and treat children with autism, will help us conceptualize and appreciate the tremendous advances in understanding this disorder. (Details regarding assessment will be found in the next chapter.)

Early Observations of Autistic-like Behaviors

Ever since autism was introduced as a distinct nosological category in the psychiatric literature more than 60 years ago, efforts have been made to historically recount the existence and observations of the disorder.

Descriptions of individuals with features of autism have been reported as early as the mid 1700s (Itard's Victor, "the wild boy of Aveyron"). It was not until the 1940s that the term *autism* was applied to these children (Kanner), drawing from work in schizophrenia (Bleuler). *Autism* and *autistic* stem from the Greek word *autos*, meaning "self." The term *autism* originally referred to a basic disturbance, an extreme withdrawal of oneself from social life, or aloneness. The common feature of this disturbance was that the children seemed unable to develop normal relationships with other people, and that the symptoms appeared from birth.

Among the modern historians who studied the evidence of features of autism in individuals, Professor Uta Frith made a significant contribution in documenting the existence of autism-like features in historical data from Europe. In her works *Autism: Explaining the Enigma* (1991) and *Autism in History: The Case of Hugh Blair of Borgue* (2000), Frith documented two famous cases of individuals with autistic-like symptoms, one in eighteenth-century Scotland, the other one in eighteenth-century France.

Hugh Blair lived in Scotland, and at the age of 39, in 1747, he appeared in court in a case regarding his mental capacities to contract a marriage. Frith analyzed documents, and based on these materials, proposed that Blair displayed symptoms that today would be classified as autism-like, including odd mannerisms, repetitive language, echolalia, collecting objects, poor social relationships, and abnormal gaze.

The second autistic-like case that Frith described was that of Victor, the wild boy of Aveyron. Victor was found in the woods at the age of 12 (1797), and could not speak, but produced bizarre noises, had very poor social skills, and displayed overactive and impulsive behaviors. These characteristics were described by Jean Marc Gaspard Itard, the physician who took care of the boy. Itard's description suggests autistic symptoms, such as impairments in reciprocal social interaction, sensory difficulties, lack of imaginative play, and presence of stereotypies. However, the argument for interpreting Victor's symptoms as an autism-like case is confounded by his being a "feral" child and thereby likely to be suffering from attachment impairments.

Disparate reports of autistic-like behaviors were made throughout the eighteenth and nineteenth centuries. In 1809, John Haslam published *Cases of Insane Children*, in which he presented the symptoms of a seven-year-old boy who had social skills problems, expressive language difficulties, abnormal gaze, echolalia, and solitary play, all suggestive of an autism-like disorder. Also, Henry Maudsley in the 1879 edition of *The Pathology of Mind* described "The insanity of early life" of children who were latere referenced by Leo Kanner as "autistic". Despite the existence of such reports, it was only in the mid–twentieth century that the neuropsychiatric category of "autism" was established.

Leo Kanner (1894–1981): The Introduction of the Concept of "Autism"

The critical point in the scientific history of autism was in 1943, when Leo Kanner published *Autistic Disturbances of Affective Conduct*, a groundbreaking paper that described the symptoms of 11 children presenting similar behaviors that had not been previously recognized. The pattern of these symptoms formed a characteristic presentation that was distinct from that of any then-recognized disorder in the medical literature.

- Disturbances in speech acquisition, difficulty with using speech, echolalia, stereotypy, and obsessive insistence on sameness
- The majority of the cases were boys; only three out of the eleven children were girls
- The presence of macrocephaly in five of the eleven children
- All the children in the group had "an innate inability to form the usual biologically provided affective contact with people"

To define the newly identified syndrome, Kanner used the term "autism," drawing inspiration from Bleuler's influential work in schizophrenia. Several historians consider that this choice of "autism" was an unfortunate one, as it led to confusion between autism and schizophrenia. Based on Kanner's terminology, autism was considered for years a psychosis, and child psychiatrists were using "childhood schizophrenia" and "child psychosis" in autism as "interchangeable diagnoses."

Over the next 30 years following his initial descriptions of autism, Kanner and his collaborator, Leon Eisenberg, followed more than a hundred cases of children suspected of having autistic symptoms. They conducted comparisons of these cases with those of children with aphasia and communication issues. Based on this work, in 1956, Eisenberg and Kanner proposed two fundamental criteria for diagnosing autistic disorder that were observed to occur from the beginning of life:

- Inability of the autistic child to relate in an ordinary way to people and situations; and
- Inability to learn to speak, or to convey meaning to others by means of language.

Hans Asperger (1906–1980): Identification of Asperger's Disorder

A parallel line of inquiry to that of Kanner and Eisenberg is represented by the work of Hans Asperger. On October 8, 1948, Hans Asperger, who was working at that time in Vienna University Hospital, gave a lecture based on his clinical studies in which he described the "autistic psychopaths." In 1944, Asperger had independently described a condition resembling Kanner's 1943 "autism," which Asperger named "autistic psychopathy," featuring:

- Difficulties in social integration, and
- Oddities of speech and gaze.

According to historical studies, Asperger's paper was not known by the international medical community, as it was written in German in the specific context of World War II. In 1981, Lorna Wing published a seminal paper titled "Asperger's Syndrome: A Clinical Account," in which she acknowledged the contribution of Hans Asperger, and proposed a diagnostic entity that she termed "Asperger's syndrome."

Kanner and Asperger: Similarities and Differences

In *Autism and Pervasive Developmental Disorders*, Fred Volkmar and Catherine Lord (2004) distinguished important points of differentiation and similarities between Kanner's and Asperger's descriptions. These are summarized in Table 1.1.

In concluding their comparison of Kanner's and Asperger's descriptions, Volkmar and Lord pondered whether, despite the relevant differences, it was "scientifically and clinically helpful to classify individuals with these traits into separate categories of autism or Asperger's disorder, or whether it would be better to treat them as parts of a greater continuum." The utility of the "greater continuum" has led to the category of autism spectrum disorder to be proposed for DSM-5.

According to DSM-IV-TR, the category of "pervasive developmental disorders" subsumes autistic disorder and Asperger's disorder, as well as two other conditions: childhood disintegrative disorder and Rett's disorder.

Childhood Disintegrative Disorder

In 1908 in Vienna, Theodore Heller described a condition that he initially called "dementia infantilis," currently known as childhood disintegrative disorder. What Heller was describing were children previously normal and typical in their development who were starting to lose developmental gains and to present "autistic-like" features. Heller stated that that affected children may lose the mental-intellectual functioning and may be at increased risk of seizures. Today this condition is considered very uncommon, with most recent reports indicating a prevalence of just two out of 100,000. Some estimates suggest that only about 100 cases have been reported since Heller's original description in 1908.

Childhood disintegrative disorder is a diagnosis in both DSM-IV-TR and International Classification of Diseases-10 (ICD-10). It is a condition difficult to distinguish from autism once it develops, and is characterized by a dramatic worsening of developmental status while the child presents

Table 1.1. Similarities and Differences—Kanner vs. Asperger

Autism (Kanner)	Asperger's Disorder
• suggested that the condition was congenital	• described the syndrome as clinically apparent after the age of three or four years
• language skills tend not to be advanced, or the individuals affected are even nonverbal	• language skills are usually an area of strength
• in autism the verbal IQ is lower, or on a par with nonverbal IQ	• associated with higher verbal IQ

autistic-like behaviors. It has been proposed that the disorder be subsumed under the autism spectrum disorder category in DSM-5. By incorporating a new dimension of presence/absence of regression in ASD, DSM-5 will offer the criterion for capturing cases with profound regression that is a characteristic of childhood disintegrative disorder.

Rett's Disorder

In 1966, Andreas Rett, an Austrian neurologist, described an unusual syndrome present exclusively in girls, characterized by a brief period of normal development followed by microcephaly, loss of purposeful hand movements, and severe psychomotor retardation. About 80% of the children suffering from Rett's disorder also have seizures. They present with severe verbal deficits and gross motor impairments.

Today, it is considered that most cases of Rett's disorder are caused by mutations in the MeCP2 gene. This gene provides instructions for making a protein: methyl CpG binding protein 2 (MeCP2) that plays a role in forming synapses and regulating the expression of other genes in the brain, and also controlling the production of other proteins in nerve cells. In more than 90% of the cases the mutation is de novo; that is, not inherited from either parent.

Rett's disorder is classified by DSM-IV-TR as a pervasive developmental disorder due to its characteristic autistic-like behaviors and cognitive impairment. The DSM-5 work group is recommending that this disorder be removed from the ASD category.

Refuting the "Psychogenic Theory" of Autism

In the early descriptions of autism, Kanner discerned a biological under-lying cause for the condition as well as a genetic risk for autism. At that time, however, there were no means to scientifically prove the genetic or biological factors. Kanner was also concerned with the psychological risks associated with autism, and in this respect he emphasized three relevant areas: social isolation, insistence on sameness, and abnormal language skills.

Kanner remarked that parents of children with autism were generally intelligent and of higher social status, aspects that subsequently proved to be the result of biases in his perception. By examining the family functioning of children with autism, Kanner described "the mechanization of human relationships" in the respective families' environment, and he suspected a lack of parental warmth in their interactions with the child. He hypothesized that autistic children received inadequate parenting and were seeking affection and comforting in their solitude.

Following these initial psychogenic hypotheses, a major trend in psychodynamic research on autistic children developed. Gutenberg, for instance, hypothesized that autism was "a disorder of emotional development" that "disturbs the child's progression through developmental stages." As the psychodynamic and psychoanalytical research in autism expanded, many hypotheses pointed toward the lack of nurturing mothering of the autistic children. In 1952, Mahler proposed that autistic children did not differentiate their mothers from inanimate objects, and therefore could not establish emotional ties with others.

Throughout the 1950s and 1960s, as the field grew, a popular hypothesis stated that children with autism suffered from nonspecific vulnerabilities that, in the absence of adequate environmental support, determined the autistic symptoms. Bruno Bettelheim wrote about cold, unresponsive parents and questioned whether this parenting style could cause or unmask a child's autistic disorder. In 1967, Bettelheim advanced the idea in *An Empty Fortress* that "any biological abnormalities present in children with autism were effects rather than causes of the disorder" and hypothesized that autism was a reaction to "emotional deprivation." He compared the emotional deprivation that he suspected with the trauma and deprivation suffered by victims of concentration camps, of which he was a survivor himself. Researchers such as Gary Mesibov, Victoria Shea, Lynn Adams, and Laura Klinger (1998) suggested that in fact this personal experience of Bettelheim's may have contributed to his emphasis on the emotional factors resulting in biological consequences and causing autistic behaviors.

Today it is considered that these theories unjustly burdened parents of children with autism who were looking for treatment, supports, and resources. The psychogenic etiology of autism, which postulated that sub-optimal parenting styles were responsible, was decisively refuted by Michael Rutter. In 1967, Rutter published his research comparing autistic children and children with difficulties in bonding due to long-term institutionalization who did not develop autistic-like behaviors. In 1979, Rutter in collaboration with Dennis Cantwell and Lorian Baker, demonstrated that parents of children with autism and parents of children with dysphasia were no different in their intensity and frequency of positive interactions, quality family interactions, and type or degree of mother–child interactions.

The "psychogenic theory" of autism was popular and widely accepted until Bernard Rimland published his book *Infantile Autism: The Syndrome and Its Implications for a Neural Theory of Behavior* (1964). In it, Rimland proposed that a biological cause was responsible for this condition, and recommended the identification of neurological causal factors. Rimland postulated deficits in certain neurological and cortical functions and developed a behavioral questionnaire that aimed at differentiating infant autism from other disorders. He also tried to identify biochemical markers and studied the patients' response to mega-vitamin therapy. Neither his biochemical findings nor the mega-vitamin therapy findings could be confirmed by other studies, however.

Current researchers in many disciplines such as psychiatry, neurology, genetics, pediatrics, neuroimaging science, and neurofunctional and neuropsychological testing have tried to identify the etiology and persistent deficits present in individuals with autism. These studies explore the connection between deficits and underlying causes. Other chapters in this book will review current findings in the neurobiology and genetics of autism (see Chapter 4), medical and syndromic etiology and workup (see Chapter 3), neuropsychological and executive functioning deficits and theory of mind (see Chapter 12), and behavioral theories (see Chapter 5). Current thinking suggests a number of possible theories regarding the nature of autism. For example, Simon Baron-Cohen (1995, *Mindblindness: An essay on autism and theory of mind*) described his "Theory of Mind" the difficulty that the individual with autism has with inferring the mental states of other people. Others have posited an "executive function deficit," described as the difficulty an individual with autism has with acquiring problem-solving skills, setting future goals, controlling impulses, inhibiting irrelevant signals or stimuli, planning and organizing, and displaying flexibility of thought and action.

Summary of Key Historical Figures

- 1797: Itard's Victor, the wild boy of Aveyron, reported by Professor Frith, documenting the existence of autism-like features.
- 1908: Heller described "dementia infantilis," currently known as "childhood disintegrative disorder."
- 1943: Kanner's *Autistic Disturbances of Affective Conduct* used term "autism" from Bleuler's works in schizophrenia—"autism" referred to extreme withdrawal from social life or aloneness.
- 1944: Asperger described a condition resembling Kanner's 1943 "autism," which he named "autistic psychopathy."
- 1967: Bettelheim wrote *An Empty Fortress* about cold, unresponsive parents, and questioned parenting style as a psychogenic cause.
- 1964: Rimland's book *Infantile Autism: The Syndrome and Its Implications for a Neural Theory of Behavior* proposed that a biological cause was responsible.
- 1967: Rutter decisively refuted the psychogenic etiology of autism.

History of "Autism" and "Pervasive Developmental Disorder" as Diagnostic Categories in the Diagnostic and Statistical Manual of Mental Disorders

DSM-I (1952) and DSM-II (1968)

DSM-I (1952) and DSM-II (1968) had no category for autism. The terms *childhood schizophrenic reaction* or *schizophrenia, childhood type* were broadly applied to all children with severe psychiatric disturbances, and the manual mentioned autism as symptoms of these conditions.

DSM-III (1980)

Infantile autism was officially included as a diagnosis in DSM-III within a new class of disorders. The pervasive developmental disorders were characterized by "distortions in the development of multiple basic psychological functions that are involved in the development of social skills and language, such as attention, perception, reality testing, and motor movement."

It contained provisions for individuals who had a "lifetime" diagnosis of autism, "residual autism," and an "atypical" category.

Diagnostic Criteria for Infantile Autism (DSM-III)

A. Onset before 30 months of age
B. Pervasive lack of responsiveness to other people (autism)
C. Gross deficits in language development
D. If speech is present, peculiar speech patterns such as immediate and delayed echolalia, metaphorical language, pronominal reversal
E. Bizarre responses to various aspects of the environment; e.g., resistance to change, and peculiar interest in or attachments to animate or inanimate objects
F. Absence of delusions, hallucinations, loosening of associations, and incoherence as in Schizophrenia.

DSM-III-R (1987)

In DSM-III-R, the criteria for autistic disorder were broadened. The "residual" category was eliminated, and diagnosis could be made in individuals at any age or development level. The PDD NOS diagnosis was included in the PDD class to represent "sub-threshold" presentations.

Diagnostic Criteria for Autistic Disorder (DSM-III-R)

A. Qualitative impairment in reciprocal social interaction
B. Qualitative impairment in verbal and nonverbal communication and in imaginative activity
C. Markedly restricted repertoire of activities and interests
D. Onset during infancy or early childhood
   Specify if childhood onset (after 36 months of age)

DSM-IV (1994) and DSM-IV-TR (2000)

Fred Volkmar and his collaborators conducted a large multi-site field trial for DSM-IV. This included ratings of nearly 1000 cases. The results of this large field trial produced an increased convergence between DSM and ICD definitions of autism, and the revised diagnosis criteria allowed for a more accurate identification and a reduction of high false-positive rates that were observed when using the DSM-III-R system. It also provided support for the inclusion of Rett's disorder, childhood disintegrative disorder, and Asperger's disorder in the PDD class.

Diagnostic Criteria for Autistic Disorder (DSM-IV-TR)

1. Qualitative impairment in social interaction
2. Qualitative impairments in communication
3. Restricted, repetitive, and stereotyped patterns of behavior, interests, and activities
4. Delays or abnormal functioning in at least one of the following areas, with onset prior to age 3 years: (1) social interaction, (2) language as used in social communication, or (3) symbolic or imaginative play
5. The disturbance is not better accounted for by Rett's disorder or childhood disintegrative disorder

Future Directions—DSM-5

At the time of publishing this book, the DSM-5 Task Force and Work Group's Proposed Draft Revisions to DSM Disorders and New Criteria are under review, in preparation for the fifth edition of Diagnostic and Statistical Manual of Mental Disorders. The DSM-5 Proposed Draft Revisions to DSM Disorders and New Criteria are defining a new category: *autism spectrum disorder*, which includes autistic disorder (autism), Asperger's disorder, childhood disintegrative disorder, and pervasive developmental disorder—not otherwise specified.

It is proposed that a single diagnostic category be used while including clinical specifiers (e.g., severity, verbal abilities, and others) and associated features (e.g., known genetic disorders, epilepsy, intellectual disability, and others). Considering that deficits in communication and social behaviors are inseparable and more accurately considered as a single set of symptoms with contextual and environmental specificities, the three DSM-IV-TR domains become two in DSM-5:
1. Social and communication deficits
2. Fixated interests and repetitive behaviors
The diagnosis is requiring that both criteria to be completely fulfilled.

Diagnostic Criteria for Autism Spectrum Disorder (DSM-5)

Must meet criteria 1, 2, and 3:
1. Clinically significant, persistent deficits in social communication and interactions, as manifested by all of the following:
   a. Marked deficits in nonverbal and verbal communication used for social interaction
   b. Lack of social reciprocity
   c. Failure to develop and maintain peer relationships appropriate to developmental level
2. Restricted, repetitive patterns of behavior, interests, and activities, as manifested by at least TWO of the following:
   a. Stereotyped motor or verbal behaviors, or unusual sensory behaviors
   b. Excessive adherence to routines and ritualized patterns of behavior
   c. Restricted, fixated interests
3. Symptoms must be present in early childhood (but may not become fully manifest until social demands exceed limited capacities)

Further Reading

1. American Psychiatric Association (2000). *Diagnostic and Statistical Manual of Mental Disorders*, fourth edition, text revision (DSM-IV-TR). Washington, D.C.

2. American Psychiatric Association (2011). DSM-5 Workgroup. Retrieved from www.dsm5.org on December 17, 2010.

3. Baron-Cohen, S. (1995). *Mindblindness: An essay on autism and theory of mind*. Cambridge, MA: MIT Press/Bradford Books.

4. Frith, U. (1991). *Autism—Explaining the enigma*. Malden, MA: Wiley-Blackwell.

5. Gilderhus, M. T. (2006). *History and historians: A historiographical introduction*, sixth edition. New York: Prentice Hall.

6. Kanner, L (1943). Autistic disturbances of affective contact. *The Nervous Child* 2:217–250.

7. Lyons, V., Fitzgerald. M. (2007). Asperger (1906–1980) and Kanner (1894–1981), the two pioneers of autism. *Journal of Autism and Developmental Disorders*. *37*(10): 2022–2023.

8. Mesibov, G., Adams, L., & Klinger, L. (1998). *Autism: Understanding the disorder (Clinical Child Psychology Library)*, 1st edition. New York: Springer.

9. Rutter, M (1971). Causes of infantile autism: Some considerations from recent research. *Journal of Autism and Childhood Schizophrenia, I*(1): 20–32

10. Rutter, M. (1978). Diagnosis and definition of childhood autism. *Journal of Autism and Childhood Schizophrenia, 8*(2): 139–161.

11. Volkmar, F., & Lord, C. (2007). Diagnosis and definition of autism and other pervasive developmental disorders. In F. Volkmar, (Ed.). *Autism and pervasive developmental disorders, 2nd Edition*. (pp. 1–31). New York, NY: Cambridge University Press.

12. Wolff, S. (2004). The history of autism. *European Child Adolescent Psychiatry*. *13*(4): 201–208.

Questions

1. The DSM-5 diagnosis of autism is requiring which criteria to be completely fulfilled?
   a. Social and communication deficits
   b. Communication deficits
   c. Fixated interests and repetitive behaviors
   d. a and c

2. In 1956, Eisenberg and Kanner proposed which two of the following fundamental criteria for diagnosing the autistic disorder?
   a. The withdrawal to fantasy
   b. The inability of the individual with autism to relate in an ordinary way to people and situations
   c. Cold, unresponsive parents
   d. The inability to learn to speak, or to convey meaning to others by means of language.
   e. b and d

3. Which one of the following features is *NOT* characteristic in Asperger's original report on autism?
   a. He described the syndrome as clinically apparent after the age of three or four years
   b. Language skills are usually an area of strength
   c. Associated with higher ver bal IQ
   d. Associated with microcephaly

4. Which one of the following is *NOT* a diagnostic criterion for infantile autism according to DSM-III (1980)?
   a. Onset before 30 months
   b. Gross deficits in language development
   c. Loosening of associations
   d. Pervasive lack of responsiveness to other people

5. A number of possible theories regarding autism include which of the following?
   a. Theory of Mind, the difficulty that the individual with autism has with inferring the mental states of other people
   b. An executive-function deficit, described as the difficulty an individual with autism has with acquiring problem-solving skills, setting future goals, controlling impulses, inhibiting irrelevant signals or stimuli, planning and organizing, and displaying flexibility of thought and action
   c. Autism as a reaction to "emotional deprivation"
   d. a and b

Answers

1. d. (a and c)
Considering that deficits in communication and social behaviors are inseparable and more accurately considered as a single set of symptoms with contextual and environmental specificities, the DSM-IV-TR's three domains become two in DSM-5:
a. Social/communication deficits
c. Fixated interests and repetitive behaviors
The diagnosis is requiring that both criteria be completely fulfilled.

2. e. (b and d.)
In 1956 Eisenberg and Kanner proposed two fundamental criteria for diagnosing the autistic disorder:
b. the inability of the autistic patient to relate in an ordinary way to people and situations; and
d. the inability to learn to speak, or to convey meaning to others by means of language.
These two symptoms were observed to occur from the beginning of life.

3. d. is not true.
Asperger described the syndrome as clinically apparent after the age of three or four years, with good language skills that are usually an area of strength and associated with higher verbal IQ.

4. c. is not true.
The diagnostic criteria for infantile autism in the DSM-III (1980) include the following:
A. Onset before 30 months of age
B. Pervasive lack of responsiveness to other people (autism)
C. Gross deficits in language development
D. If speech is present, peculiar speech patterns such as immediate and delayed echolalia, metaphorical language, and pronominal reversal
E. Bizarre responses to various aspects of the environment; e.g., resistance to change, peculiar interest in or attachments to animate or inanimate objects
F. Absence of delusions, hallucinations, loosening of associations, and incoherence as in schizophrenia.

5. d. (a and b).

Recognition of Autism Spectrum Disorder— Early Identification and Diagnosis

John J. McGonigle, Virginia Martin, and Martin J. Lubetsky

Early Identification: First Signs and Red Flags
    (See Chapter 7 for Early Childhood Interventions) 22
Evaluation Algorithms and Assessment of ASD 26
Autism Assessment and Diagnosis 32
Summary 35
Further Reading and References for Rating Scales and
    Testing Instruments 36
Questions 38
Answers 39

Early and accurate diagnosis of autism spectrum disorder is critical not to only early intervention and more successful outcomes for children and their families, but for long-range planning and support through the developmental years and adulthood. Recent studies and reports from the Centers for Disease Control (CDC, 2009; Cox & Shaw, 2010) have shown an increase in the prevalence of children diagnosed with an ASD to one in 110, emphasizing the need to sharpen the focus on early identification and improve diagnostic assessment and interventions. The reported increase is thought to be attributable to several factors. First, there have been changes in diagnostic practices, including the inclusion of Asperger's disorder in DSM-IV and a broadened definition of PDD (allowing the diagnosis of ASD to be applied more widely than before). Second, there is greater public awareness of ASD and more case-finding and earlier diagnoses. Finally, there has been a tendency to diagnose many children with intellectual disability as PDD. While some still question that the rise in the incidence of ASD is due to factors such as the use of thimerosal or mercury contained in childhood immunizations, there is no scientific evidence to support that these are related to ASD. The possible roles of other, yet unclear, environmental factors have also been posited. However, no evidence currently exists to support any association between ASD and a specific environmental exposure.

Whether diagnosis is accurately made in childhood, adolescence, or adulthood, the access to quality assessment and evidenced-based treatments have been shown to be critical variables for positive developmental outcomes. This chapter will provide an overview of the early identification: first signs and red flags, evaluation algorithms and practice parameters, assessment approaches and DSM-IV-TR diagnosis of ASD. The salient points to be emphasized include:

- Practitioners need to be aware of early identification and warning signs for children at risk for ASD (including the siblings of children already identified with ASD).
- Early identification requires training of practitioners who see young children, including pediatricians, nurse practitioners, and early intervention, Head Start, and preschool workers.
- Multidisciplinary teams need to be involved in the comprehensive assessment of children with ASD.
- Early diagnosis requires experienced professionals who take a developmental perspective in the diagnostic assessment process—clinical psychologists, developmental behavioral pediatricians, pediatric neurologists, and child and adolescent psychiatrists.
- Clinicians need to use evidenced-based and recommended best-practice assessments.
- Evaluations can take place and can be completed in a variety of settings (i.e., clinic, home, school, and community).
- Diagnostic and treatment services need to be available across the lifespan, including toddlers, preschoolers, latency-age children, adolescents, and adults.

Early Identification: First Signs and Red Flags (See Chapter 7 for Early Childhood Interventions)

Child development is quite variable, with a range of skills developing at different rates. Wide individual variations in the rate of skill acquisition can make identification of early signs of ASD even more challenging for a clinician. Often parents do not see how their child differs from others, especially if it is their first child. For parents who are concerned about their child's development, it may be difficult to persuade professionals to pursue a more detailed assessment. In spite of some parents' identifying their concerns prior to their child's third year, many children are not diagnosed with ASD until they reach school age (Howlin & Asgharian, 1999). The CDC (2009) reports the median age for a diagnosis of ASD to be between 4.5 and 5.5 years. Also, a recent report noted a disparity in age of diagnosis based upon race, in which children who were African American and had low socioeconomic status were diagnosed later than children who were Caucasian and from low socioeconomic status (Mandell, et. al., 2002). Research has shown that early identification and early intervention results in improvement in developmental progress and language as well as reduction of challenging behaviors (Eaves & Ho, 2004; Howlin, 2005; Lord, Wagner, et. al., 2005; Matson, 2006).

Some early social communicative language difficulties that may be signs of ASD include:

- Avoiding eye contact (not studying the mother's face);
- Not responding to parents' voice and appearing to be deaf (vs. being easily stimulated by and appearing to recognize sounds);
- Lack of facial responsiveness and socially directed smiling (vs. responding with a range of affect to pleasant social stimuli);
- Starting to develop language and then abruptly stopping (vs. continuous growth in vocabulary and grammar);
- Not being able to ask for something to indicate an interest (vs. being able to point to or ask for a desired object or to indicate an interest) (APA, 2000; Baron-Cohen et. al, 2000); and
- Failure to engage in pretend games (vs., for example, being able to pretend to make a cup of tea with a toy cup and teapot) (Baron-Cohen et. al, 2000).

The first step to take if there are concerns regarding possible ASD symptoms is surveillance. This may be done by a pediatrician, healthcare professional, or mental health clinician. Surveillance includes a brief review of the parents' concerns, family history, and any atypical behaviors or developmental delays. Pediatricians may make use of the *Learn the Signs—Act Early* campaign through the Center for Disease Control, or *First Signs for Practitioners*, which provides pamphlets, brief reading materials, and rating scales for parents or others who come into contact with young children. These materials describe general developmental milestones to watch for in young children (starting at seven months until the end of four years). They also include questions to ask the child's doctor or nurse. These materials are available in English and Spanish. The training program includes a videotape, workbook, handouts, and examples of available screening tools.

First Signs (First Signs, Inc., 2004) is an organization started to encourage screening for signs and symptoms that could be indicative of an ASD. These "Red Flags" include:
- No big smiles or other warm, joyful expressions by six months or thereafter;
- No back-and-forth sharing of sounds, smiles, or other facial expressions by nine months or thereafter;
- No babbling by 12 months;
- No back-and-forth gestures, such as pointing, showing, reaching, or waving, by 12 months;
- No words by 16 months;
- No two-word meaningful phrases (without imitating or repeating) by 24 months;
- ANY loss of speech or babbling or social skills at ANY age.

The Center for Disease Control (CDC–www.cdc.gov/actearly) has printed a handout for public use to promote the early identification of signs of ASD. This *Learn the Signs—Act Early* handout states: "As they grow, children are always learning new things. These are just some of the things you should be looking for as your child grows. Because every child develops at his or her own pace, your child may reach these milestones slightly before or after other children the same age. Use this as a guide, and if you have any concerns, talk with your child's doctor or nurse." The pediatrician or clinician may discuss the developmental or behavioral concerns with the family to determine if the next step (referral) is necessary. Below is the CDC list of "early signs" for both younger and older children.

Early signs of an ASD in younger children may include:
- No babbling or pointing or other gestures by age 12 months
- No single words by 16 months
- No two-word spontaneous (not echolalic) phrases by 24 months
- Loss of language or social skills at any age
- Lack of joint attention
- The child having a sibling with an ASD
- Atypical behaviors consistent with an ASD (i.e., stereotyped behaviors, atypical interests, very limited social interest)

Early signs of an ASD in older children may include:
- Pragmatic language impairment
- Difficulty taking the perspective of others
- Obsession with facts, details, collections
- Lack of true friendships, relationships
- Child viewed as "odd" or "eccentric" by peers
- Appears to lack empathy

Research suggests that 75% to 88% of children with ASD show signs of this condition in the first two years of life, with 31% to 55% displaying symptoms in their first year (Young & Brewer, 2002). The substantial cognitive and behavioral gains made during the normal development of young children and the findings that intensive early intervention results in improved outcomes for children with ASD (Ozonoff & Rogers, 2003; Rogers, 2001; Rogers, 1998), have led to a consensus that early intensive intervention is essential (Mastergeorge et al., 2003).

Assessments for ASD are completed in a variety of settings, and it is extremely important that any ASD evaluation involve the combining of information from multiple sources (Risi et al., 2006). Teams and systems are typically involved in the diagnostic assessment for ASD. To make an accurate diagnosis, the team must view children in the context of their functional developmental level, including cognitive, language, adaptive, social, and emotional skills. Other factors to take into consideration include the context in which the child is observed—with family, in a home setting, at school, in a clinic—and the person who is providing the information.

"A Review of the State of Science for Pediatric Primary Healthcare Clinicians" was recently published in *The Archives of Pediatric Adolescent Medicine*, which suggested the use of a systematic approach to the assessment and treatment of children with ASD and the children who fail routine developmental screenings (Barbaresi et al., 2006). Also, a recent study in the *Journal of Pediatrics* suggested an algorithm for surveillance and screening in identifying infants and young children with developmental disorders (2006). In fact, screenings are now recommended by American Academy of Pediatrics at the 18- and 24-month well-child visit. Pediatricians should administer a standardized autism screening tool on all children who present developmental delays. It is vital that examiners use valid and reliable tools to supplement their skilled clinical observations and clinical judgment.

Practice Parameters for the assessment of ASD have been published by the following:
- American Academy of Pediatrics (Johnson et al., 2007)
- American Academy of Neurology (Filipek, et al., 2000; Pinto-Martin & Levy, 2004; Ozonoff, 2005)
- American Academy of Child and Adolescent Psychiatry (Volkmar et al., 1999).

Evaluation Algorithms and Assessment of ASD

In order to clarify what to look for in early child development, early signs of ASD will be reviewed. The screening and evaluation process will be described first. There have been many evaluation algorithms developed to guide both the screening and the diagnosis of children suspected to have ASD. Two algorithms will be presented here. The first was developed by the Council on Children with Disabilities in Pediatrics (2007) as an algorithm for identifying infants and children with developmental disorders. Figure 2.1 details the specific steps of the algorithm.

A second algorithm, developed by the Pennsylvania Autism Diagnostic Workgroup as a three-stage screening and evaluation process, has been recommended for use across the state. Stage 1 involves a basic screening of the child (e.g., M-CHAT, SCQ, medical/developmental history). Based on Stage 1, the evaluation team will determine what type of evaluation is appropriate and, if necessary, refer the child to Stage 2 for more-comprehensive evaluations (e.g., cognitive, emotional, language, adaptive, play, social, sensory, behavioral). Following the Stage 2 comprehensive evaluations, if the ASD diagnosis is not confirmed or there continue to be remaining questions, then Stage 3, specialized diagnostic instruments, will be completed (Pennsylvania Bureau of Autism Services Department of Public Welfare Task Force Report, 2004).

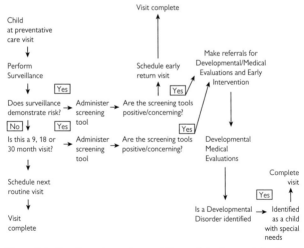

Figure 2.1. Identifying infants and young children with developmental disorders in the medical home: An algorithm for developmental surveillance and screening (*Pediatrics* 2006, *118*(1) 405–420).

Stage 1: screening

Demographic information and concerns from the parent, caregiver, or teacher should be obtained. The process involves review of the child's records, interviews with parents, observations of the child, and the administration of various developmental assessments. For children for whom there is a question of an ASD diagnosis, a brief ASD-specific questionnaire should be completed. This is usually completed at the primary care physician/pediatrician's office or at preschool. Options include:

- Checklist for Autistic Toddlers (CHAT)
- Modified Checklist for Autism in Toddlers (M-CHAT)
- Social Communication Questionnaire (SCQ)
- Social Responsiveness Scale (SRS)

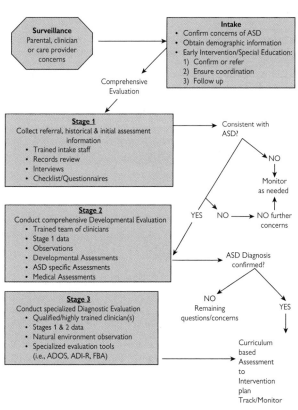

Figure 2.2. Algorithm from Pennsylvania Expert Autism Diagnostic Workgroup.

- Screening Tool for Autism at Two-Year-Olds (STAT)
- Asperger's Syndrome Diagnostic Scale (ASDS) over 4
- Autism Spectrum Screening Questionnaire (ASSQ)
- Gilliam Autism Rating Scale, Second Edition (GARS-2)
- Asperger's Syndrome Diagnostic Scale (ASDS)
- Childhood Autism Rating Scale 2 (CARS 2)
- Pervasive Developmental Disorder Screening Test (PDDST)

One screening instrument that is recommended is the M-CHAT. The Modified Checklist for Autism in Toddlers (Robins et al., 1999, 2001) is available for free download for clinical, research, and educational purposes. There are two authorized websites: the M-CHAT and supplemental materials can be downloaded from www.firstsigns.org or from Dr. Robins' website, at: http://www2.gsu.edu/~wwwpsy/faculty/robins.htm.

The M-CHAT is validated for screening toddlers between 16 and 30 months of age, to assess risk for ASD. The M-CHAT can be administered and scored as part of a well-child check-up to assess the risk for ASD. The M-CHAT can be scored in less than two minutes. There are 23 items, and children who fail more than three items total or two critical items (particularly if these scores remain elevated after the follow-up interview) should be referred for diagnostic evaluation by a specialist trained to evaluate ASD in very young children.

Stage 2: diagnostic evaluation

For children who fail routine developmental screening, specific diagnostic assessment for ASD should be performed. Ideally, an ASD diagnostic evaluation includes professionals from a wide range of disciplines, including some but not necessarily all of the following:

- Developmental behavioral pediatrician
- Child neurologist
- Pediatric nurse practitioner
- Child and adolescent psychiatrist
- Child psychologist
- Speech and language specialist
- Teacher
- Board certified behavior analyst
- Occupational and physical therapists
- Medical geneticist
- Physical medicine and rehabilitation physician
- Nutritionist
- Medical social worker

The assessment should include a detailed evaluation of the child's developmental history and family history, current presentation (specifically, the presentation of the core features of ASD), and course of the disorder (onset and regressions). It is vital that examiners use valid and reliable tools to supplement their skilled clinical observations and clinical judgment. Comprehensive evaluation should include assessments across all domains.

Domain Assessments

Regardless of the instruments used, the following domains should be assessed as the child's status in each domain is summarized in the evaluation report:

- Cognitive skills
- Language skills
- Adaptive behavior skills
- Developmental/academic skills
- Play skills
- Social interaction skills
- Sensory-motor skills
- Behavioral/emotional adjustment.

Cognitive Assessments

The professional should be experienced in assessing children with neurodevelopmental disabilities, including ASD. Psychological evaluations for ASD should:

- Be appropriate for the mental and chronological age of the child
- Provide independent measures of verbal and nonverbal abilities
- Provide an overall index of ability
- Assess the child's ability to remember, solve problems, and develop concepts
- Measure motor and visual motor skills
- Assess social cognition
  Infant and pre-school tests:
- Bayley Scales of Infant Development II (1–42 months)
- Batelle Developmental Inventory (BDI) (birth to 8 years)
- Differential Abilities Scale (DAS) (2–18 years)
- Wechsler Preschool and Primary Scale of Intelligence (WPPSI)
- Kaufman–Assessment Battery for Children (K-ABC) (2–12)
- McCarthy Scales of Children's Ability (MSCA)
- Stanford Binet Intelligence Scales, Fifth Edition (2–85)
- Wechsler Intelligence Scale for Children–IV (6–16)
- Woodcock Johnson Cognitive Abilities III (2–80)

Speech and language assessments (see chapter on speech and language)

Assessment areas should include:

- Receptive and expressive abilities in all aspects of language: syntax and semantics
- Pragmatics: speech articulation–phonology, oral-motor skills (including feeding), voice quality, prosody (i.e., rate, rhythm, melody, tone), atypical verbal behavior (echolalia, perseverative speech).

Occupational and physical therapy evaluations

Assessments of sensory processing related to auditory, visual, tactile, vestibular, gustatory, and olfactory systems that may be associated with deficits in attention, arousal, behavior, and emotion.

Stage 3: expert diagnostic confirmation

Stage 3 evaluations are only necessary for children whose diagnostic status is still unclear at the end of Stage 2, or when the treatment team would like further clarification of the child's strengths and weaknesses to help guide treatment. In Stage 3, a diagnostic evaluation for autism may be conducted by a single clinician who has specialized training in formal diagnostic evaluations (e.g., a licensed psychologist, developmental/behavioral pediatrician, or child psychiatrist) and extensive clinical experience. The team of

> **Medical Evaluations (see Chapter 3 on medical and behavioral health evaluation)**
>
> *Provide general heath profile*
> - Rule out hearing impairment or medical conditions that are expressed in autistic features
> - Identify co-occurring medical conditions often associated with ASD: seizure disorder, metabolic disorders
> - Consider the need for sub-specialty evaluation: geneticist, pediatric neurologist, sleep specialist, nutritionist
>
> *Physical examination*
> - Assess for dysmorphic features and neurocutaneous abnormalities
> - Neurological exam: gait, muscle tone, reflex, etc.

clinicians should be led or supervised by a physician or psychologist licensed to make a diagnosis of autism.

Stage 3 evaluations will often involve administration of very specialized instruments, such as the ADI-R (Autism Diagnostic Interview–Revised) and the ADOS (Autism Diagnostic Observation Schedule). Caution must be taken to assure appropriate training and supervision of personnel who will administer these complex tools (Mazefsky & Oswald, 2006). The evaluation should include observation of the child and family in different settings. If observations in a school setting are not possible, and providing HIPPA regulations are followed, a videotape of typical behavior of the child will provide valuable information.

Indirect Diagnostic Assessment: ADI-R Interview

Developed by Rutter, Le Couteur, and Lord (2003), the *Autism Diagnostic Interview–Revised* (ADI-R), along with the *Autism Diagnostic Observation Schedule* (ADOS), is currently considered the "gold standard" for the diagnostic interview that yields the most reliable and valid diagnosis of ASD. The ADI-R employs a semi-structured interview format to elicit the information needed to diagnose autism. The interview's primary focus is on the three core domains of autism (i.e., language/communication, reciprocal social interactions, and restricted, repetitive, and stereotyped behaviors and interests). The ADI-R requires a trained interviewer and caregiver familiar with both the developmental history and the current behavior of the child. The individual being assessed must have a developmental level of at least two years

Direct Diagnostic Observation: ADOS

The *Autism Diagnostic Observation Schedule* (ADOS) (Lord et al., 2000) is considered to be part of the "gold standard" in the diagnosis of ASD. The ADOS is a standardized, semi-structured interactive play assessment of social behavior. By making use of "planned social occasions," the ADOS facilitates observation of the social, communication, and play or imaginative use of material behaviors related to the diagnosis of ASD.

Autism Assessment and Diagnosis

DSM-IV-TR diagnostic criteria (see Chapter 1 for historical perspective and DSM)

ASD is reported to occur across all racial, ethnic, and economic groups, and the ASD diagnosis is four times more common for boys than in girls. Research by Zwiagenbaum, Bryson, Rodgers, Roberts, and Szatmari (2005) and Rogers (2001) indicates that some parents become concerned with their child's development or behavior around the age of 15 to 18 months. They may speak to their healthcare professional at that time, or may delay the discussion in an effort to give their child time to "catch up" developmentally. Other parents note differences in their child somewhat later, when more social demands are placed on the child (i.e., in preschool). Still others become concerned with their child's behavior and social interactions later as the social demands of elementary or high school elicit questions of a possible ASD. A child's pediatrician, healthcare provider, or teacher may express concern to the parents first, based on the quality of their child's interactions, or the way that they communicate. This may prompt families to pursue further evaluation of potential symptoms of an ASD.

The DSM-IV-TR (Diagnostic and Statistical Manual in the current text, revised fourth edition), identifies ASD as a pervasive developmental disorder with five subtypes (DSM-IV-TR, APA, 2000). The first subtype is autistic disorder, in which individuals who do not have mental retardation (now referred to as intellectual disability) are described as having high-functioning autism. The specific criteria to make the diagnosis of autistic disorder require "onset prior to age three years and delays or abnormal functioning in social interaction, language as used in social communication, and symbolic or imaginative play, with a total of six or more items."

DSM-IV-TR Autistic Disorder diagnosis*

A. A total of six (or more) items from (1), (2), and (3), with at least two from (1), and one each from (2) and (3):

    (1) Qualitative impairment in social interaction, as manifested by at least two of the following:

        (a) marked impairment in the use of multiple, nonverbal behaviors such as eye-to-eye gaze, facial expression, body postures, and gestures to regulate social interaction

        (b) failure to develop peer relationships appropriate to developmental level

        (c) a lack of spontaneous seeking to share enjoyment, interests, or achievements with other people (e.g., by lack of showing, bringing, or pointing out objects of interest)

        (d) lack of social or emotional reciprocity

    (2) Qualitative impairments in communication as manifested by at least one of the following:

        (a) delay in, or total lack of, the development of spoken language (not accompanied by an attempt to compensate through alternative modes of communication such as gestures or mime)

        (b) in individuals with adequate speech, marked impairment in the ability to initiate or sustain a conversation with others

      (c) stereotyped and repetitive use of language or idiosyncratic
language
      (d) lack of varied, spontaneous make-believe play or social imitative
play appropriate to developmental level
  (3) Restricted repetitive and stereotyped patterns of behavior,
interests, and activities, as manifested by at least one of the
following
      (a) encompassing preoccupation with one or more stereotyped
and restricted patterns of interest that is abnormal either in
intensity or in focus
      (b) apparently inflexible adherence to specific, nonfunctional
routines or rituals
      (c) stereotyped and repetitive motor mannerisms (e.g., hand or
finger flapping or twisting, or complex whole-body movements)
      (d) persistent preoccupation with parts of objects
B. Delays or abnormal functioning in at least one of the following areas,
with onset prior to age three years: (1) social interaction, (2) language
as used in social communication, or (3) symbolic or imaginative play
C. The disturbance is not better accounted for by Rett's disorder or
childhood disintegrative disorder.

DSM-IV-TR Asperger's Disorder diagnosis*

The essential features of Asperger's disorder are severe and sustained impairment in social interaction (criterion A); and the development of restricted,
repetitive patterns of behavior, interests, and activities (criterion B); which
must cause clinically significant impairment in functioning (criterion C). There
are no clinically significant delays in language (criterion D) or cognitive
development (criterion E).

A. Qualitative impairment in social interaction, as manifested by at least
two of the following:
  (1) marked impairment in the use of multiple, nonverbal behaviors such
as eye-to-eye gaze, facial expression, body postures, and gestures to
regulate social interaction
  (2) failure to develop peer relationships appropriate to developmental
level
  (3) a lack of spontaneous seeking to share enjoyment, interests, or
achievements with other people (e.g., by lack of showing, bringing,
or pointing out objects of interest)
  (4) lack of social or emotional reciprocity
B. Restricted repetitive and stereotyped patterns of behavior, interests,
and activities, as manifested by at least one of the following:
  (1) encompassing preoccupation with one or more stereotyped
and restricted patterns of interest that is abnormal either in
intensity or in focus
  (2) apparently inflexible adherence to specific, nonfunctional
routines or rituals
  (3) stereotyped and repetitive motor mannerisms (eg, hand or
finger flapping or twisting, or complex whole-body movements)
  (4) persistent preoccupation with parts of objects
C. The disturbance causes clinically significant impairment in social,
occupational, or other important areas of functioning.

D. There is no clinically significant general delay in language (e.g., single words used by age two years, communicative phrases used by age three years).
E. There is no clinically significant delay in cognitive development or the development of age-appropriate self-help skills, adaptive behavior (other than in social interaction), and curiosity about the environment in childhood.
F. Criteria are not met for another specific pervasive developmental disorder or for schizophrenia.

DSM-IV-TR Pervasive Developmental Disorder–Not Otherwise Specified (including atypical autism) diagnosis*

This category should be used when there is a severe and pervasive impairment in the development of reciprocal social interaction associated with impairment in either verbal or nonverbal communication skills or with the presence of stereotyped behavior, interests, and activities, but the criteria are not met for a specific pervasive developmental disorder, schizophrenia, schizotypal personality disorder, or avoidant personality disorder. For example, this category includes "atypical autism"—presentations that do not meet the criteria for autistic disorder because of late age at onset, atypical symptomology, subthreshold symptomology, or all of these.

*(Source: American Psychiatric Association. *Diagnostic and Statistical Manual of Mental Disorders*, Fourth Edition, Text Revision (DSM-IV-TR), Washington, D.C.: American Psychiatric Publishing, 2000)

Summary

Screening and early identification, multidisciplinary assessment, and quality diagnosis of ASD is critical to early intervention and more successful outcomes for children and their families. This chapter has reviewed early identification: first signs, red flags, evaluation algorithms and practice parameters, diagnostic instruments, and DSM-IV-TR diagnostic criteria.

It is important to emphasize that early identification requires training of practitioners, clinicians and support staff that see young children. Similarly, early diagnosis requires training of professionals who can participate in the diagnostic process. Appropriate evidenced-based and best-practice assessment requires a multidisciplinary team approach with observation and information from a variety of sources. Whether the diagnosis of ASD is accurately made in childhood, adolescence, or adulthood, the access to comprehensive assessment and appropriate treatment needs to be available to the individual and family. Early, accurate diagnosis leads to early treatment and intervention and improved quality of life for people with ASD.

Key Fact Box

- Early and accurate diagnosis of ASD is critical to early intervention and more successful outcomes for children and their families.
- Recent studies and reports from Center for Disease Control (2009) have shown an increase in the prevalence of children diagnosed with an ASD, to one in 110.
- ASD is reported to occur in all racial, ethnic, and economic groups.
- ASD diagnosis is four times greater for boys than for girls.
- Some parents become concerned with their child's development or behavior around the age of 15 to 18 months.
- Screenings are now recommended by American Academy of Pediatrics (AAP) by the 18-month and by the 24-month well-child visit.
- The M-CHAT is validated for screening toddlers between 16 and 30 months of age to assess risk for ASD.
- The team should include professionals with extensive experience, training, and skill in conducting pediatric, functional, cognitive, educational, communication, behavioral, and sensory-motor evaluations.
- Stage 3 evaluations will often involve the administration of very specialized instruments, such as the ADOS (Autism Diagnostic Observation Schedule).

Further Reading and References for Rating Scales and Testing Instruments

1. Allen, C.W., Silove, N., Williams, K., & Hutchins, P. (2007) Validity of the Social Communication Questionnaire in assessing risk of autism in preschool children with developmental problems. *Journal of Autism and Developmental Disorders*, 37, 1272–1278.

2. America Psychiatric Association (2000). *Diagnostic and Statistical Manual of Mental Disorders*, 4th ed. (DSM-IV-TR). Washington, D.C.: American Psychiatric Association.

3. Barbaresi, W. J., Katusic, S. K., & Voigt, R. (2006). A review of the state of the science for primary health care clinicians, *Archives of Pediatric Adolescent Medicine*, 160:1167–1175, Retrieved March 8, 2008, from online website: http://www.archpediatrics.com.

4. Baron, S. (2005). Test review: Wechsler Intelligence Scale for Children–Fourth Edition (WISC-IV). *Child Neuropsychology* 11:471–475.

5. Brock, S. (2006). *The identification of Autism Spectrum Disorder: A primer for the school psychologist.* Sacramento: California State University. Online website: http://www.csus.edu/indiv/b/brocks

6. California Department of Developmental Services (2002). *Autistic spectrum disorders: Best practice guidelines for screening, diagnosis and assessment.* Sacramento, CA. Retrieved February 11, 2007, from http://www.ddhealthinfo.org.

7. Constantino, J. N., Davis, S. A., et al. (2003). Validation of a brief quantitative measure of autistic traits: Comparison of the Social Responsiveness Scale with the Autism Diagnostic Interview–Revised. *Journal of Autism and Developmental Disorders* 33(4): 427–433.

8. Counsel on Children With Disabilities, Section on Developmental Behavioral Pediatrics, Bright Futures Steering Committee and Medical Home Initiatives for Children With Special Needs Project Advisory Committee. Identifying infants and young children with developmental disorders in the medical home: An algorithm for developmental surveillance and screening. *Journal of Pediatrics*, 118(1): 405–420. Retrieved April 4, 2007, from American Academy of Pediatrics online website: http://www.pediatrics.org/cgi/content/full/118/1/405.

9. Cox, A, & Shaw, C. (2010). National Professional Development Center on ASD: Promoting evidence-based practices in early identification and intervention. Presentation at Act Early Regional Summit. Philadelphia, PA, March 26, 2010. National Professional Development Center on Autism Spectrum Disorder, FPG Child Development Institute, The University of North Carolina at Chapel Hill.

10. Dumont-Mathieu, T., & Fein, D. (2005). Screening for autism in young children: The Modified Checklist for Autism in Toddlers (M-CHAT) and other measures. *Mental Retardation and Developmental Disabilities Research Reviews* 11: 253–262.

11. Eaves, L. C., Wingert, H. D., et al. (2006). Screening for Autism Spectrum Disorder with the Social Communication Questionnaire. *Developmental and Behavioral Pediatrics* 27(2): S95–S103.

12. Filipek, P. A., Accardo, P. J., Asshwal, S., Baranek, G. T., Cook, E. H., Dawson, G., et al. (2000). Practice parameter: Screening and diagnosis of autism. *Neurology* 55: 468–479.

13. Fombonne, E. (2001). Is there an epidemic of autism? *Pediatrics* 107:411–412.

14. Howlin, P., & Asgharian, A. (1999). Diagnosis in autism and asperger syndrome: Findings from a survey of 770 families. *Developmental Medicine and Child Neurology* 41: 834–839.

15. Howlin, P., & More, A. (1997). Diagnosis in autism: Survey of over 1200 patients in the U.K. *Autism* 1(22): 135–162.

16. Johnson, C. P., Myers, S. M., & Council on Children with Disabilities–American Academy of Pediatrics (2007). Identification and evaluation of children with Autism Spectrum Disorder. *Pediatrics*, 120(5), 1183–1215.

17. Loftin, R., & Lantz, J. (2003). Cognitive assessment of children with Autism Spectrum Disorder. *The School Psychologist* 57(3): 105–108.

18. Lord, C., Risi, S., Lambrecht, L., Cook, E. H., Leventhal, B. L., DiLavore, P., Pickles, A., & Rutter, M. (2000). The Autism Diagnostic Observation Schedule–Generic: A standard measure of social and communication deficits associated with the spectrum of autism. *Journal of Autism and Developmental Disorders* 30(3): 205–223.

19. Mazefsky, C. A., & Oswald, D. P. (2006). The discriminative ability and diagnostic utility of the ADOS-G, ADI-R, and GARS for children in a clinical setting. *Autism* 10(6): 533–549.

20. Newschaffer, C. J., Fallin, D., & Lee, N. L. (2002). Heritable and non-heritable risk factors for Autism Spectrum Disorder. *Epidemiologic Reviews* 24: 137–153.

21. Ozonoff, S., Goodlin-Jones, B. L., & Solomon, M. (2005). Evidence-based assessment of Autism Spectrum Disorder in children and adolescents. *Journal of Clinical Child and Adolescent Psychology* 34(3): 523–540.

22. Pennsylvania Autism Assessment and Diagnosis Expert Work Group (2007). Supporting quality diagnostic practices for persons with suspected Autism Spectrum Disorder. Document retrieved February 11, 2007, from Pennsylvania Department of Public Welfare: http://www.padpw.pa.us.
23. Pinto-Martin, J., & Levy, S. E. (2004). Early diagnosis of Autism Spectrum Disorder. *Current Treatment Options in Neurology* 6: 391–400.
24. Rogers, S. (2001). Diagnosis of autism before the age of three. *International Review of Research in Mental Retardation* 23: 1–31.
25. Risi, S., Lord, C., Gotham, K., Corsello, C., Chrysler, C., Szatmari, P., et al. (2006). Combining information from multiple sources in the diagnosis of Autism Spectrum Disorder. *Journal of the American Acadent of Child and Adolescent Psychiatry* 45(9): 1094–1103.
26. Robins, D. L., Fein, D., et al. (2001). The Modified Checklist for Autism in Toddlers: An initial study investigating the early detection of autism and pervasive developmental disorders. *Journal of Autism and Developmental Disorders* 31(2): 131–144.
27. Rutter, M., Bailey, A., & Lord, C. (2003). *Social communication questionnaire*. Los Angeles, CA: Western Psychological Services.
28. Simonoff, E. (1998). Genetic counseling in autism and pervasive developmental disorders. *Journal of Autism and Developmental Disorders* 28: 447–456.
29. Zwiagenbaum, L., Bryson, S., Rodgers, T., Roberts, W., Brian, J., & Szatmari, P. (2005). Behavioral manifestations of autism in the first year of life. *International Journal of Neuroscience* 23: 143–152.
30. Volkmar, F., Cook, E. H., Jr., Pomeroy, J., Realmuto, G., & Tanguay, P. (1999). Practice parameters for the assessment and treatment of children, adolescents, and adults with autism and other pervasive developmental disorders. *Journal of the American Academy of Child & Adolescent Psychiatry*, 38, 32s–54s.

Questions

1. The combination of which three features meets the diagnostic criteria for an ASD diagnosis?
   a. Impairments in social interaction, absence of gestures, attention deficit
   b. Impairments in communication, self-stimulatory behaviors, tantrums
   c. Impairments in social interaction, impairments in communication, and restricted and repetitive patterns of behavior
   d. Impairments in communication, cognitive delay; no eye contact
   e. None of the above

2. Which of the following is NOT a common presenting sign specific to ASD?
   a. Not responding to his/her name
   b. Not pointing to show objects to others
   c. Lack of social interest in other children
   d. Delayed or unusual communication
   e. Night seizures

3. Current rates show that ASD occurs in one out of every
   a. 180 children
   b. 110 children
   c. 250 children
   d. 500 children

4. Examples of screening tools, rating scales, or structured assessments used to assess for ASD include which of the following?
   a. M-CHAT
   b. ADOS
   c. GARS2
   d. CARS
   e. All of the above

5. The "red flags" for early identification of ASD include which of the following?
   a. No big smiles or other warm, joyful expressions by six months or thereafter
   b. No back-and-forth sharing of sound, smile, or other facial expression by nine months or thereafter
   c. No babbling by 12 months
   d. No back-and-forth gestures, such as pointing, showing, reaching, or waving, by 12 months
   e. All of the above

Answers

1. c. Impairments in social interaction, impairments in communication, and restricted and repetitive patterns of behavior (per DSM-IV-TR).

2. e. Night seizures are not, all of the others are correct: Not responding to his/her name; Not pointing to show objects to others; Lack of social interest in other children; Delayed or unusual communication.

3. b. 110 children (CDC 2009).

4. e. All of the above: M-CHAT (Modified Checklist for Autism in Toddlers screening tool in pediatrician's office), ADOS (Autism Diagnostic Observation Schedule performed by experienced, trained clinician), GARS2 (Gilliam Autism Rating Scale, Second Edition), CARS (Childhood Autism Rating Scale)

5. e. All of the above: No big smiles or other warm, joyful expressions by six months or thereafter; No back-and-forth sharing of sound, smile, or other facial expression by nine months or thereafter; No babbling by 12 months; No back-and-forth gestures, such as pointing, showing, reaching, or waving, by 12 months

Medical Evaluation and Comorbid Psychiatric Disorders

**Carla A. Mazefsky, Robyn Filipink,
Jodi Lindsey, and Martin J. Lubetsky**

Basic Medical History 44

Family History 45

Physical Exam 46

Laboratory Workup 46

Testing 47

Referrals 47

Additional Clues on the Examination or History 48

ASD and Immunizations 50

Optimize Pediatric Office Visits with Children with ASD 52

Overview of Assessment of Psychiatric Comorbidity in ASD 56

General Issues in the Assessment of Psychiatric Disorders in
    ASD 58

Diagnosing Specific Psychiatric Disorders in ASD Populations 68

Summary 78

Further Reading 80

Questions 82

Answers 83

A thorough assessment of children with autism spectrum disorder includes the evaluation of any medical and developmental history or findings. In completing a medical evaluation, it is important to review many areas in the child's, mother's, and family's history in order to identify associated symptoms that might require further evaluation, laboratory testing, referral, or treatment. Research is providing more understanding about the genetic or metabolic etiology of ASD (see below, and Chapter 4 on neurobiology), which can help clarify the diagnosis or confirm other disorders. Some genetic syndromes may have an increased prevalence of ASD diagnosis. Having a diagnosis of ASD increases the risk for seizures and intellectual disability. Some of the areas identified in medical and developmental history below are further discussed in Chapter 2, which covers early identification and first signs or red flags. As part of the comprehensive medical assessment, it is important to identify the individuals with ASD who have behavioral and emotional symptoms that correlate with a comorbid psychiatric disorder. This chapter will review medical evaluation and psychiatric comorbidities for individuals with ASD.

Basic Medical History

The basic medical history should include the following areas of interest.

- *Birth history: identify risk factors or associations for ASD*
  Mother's age, number of total pregnancies and live births, pregnancy problems (drug or alcohol use, infections, hemorrhaging, diabetes, medication use, assisted technologies), any concerns on ultrasound or on screening tests, gestational age at delivery, delivery complications, and birth weight.
- *Early development: determine global delay vs. isolated language delay. The following are general guidelines regarding typical development*
  Motor: sitting (6 months), crawling (8 months), walking (12 months)
  Language: cooing (3 months), babbling (6 months), first words (12 months), 2–3-word phrases (24 months), 2-step commands (24 months)—ASD (excluding Asperger's disorder) has early language and communication impairment.
  Any regression in skills should be identified (assess if associated with illness, vomiting, fever).
- *General growth: review growth charts*
  Document height, weight, and head circumference.
  - Severe growth retardation can be associated with metabolic disease as well as multiple system involvement.
- *Sleep: identify common sleep issues and signs of sleep apnea or seizures*
  Difficulties with sleep initiation, frequent awakenings, snoring and pauses in breathing, unexplained bruising, tongue biting, or new nocturnal enuresis.
  - Sleep disruption may correlate with seizures, since ASD has increased risk of seizures (see neurological list below).
- *Gastrointestinal (GI): identify failure to thrive, diarrhea, constipation, indigestion, gas, burping, vomiting*
  - Children with ASD may have early GI symptoms that are missed due to communication impairment and challenging behaviors (see Chapter 9 on feeding and toileting issues). Challenging behaviors may reflect the child's discomfort or pain that is not communicated due to language limitations.
- *Neurological: identify signs or symptoms for seizures that affect up to one third of individuals with ASD (one peak under age five and a second peak in adolescence)*
  - Regression in speech can be a sign of Landau-Kleffner syndrome; regression in skills or behavior after fever or illness can be a sign of a metabolic or mitochondrial disease; abnormal movements such as stereotypies or tics are common in ASD (if motor and vocal tics last more than one year, then symptoms meet Tourette syndrome diagnosis); tremor can be secondary to medications, but can also be associated with metabolic or mitochondrial disease or pediatric neurotransmitter disorders. Staring and freezing episodes, convulsions, or symptoms during sleep (tongue- or cheek-biting, bruising, nocturnal enuresis) can be signs of seizure; deafness, muscle weakness, or significant hypotonia can be a sign of a metabolic or mitochondrial disorder.
- *Menstrual: identify changes during puberty and menses, pain or discomfort, mood changes*

Explore signs of premenstrual dysphoric disorder (PMDD) and pre-menstrual symptoms (PMS), hygiene issues, and contraception use.
  • Girls with ASD may have difficulty communicating menstrual discomfort and pain, which may result in their displaying challenging behaviors. Teaching them hygiene care may be more difficult.
• *Behavioral/psychiatric: Diagnosis given or suspected, medication list to clarify diagnosis*
Attention deficit hyperactivity disorder (ADHD), disruptive behavior disorder/oppositional defiant disorder (ODD)/conduct disorder, anxiety, obsessive-compulsive disorder (OCD), depression, or bipolar disorder (see the second section of this chapter).
  • Challenging behaviors may make it difficult to sort out whether they are due to ASD or a comorbid psychiatric disorder—which may require additional diagnosis and a different focus of treatment (see section below, as well as Chapter 5 on functional behavior assessment and Chapter 12 on interventions).

Family History

A thorough family history should be taken, covering any known relatives (up to third generation) with:
• autism (twin siblings have a high rate of concordance)
• intellectual disability (almost two thirds of individuals with ASD also have ID)
• known genetic syndromes (Fragile X syndrome, tuberous sclerosis complex—see below)
• metabolic disorders
• epilepsy
• appears eccentric or socially awkward
Symptoms in family members who have gray zone allele, pre-mutations allele, or full mutation fragile-X syndrome include anxiety, learning disorders, thyroid disease, migraine, infertility, primary ovarian insufficiency, tremor and ataxia, or cognitive difficulties resembling Alzheimer's disease (see below).

Physical Exam

Dysmorphic features increase concern that there is a genetic etiology; skin findings evaluate for phacomatoses; multiple body-system involvement suggests mitochondrial disease; focal neurological exam or abnormal head circumference lead to MRI; signs of seizure lead to EEG.

- Growth measurements: head circumference (microcephaly or macrocephaly), weight, height
- Dysmorphic features: ear size and structure, nose size, face shape, size, coarseness of features, teeth, size of hands and feet, and finger and toe abnormalities
- Skin/examined under Wood's lamp: hyper- or hypopigmented skin lesions, axillary or inguinal freckling (Wood's ultraviolet light useful in diagnosing certain conditions seen on skin, such as tuberous sclerosis)
- General: cardiac, pulmonary, GI, orthopedic abnormalities
- Neurological: cranial nerves, muscle (hypotonia, spasticity), sensory, deep tendon reflex, gait (toe walking) and balance (ataxia), adventitious movements (chorea, tremor, tic, stereotypy, dystonia).

Laboratory Workup

A basic genetic screening assesses commonly associated conditions. A more detailed and specific evaluation is based on family history, a physical exam, and concern for metabolic or mitochondrial disease.

These tests are usually ordered by the evaluating pediatrician, developmental behavioral pediatrician, neurologist, or geneticist, or per their consultation with the child and adolescent psychiatrist. The psychiatrist may order lead level tests based on pica history; DNA testing for Fragile X (for ASD diagnosis or family history of Fragile X); and high-resolution chromosome analysis by G-banding have the highest yield in determining etiology in children with ASD (Johnson et al., 2007). Chromosomal/cytogenetic microarray (CMA) has been proposed to replace high-resolution karyotyping (Shen et al., 2010, Manning et al., 2010). See Table 3.1 for description of neuro-metabolic disorders and ASD: onset, prevalence of ASD associated with metabolic disease, and diagnostic testing.

- Lead level—suspected pica (*pica* is described as the eating of non-food substances such as paint, dirt, crayons, coins, etc.; and some substances may contain lead. Lead toxicity is suspected of causing learning and behavior problems, and when detected, can be treated by chelation)
- High-resolution chromosome analysis–detects chromosomal aneuploidy in 5% ASD
- Array Comparative Genomic Hybridization (aCGH) (microarray, oligoarray)—detects deletion/duplication syndromes and Copy Number Variants (CNVs) estimated to identify 7%–10% of ASD
- FMR1 molecular genetic testing (Southern blot, PCR) for Fragile X–associated disorders—identifies gray zone (45–54 repeats), pre-mutation (55–199 repeats), and full mutation (> 200 repeats) with and without mosaic pattern for repeat number and methylation patterns
- Metabolic/mitochondrial workup:

1st tier: complete metabolic panel, lactate, pyruvate, ammonia, uric acid, CPK, serum amino acids, total/free carnitine, acylcarnitines, urine organic acids, urine creatine/GAA
2nd tier: POLG 1, Mito 3000 panel, 7-dehydrocholesterol, urine mucopolysaccharides/oligosaccharides, MRI/MRS.

If dysmorphic features and history are specific to a syndrome, specific testing is recommended. If the examiner strongly suspects Angelman syndrome, then test through methylation studies.

Testing

EEG—"there is no evidence to support universal screening EEG unless [there is] a clinical indication of seizures or clear language regression" (Johnson et al., 2007).
MRI—"screening MRIs on all children who present with ASD are not necessary" (Johnson et al., 2007).

Referrals

Consider referral to genetics/metabolic genetics or neurology specialists, if there is significant family history of such, dysmorphic features, or you suspect metabolic/mitochondrial disease. Additional evaluations may include: audiologic testing, speech and language evaluation, psychoeducational/neuropsychological testing, and occupational/physical therapy evaluation.

If there is concern about pain (e.g., challenging behaviors which may be correlated with pain such as tooth or stomach) or other healthcare issues, then consider referral to dentist or gastroenterologist. The child and adolescent psychiatrist may order any of these referrals directly or after consultation with the pediatrician or neurologist. (See helpful recommendations in Volkmar & Wiesner's book *Healthcare for Children on the Autism Spectrum: A Guide to Medical, Nutritional and Behavioral Issues*).

Additional Clues on the Examination or History

See Table 3.2 for descriptions of genetic syndromes and ASD: gene[s] associated with the syndrome, percentage of patients with ASD who have the syndrome, and percentage of patients with the syndrome who have an ASD.

- Microcephaly: Rett or atypical Rett syndrome (MECP2, CDKL5/STK9, FOXG1)
- Microcephaly and self-injurious behavior: 2,3 syndactyly: Smith-Lemli-Opiz syndrome
- Macrocephaly: PTEN mutations, Sotos syndrome, neurofibromatosis, Fragile X syndrome
- Brain malformation, epilepsy, ID: Aristaless-related homeobox gene (ARX) mutation
- Large ears, hyperextensibility of joints, long face, ID, anxiety: Fragile X syndrome
- Facial weakness, limited abduction of eye: Moebius syndrome
- Coarse facies: Sanfilippo syndrome
- Movement disorder: succunic semialdehyde dehydrogenase deficiency, creatine deficiency syndromes
- Epilepsy or abnormal EEG: Fragile X syndrome, urea cycle disorders, creatine deficiency syndrome, adenylosuccinase deficiency, dihydrpyrimidine dehydrogenase deficiency, Angelman syndrome

---

Neurogenetic syndromes associated with ASD may include:

- Fragile X Syndrome (FXS)—the most common identifiable cause of ASD and the most common inheritable cause of ID. Expansion CGG repeat disorder of FMRI gene on Xq27.3 chromosome. Phenotype present in only 30%–50% of patients: includes ID, macrocephaly, long and narrow face, large protruding ears, prominent jaw and forehead, broad nose, large testicles (macroorchidism), hypotonia, large hands and joint hyperextensibility, and mitral valve prolapse. Estimated that 20% may have epilepsy. Fragile X–associated disorders include FX tremor ataxia syndrome, FX primary ovarian syndrome and FXS. Pathological CGG repeats: gray zone (45–54), pre-mutation (55–199) and full mutation (200+). May have mosaicism for repeat number and methylation pattern. Refer any patient with a repeat of 45 and above to an FXS clinic for long-term medical surveillance and care, and behavioral and educational support. Thirty percent of individuals with FXS demonstrate characteristics of ASD. (www.fragilex.org, www.fraxa.org).
- Tuberous Sclerosis Complex (TSC)—a neurocutaneous disorder characterized by ID (at least 50%–60%), hypopigmented macules (Wood's lamp ultraviolet light skin visualization), hamartomas (benign tumors or "tubers") in the brain and central nervous system, skin, kidneys, eyes, heart, and lungs; and facial fibroangiomata (formerly called adenoma sebaceum). Intracerebral lesions may result in seizures in up to 80% of patients. Autosomal dominant disorder caused by mutations in TSC1 (9q34 chromosome) or TSC2

(16p13.3 chromosome). Seventeen to 65% of individuals with
TSC demonstrate characteristics of ASD. Refer to TS Clinic for
long-term care.
- Angelman Syndrome—associated with loss of maternally expressed
ubiquitin-protein ligase gene (UBE3A) on 15q, most often through
deletion (90% detected through methylation analysis and UBE3A
sequence analysis). Smaller percentage caused by mutation of maternal
copy, paternal uniparental disomy, or translocation. Wide-based ataxic
gait and frequent laughing/smiling; referred to as the "happy puppet
syndrome"; general developmental delay, often nonverbal, hypotonia,
seizures (up to 80%), progressive spasticity, and sleep disturbance.
Often patients are fair-skinned and have light-colored hair.
- Rett Syndrome—consider in all females who demonstrate autistic-like
regression, especially with "hand-wringing" stereotypic movements,
progressive microcephaly, abnormal breathing patterns, and seizures.
Can cause profound ID. DNA testing for mutation of methyl CpG-
binding protein 2 (MECP2) gene positive in approximately 80% of
cases. Deletion and duplication of gene also present in males with the
same symptoms, especially ID. Atypical Rett syndrome is associated
with early-onset epilepsy in mutation of gene CDKL5/STK9, and
severe hypotonia and developmental delay within the first few months
of life in mutation of gene FOXG1.

ASD and Immunizations

Numerous studies have failed to demonstrate a causal relationship between immunizations, particularly thimerosal-containing vaccines, and ASD, including a case-control study from the journal *Pediatrics* that demonstrated no increased risk of ASD in relation to either a prenatal or early-life exposure to ethylmercury from thimerosal-containing vaccines (Price et al. 2010).

Other studies have attempted to evaluate the difference of immune-mediated or antibody responses to particular vaccines, such as the measles component of the MMR vaccine, and have also failed to demonstrate a significant difference in outcomes related to an ASD. (Baird et al. 2008).

A large debate over this hypothesis of a causal relationship between the thimerosal-containing vaccines and the immune-mediated response and ASD began in relation to a study by Wakefield et al. (1998). This study subsequently was fully retracted in 2010 by the *Lancet*, and many of the authors withdrew their names from the study (Editors of *Lancet*, 2010).

Despite the lack of significant evidence to support a causal relationship between vaccinations and ASD, it is important to note any clinical correlation in a child with an ASD with any regression in language or other developmental milestones that occur in association with an immunization, especially with fever or seizure, as this may suggest a possible underlying neuro-metabolic or mitochondrial disorder that is currently undiagnosed.

Optimize Pediatric Office Visits with Children with ASD

- Child with ASD may not look ill, but may display challenging behaviors
- Challenging behaviors may reflect pain that is not communicated verbally
- Challenging behaviors may reflect the child's difficulty with communication, changes, new places, new situations, new experiences, new sounds, new smells, and new people
- The child with ASD may display injuries that could reflect self-injurious behaviors, limited pain sensation, and lack of sense of danger
- Be alert to one's own safety and the child's personal space in order to avoid being injured by the child's reaction to physical exam and potential head butt, bite, kick, spit, punch, pull hair, bolt, etc
- Consider an advance telephone conference with the parent (or advance form completion) to:
  - obtain history
  - ask for the parent's advice on how to make the appointment easier for the child
  - ask the parent to bring reinforcers for the child
  - ask the parent to bring another adult to help with the child while history is obtained
  - suggest that the parent prepare the child with a medical social story
  - if blood draw will be done, consider prescribing an anesthetic cream for the parent to apply in advance
- Prepare the exam room for safety and limited stimulation
- Try to limit any wait time in the waiting room by scheduling appropriately

  (See these suggestions and more information in *Autism Physician Handbook*, Help Autism Now Society (HANS), 2007, Salem, OR.)

Table 3.1 – Neuro-metabolic Disorders and ASD

Neuro-metabolic Disorders	Onset	Prevalence of ASD associated with metabolic disease	Diagnostic Testing
Phenylketonuria	Neonatal	5.7%	Quantitative plasma amino acid analysis
Adenylocsuccinase Deficit	Within first year	~50% display autistic features	Presence of succinyl aminoimidazole, carboxamide riboside, and succinyl adenosine in urine and cerebrospinal fluid
Creatine Deficiency Syndromes	3 mos–2 yrs		Blood and urinary concentrations of creatine and guanidinoacetate; ratio of creatine/creatinine; gene mutations; brain MR spectroscopy
Inborn Errors of Cholesterol Biosynthesis	After infancy	50% to 86%	Abnormal sterol pattern (Low plasma and tissue cholesterol concentrations with increased plasma and tissue 7–dehydrocholesterol reductase and its metabolite in Smith-Lemli-Opitz syndrome or known gene mutation on chromosome 11q12-q13)
Biotinidase Deficiency	3–12 mos		Serum biotinidase deficiency → sequence of gene
Infantile Ceroid Lipofuscinosis	> 2 yrs		Palmitoyl protein thioesterase 1 enzyme activity, histopathologic examination demonstrates inclusion on lymphocytes on brain
Sanfilippo Syndrome	Within first year		Quantitative urinary glycosaminoglycan analysis; mutation analysis

(continued)

Table 3.1 – Neuro-metabolic Disorders and ASD (continued)

Neuro-metabolic Disorders	Onset	Prevalence of ASD associated with metabolic disease	Diagnostic Testing
Histidinemia	Birth		Elevated blood histidine, increased urinary excretion of histidine and its transamination products
Succinic Semialdehyde Dehydrogenase Deficiency	> 3 mos		Accumulation of γ-hydroxybutyrate in urine, serum, and cerebrospinal fluid; enzymatic deficiency in lymphocytes and cultured lymphoblasts
Dihydropyrimidine Dehydrogenase Deficiency	Within first year		Increased uracil and thymine on organic acid analysis by gas chromatography–mass spectrometry

Source, Table 3.1: Reproduced with minor modifications from Manzi, B., Loizzo, A. L., Giana, G., & Curatolo, P. (2008). Autism and metabolic diseases. *Journal of Child Neurology,* 23(3), 307–314.

Table 3.2 – Genetic Syndromes and ASD

Genetic Syndrome	Gene[s] associated with the syndrome	Percentage of patients with an ASD that have the syndrome	Percentage of patients with the syndrome that have an ASD
Fragile X syndrome	FMR1	2%–5%	20%–40%
Tuberous sclerosis	TSC1, TSC2	3%–4%	43%–86%
15q duplication Angelman/ Prader Willi syndrome	UBE3A GABAr cluster	1%–2%	> 40%
16p11 deletion	PCKB1	1%	High
22q deletion	SHANK3	1%	High
2q37 deletion	KIF1A, GBX2	Unknown	50%
Joubert syndrome	AHI1	Unknown	40%
Timothy syndrome	CACNA1C	Unknown	60%–70%
Cortical dysplasia–focal epilepsy syndrome	CNTNAP2	Rare	70%

Table 3.2: Excerpted from Benvenuto, A., Manzi, B., Alessandrelli, R., Galasso, C., & Curatolo, P. (2009). Recent advances in the pathogenesis of syndromic autism. *International Journal of Pediatrics*, DOI: 10.1155/2009/198736.

For additional information on ASD and genetics see: Moss, J., & Howlin, P. (2009). Autism Spectrum Disorder in genetic syndromes: Implications for diagnosis, intervention and understanding the wider autism spectrum disorder population. *Journal of Intellectual Disability Research*, 53(10), 852–873.

Overview of Assessment of Psychiatric Comorbidity in ASD

Psychiatric comorbidity is now acknowledged as quite common in ASD (e.g., Matilla et al., 2010; Matson & Nebel-Schwalm, 2007). For example, using a structured psychiatric interview developed specifically for ASD populations, 72% of children with ASD across a range of intellectual abilities were found to have two or more comorbid diagnoses (Leyfer et al., 2006). However, firm prevalence rates for the various disorders are unavailable at this time, due partly to a lack of large-scale epidemiological studies and partly to widely varying methods of assessment and participant samples across studies. What is clear, however, is that psychiatric comorbidity increases the level of impairment for a significant majority of the population, including increases in behavioral problems, exacerbation of social impairment, and general deterioration in functioning. Therefore, it is critical to remain aware of potential comorbid diagnoses and to complete further assessment should there be any potential concerns.

General Issues in the Assessment of Psychiatric Disorders in ASD

Diagnosing psychiatric conditions in individuals with ASD is quite a challenge for many reasons. The Key Facts box below summarizes a few of the main complications.

> **Key Fact Box 3.1 – General Factors Complicating the Diagnosis of Psychiatric Comorbidities in Individuals with ASD**
>
> - Difficulty assessing individuals across all levels of intellectual disability and language ability
> - Unclear phenomenology of psychiatric disorders in ASD, but some reason to believe that there may be different presenting symptoms and manifestations to consider
> - Scarcity of measures to diagnose or screen for psychiatric disorders that are validated or modified specifically for individuals with ASD; limited research on the measures that do exist
> - Ideal methods of assessment are time-intensive and include multiple reporters, such as parent-report, self-report, teacher-report, and clinician interview and observation
> - Debates about whether symptoms represent a separate disorder or are related to the underlying ASD
> - Difficulty distinguishing ASD-related impairment from comorbidity, especially for non-episodic disorders

Methods of Assessment

In this section, the various forms of psychiatric assessments and related issues regarding their use in ASD are summarized, including self-report questionnaires, parent/caregiver- and teacher-report questionnaires, and structured interviews. There are countless measures designed to detect psychiatric disorders used in general psychiatry that have been applied to ASD populations in research or clinical practice. However, the emphasis below is on those developed or modified specifically for use with individuals with ASD or other developmental disorders, including intellectual disabilities. Screening can occur in the primary care doctor's office, school, or vocational training setting, but most often takes place in the psychiatrist or psychologist's office.

- **Self-report questionnaires**

Self-report questionnaires are commonly used as a screening tool for psychiatric disorders in typically developing populations. This is an efficient way to detect high risk and identify patients in need of further assessment. However, there are concerns about the degree of self-awareness and understanding regarding one's own emotions in ASD, which could hamper the utility of self-report questionnaires in ASD. Furthermore, most studies that established the norms and psychometric properties for the self-report questionnaires specifically excluded children and adults with ASD. Therefore, the validity and reliability of these measures completed by individuals with ASD is unclear. A handful of studies have utilized self-report questionnaires as measure of treatment outcomes for higher-functioning individuals with ASD, but the results have been mixed. Some studies found that they were able to detect change consistent with other informants, whereas others did not.

There have not been any systematic studies of the psychometric properties of self-report questionnaires completed by children and adults with ASD, with one exception. Mazefsky, Kao, and Oswald (2011) administered four commonly used self-report psychiatric screener questionnaires to 10–17-year-old children and adolescents with ASD and without mental retardation, and compared the findings to parent-reported diagnoses based on a structured psychiatric interview. The anxiety, depression, and attention-deficit/hyperactivity disorder questionnaires resulted in many false negatives, and a questionnaire to screen for obsessive-compulsive disorder symptoms resulted in a high number of false positives (Mazefsky et al., 2011). Although perfect concordance between parent and child report would not be expected, the inability of the screening questionnaires to detect risk when a comorbid disorder was present was discouraging. The one positive finding was a high degree of internal reliability for all of the measures (Mazefsky et al., 2011), which suggests that higher-functioning individuals with ASD can understand and provide consistent responses to self-report questionnaires.

Overall at this point, however, research does not support recommending any particular self-report questionnaires for use in ASD populations. Self-report psychiatric screeners administered to individuals with ASD may yield additional valuable information, but clinicians should interpret this information carefully based on their own clinical judgments and available information from other sources, given the potential concerns about validity. It is particularly important not to stop assessing for the possibility of a psychiatric disorder when a self-report measure does not indicate risk, especially if other indicators such as a decline in functioning are present.

- **Parent or other informant questionnaires**

There are many broad-based psychiatric screening tools available with both parent- and teacher-report versions. In addition, there are many disorder-specific questionnaires with parent- and teacher-report versions. Many of these questionnaires could also be completed by other caregivers and providers, particularly for individuals in residential treatment programs. However, similar to self-report instruments, the vast majority of these measures have not been specifically validated for use with individuals with ASD, despite being widely used.

For children, the Child Behavior Checklist and Behavior Assessment System for Children are broad-based screeners that are quite commonly administered to parents of children with ASD. The same cautions exist for these measures as for the self-report measures, given a lack of systematic studies regarding their use for individuals with ASD as screeners of psychiatric problems. One additional potential concern is that some of the scales designed to detect symptoms of other disorders may be commonly elevated among children with ASD, regardless of their comorbidity status. For example, studies have shown that children with ASD diagnoses as a group tend to have very high mean scores on the social, thought, attention, and withdrawn/depressed problems scales of the Child Behavior Checklist (e.g., Mazefsky et al., 2010). Therefore, as with parent- and teacher-report questionnaires, it will be important to consider other sources of information when determining if elevations are due to comorbidity or if they are in fact detecting underlying ASD symptoms.

There is a handful of questionnaires that have been developed specifically for use in developmentally disordered or ASD populations. These are summarized in Table 3.3 below. Because they may aid in diagnostic decision-making, the table also includes some scales designed to assess problematic behaviors that do not map directly onto psychiatric diagnoses (such as the Aberrant Behavior Checklist and Behavior Problems Inventory, etc.). Many of these questionnaires may also be helpful for tracking treatment progress when treating comorbid disorders or symptoms. It should be noted that several of these measures were developed and designed for populations with intellectual disabilities and not ASD. They may be more helpful than traditional measures, especially for children and adults who have both ASD and intellectual disability. Another important caution is that none of the measures has the level of research support possessed by questionnaires used in other branches of psychiatry. The vast majority of these instruments have just one study behind their development, or have been studied only by the developer of the instrument. Therefore, practitioners using these questionnaires should remain aware of potential validity and reliability limitations.

- **Parent or other informant interviews**

Although full structured interviews are difficult to administer in practice due to their time-intensive nature, interviews provide the type of in-depth information necessary for complex differential diagnosis. Therefore, when true concern exists regarding a comorbid disorder, it would be most helpful to utilize a more structured interview format, or at least portions of a structured interview, as part of the diagnostic process.

Many different interviews have been used across psychiatric comorbidity research studies, including those developed for ASD populations and interviews modified from other existing measures for use in ASD. In addition, several interviews have been developed for individuals with developmental disabilities in general (usually targeting intellectual disabilities), and are used in ASD populations. Finally, many comorbidity studies and clinicians use interviews from general psychiatry without modifications. Although caution must again be applied when using this method, the most commonly used general psychiatry measures include the Kiddie Schedule for Affective Disorder and Schizophrenia–Present and Lifetime version (K-SADS) for children; and the adult version of this measure, the Schedule for Affective Disorders and Schizophrenia–Lifetime version—modified for the study of anxiety disorders (SADS-LA). These tools may be effective for higher-functioning individuals in the spectrum, particularly if some of the conceptual comments noted in the next section are considered during administration.

Table 3.4 below summarizes pertinent information for some of the measures that have been developed or modified specifically for use with individuals with ASD or other developmental disabilities (predominantly intellectual disability). It should be noted that all of the interviews discussed require the interviewer to be highly trained and skilled in both general psychiatry and ASD/developmentally disordered populations in order to maintain reliable and valid administration.

Table 3.3 – Rating Scales to Assess for Behavioral and Emotional Concerns in Developmentally Disabled Populations

Name of Instrument	Scores Produced	Age Range	Population Developed for and Other Notes	Availability
Aberrant Behavior Checklist (ABC)	Irritability, agitation, crying; lethargy, social withdrawal; stereotypic behavior; hyperactivity, noncompliance; and inappropriate speech	5–51 yrs+	Has separately normed community and residential versions; developed for intellectual disabilities but very widely applied in ASD research	Slosson Educational Publications, Inc.
Anxiety, Depression, and Mood Screen (ADAMS)	Manic/hyperactive behavior; depressed mood; social avoidance; general anxiety; and compulsive behavior	10–79 years	Developed for intellectual disability populations	None noted; corresponding author is Anna Esbensen: esbensen.l@osu.edu
Autism Spectrum Disorder—Comorbid for Children (ASD-CC)	Items cover depression, conduct disorder, ADHD, tic disorder, OCD, specific phobia, and eating difficulties	Children (tested on 2–16-year-olds)	Developed and normed for ASD & intellectual disability population	http://www.disabilityconsultants.org/Order.asp
Autism Spectrum Disorder—Comorbid for Adults (ASD-CA)	Anxiety/repetitive behaviors; conduct problems; irritability/behavioral excesses; attention/hyperactivity/impulsivity; and depressive symptoms	Adults	Developed and normed for ASD & intellectual disability population	http://www.disabilityconsultants.org/Order.asp

(continued)

Table 3.3 – Rating Scales to Assess for Behavioral and Emotional Concerns in Developmentally Disabled Populations (continued)

Name of Instrument	Scores Produced	Age Range	Population Developed for and Other Notes	Availability
Behavior Problems Inventory (BPI-01)	Aggressive/destructive; self-injurious behavior; and stereotyped behavior	14–91	Individuals with intellectual disability	Email Johannes Rojahn, jrojahn@gmu.edu
Developmental Behavior Checklist	Total score; disruptive/antisocial; self-absorbed; communication disturbance; anxiety; social relating; and depressive (adults only); symptom cluster information available to calculate depression and attention deficit hyperactivity scores for the parent version	Separate versions for children (4–18) and adults	Separate versions for parents/caregivers, teachers, and adults; short versions are also available, as is a version designed for daily monitoring; norms are available by intellectual disability level	Western Psychological Services or DBC@med.monash.edu.au
Psychiatric Assessment Schedule for Adults with Developmental Disabilities Checklist (PAS-ADD Checklist)	Total score; affective/neurotic disorder; possible organic disorder; and psychotic disorder	Adults	Developed and normed for intellectual disability populations; focuses on symptoms in the past 4 weeks	Pavilion Publishing; http://www.pavpub.com/pavpub/home/index.asp

Reiss Scales for Children's Dual Diagnosis	Anxiety disorder; anger/self-control; attention deficit; autism/PDD; conduct disorder; depression; poor self-esteem; psychosis; somatoform behaviors; withdrawn/isolated; total score	Ages 4–21	Has norms for children with intellectual disability and also provides information on how scores correspond to DSM-IV diagnosis when appropriate	IDS publishing; http://www.idspublishing.com/screen.htm
Reiss Screen for Maladaptive Behavior	Aggressive behavior, autism, psychosis, paranoia, depression–physical signs, depression–behavioral signs, dependent personality disorder, avoidant disorder	Ages 16 and up	Normed for mild versus severe intellectual disabilities; screens based on severity of behavior, diagnosis and rare symptoms	IDS publishing; http://www.idspublishing.com/screen.htm

Table 3.4 – Interviews Developed or Modified for use with Developmentally Disordered and ASD Populations

Name of Interview	Disorders Assessed	Age Range	Population Developed For	Information Produced	Availability	Other
Assessment for Dual Diagnosis (ADD)	All major DSM-IV-TR Axis I disorders	Adults	Mild to Moderate Intellectual disability, both institutionalized and community	Present or not with severity and duration indices	http://www.disabilityconsultants.org/Order.asp	
Autism Comorbidity Interview	All major DSM-IV-TR Axis I disorders, both current and past (except ASD)	Children and adults	ASD and/or intellectual disability and other developmental disorders	Syndromal, subsyndromal, subthreshold, or not present diagnostic status	Used by author-approved researchers and not public	
Baby and Infant Screen for Children with Autism Traits (BISCUIT)	Part I of the BISCUIT focused on autism traits and associated problems; Part 2 focused on comorbidity in developmental disabilities; Part 3 focused on problems behaviors in children with developmental delays	17–37-month olds	Infants and toddlers at risk for or with ASD	Part 2: scores for: tantrum/conduct problems; inattention/impulsivity; avoidance behavior; anxiety/repetitive behavior; and eating problems/sleeping	http://www.disabilityconsultants.org/Order.asp	Also can be used as an ASD screener

Children's Yale-Brown Obsessive-Compulsive Scale modified for Pervasive Developmental Disorders (CYBOCS-PDD)	OCD, obsessions not assessed, and additional repetitive behaviors added to list of compulsions (e.g., it is probably tapping repetitive behavior more broadly than related to OCD alone)	Children		Severity score	Contact author, Dr. Scahill, lawrence.scahill@yale.edu	Clinician-rated measure that integrates parent-report, observation, and child report
Diagnostic Assessment for the Severely Handicapped–II	Anxiety; depression; mania; PDD/autism; schizophrenia; stereotypies and tics; self-injurious behavior; elimination disorders; eating disorders; sexual disorders; organic syndromes; impulse control	Adults	Severe to profound intellectual disability	Norms and cutoffs for each subscale; DSM-IV criteria can be applied to these scores but the scores themselves do not produce diagnoses per se	http://www.disabilityconsultants.org/Order.asp	Can be used as a rating scale instead of interview

(continued)

Table 3.4 – Interviews Developed or Modified for use with Developmentally Disordered and ASD Populations (continued)

Name of Interview	Disorders Assessed	Age Range	Population Developed For	Information Produced	Availability	Other
Mood and Anxiety Semi-Structured Interview for Patients with Intellectual Disabilities (MASS)	DSM-IV generalized anxiety disorder, any anxiety disorder, major depressive episode, or manic episode	Adults	Moderate to profound intellectual disability	Present or absent mood or anxiety symptoms to meet diagnoses	Unclear; corresponding author is:	
Psychiatric Assessment Schedule for Adults with Developmental Disability (PAS-ADD 10 Interview)	ICD-10 diagnostic classes of psychotic disorders, hypomania, depression, and anxiety disorders	Adults	Intellectual disability	Uses a computer algorithm to compute ICD-10 diagnoses	Contact author Dr Steve Moss; enquiries@pasadd.co.uk	Parallel version to interview the respondent and an informant

Schedule for the Assessment of Psychiatric Problems Associated with Autism (SAPPA)	Episodic disorders including mood, anxiety, and psychotic disorders; as well as some non-episodic concerns (self-injury, stereotypies, etc)	Autism and developmental disorders	Absent, possible, probable, or definite; linked to ICD-10 Research Diagnostic Criteria	Unlisted; authors are Bolton & Rutter, 1994

Diagnosing Specific Psychiatric Disorders in ASD Populations

As noted in the beginning of this chapter, one of the main challenges in diagnosing psychiatric disorders in individuals with ASD is the possibility of different presenting symptoms and difficulty in differentiating impairment related to the underlying ASD from impairment due to a separate condition. Below, available information is summarized regarding these issues (e.g., identification of possible alternative presenting symptoms to be aware of, and information on differential diagnosis) for several disorders that are commonly considered as comorbid diagnoses in children and adults with ASD, including mood disorders (e.g., depression, bipolar disorder), anxiety, obsessive-compulsive disorder, attention-deficit/hyperactivity disorder, and oppositional defiant disorder. Many specific points are taken from the Autism Comorbidity Interview (ACI; J. Lainhart, personal communication). Disorders not discussed, such as schizophrenia, eating disorders, substance use disorders, and personality disorders, are less common in ASD.

While we do not want to miss true comorbid diagnoses, over-diagnosing comorbidity can be equally harmful. General rules of thumb in the differential diagnostic process, particularly for episodic disorders, are:

- Symptoms should differ qualitatively or quantitatively (*an important and meaningful change*) from "baseline" functioning with the ASD
  - In order to determine this, one must first establish how the individual is, *at his best* or in his *normal mood*.
  - With comorbidity, there may be new symptoms *or* a worsening of baseline behavior/emotions
  - There should be *additional* impairment related to the new or changed symptoms
- It is important to make sure that the "additional" symptoms we are applying as evidence of a comorbid disorder make sense for the child with ASD (disorder-specific examples provided in sections below).
- Symptoms counted as evidence of the existence of a comorbid disorder should co-occur temporally.

Mood Disorders

Mood disorders, such as depression and bipolar disorder, in ASD have recently begun to receive a great deal of attention (see Ghaziuddin et al., 2002, and Stewart et al., 2006, for review of depression in ASD). There are many factors that may increase risk for mood disorders in ASD. For example, there are high rates of mood disorders in parents of individuals with ASD, suggesting possible increases in genetic risk (e.g., Mazefsky et al., 2008). In addition, there are many potential psychosocial stressors that could be possible triggers. For example, higher-functioning individuals who are aware of their deficits and badly desire friends, but lack success in this area, are at particular risk. Features of depression, bipolar disorder, and catatonia are listed in the box below. It is important to remember that catatonia can be diagnosed in individuals with ASD.

However, there is a delicate balance between considering underlying emotion-regulation concerns that may be part and parcel of the ASD and concerns that are distinct and require a comorbid diagnosis and a different treatment. Although there is little research on emotion regulation in ASD, there is clear evidence that emotion regulation is highly variable and often problematic in this population, regardless of psychiatric comorbidity (Mazefsky, Pelphrey, & Dahl, under review). In fact, the extent of emotional problems can sometimes mask or overshadow other ASD symptoms, leading to a delay in receiving an ASD diagnosis. In addition, problems regulating emotions in general can lead to the appearance of "mood swings," which in turn often lead to questions of bipolar disorder (Ghaziuddin, 2005). Therefore, particularly for mood disorders, it is imperative to consider baseline functioning and not over-diagnose mood disorders when the concern may be more temperamental in nature. Given that mood disorders are episodic by definition, gathering a strong baseline understanding is of particular importance.

Depression
- Features (Ghaziuddin, 2005): Sad affect, crying spells, disturbance in sleep and appetite, increased social withdrawal and isolation, increased ritualistic behaviors, change in preoccupations or fixations (to more morbid, sad, worried), increased irritability, regression of skills/ activities of daily living, and possible psychotic symptoms.

Bipolar disorder
- Features: Mood instability, alternating depressed and elated mood, increased irritability, increased impulsivity, aggressive/destructive outbursts, and possible psychotic symptoms.

Catatonia
- Features (Dhossche & Wachtel, 2010; Kakooza-Mwesige et al., 2008): Excitement, immobility/stupor, mutism, staring, posturing/ catalepsy, grimacing, echopraxia/echolalia, stereotypy, mannerisms, verbigeration, rigidity, negativism, waxy flexibility, withdrawal, impulsivity, automatic obedience, passive obedience, ambitendency, grasp reflex, perseveration, combativeness, autonomic abnormality (body temperature, blood pressure, pulse rate, respiratory rate, inappropriate sweating).

Catatonia has been increasingly diagnosed in individuals with ASD as a comorbid syndrome, usually with mood disorder such as depression. It is important to assess for symptoms; rule out causes such as infectious, metabolic, endocrinological, neurological, or autoimmune disorders; pre- scribed medications, or recreational drugs; and to complete differential diagnosis for hyperkinetic disorders—acute dystonia, tardive dyskinesia, akathisia, withdrawal dyskinesias, tics, epilepsy, delirium; or hypokinetic disorders—Parkinsonism, neuroleptic malignant syndrome, malignant hyperthermia, serotonergic syndrome, status epilepticus.

Table 3.5 summarizes key concepts to consider regarding potential symptoms of mood disorders in ASD, including depression and bipolar disorder. Many of the concepts presented in Table 3.3 are from the Autism Comorbidity Interview (ACI; J. Lainhart, personal communication). In the second column, "baseline/differential diagnosis considerations," symptoms or concepts are noted that should be probed regarding the individual's best or normal mood. Many of the considerations noted represent possible

Table 3.5 – Special Considerations Related to the Presentation and Diagnosis of Mood Symptoms in ASD

Symptom	Baseline/differential diagnosis considerations	Potential unique manifestations in ASD
Depressed Mood	General history of restricted or flat affect	Behavioral manifestations such as increases in self-injury or aggression
Irritability; Anger	Temperamental or situational irritability; temper tantrums related to communication frustrations	
Anhedonia; boredom	General history of restricted interests	Less enjoyment from special interests; more morbid quality to special interests.
Suicidal ideation/behavior		Out of character behaviors (jumping off stairs or out a window, running into traffic) for those with limited ability for more sophisticated plans.
Insomnia, hypersomnia, decreased need for sleep	General history of sleep problems and general sleep patterns (see Chapter 14 regarding sleep in ASD)	Continuing to follow sleep routine despite sleeping more poorly.
Psychomotor agitation	Typical activity level/degree of restlessness	More frequent repetitive behaviors combined with irritability/tension; normal levels of activity for those with low baseline levels.
Guilt	Ever demonstrated understanding of the concept?	
Poor concentration; distractibility	History of inattention; slow processing time; tendency to focus on details	

Indecision	Ability and opportunities to make independent decisions	
Weight gain	Medication-related weight changes	
Elated mood	History of inappropriate affect (laughing when nothing is funny); tendency to get easily excited by things they like	More social engagement
Racing thoughts; pressured speech	Tendency to be overly verbose (especially in Asperger's), history of prosody problems (speech too fast, loud, etc), history of tangential speech	
Unusual violence	Frequency, quality, and triggers of baseline aggression	
Grandiosity	Over-attachment to important people or favorite characters from special interests	
Engagement in dangerous activities	Level of judgment/cognitive ability	

Note: The majority of the above concepts are from the Autism Comorbidity Interview (ACI; J. Lainhart, personal communication).

symptoms of the underlying ASD that should not be applied or counted as a new symptom of a comorbid mood disorder. On the other hand, there are also some ways in which mood instabilities may present differently that should not be overlooked. These potential different manifestations of concerns are also included in the final column of the table, when relevant.

Anxiety

Anxiety is considered by some to be the most common comorbid psychiatric concern in ASD (see White et al., 2009, for review of anxiety in ASD). The DSM-IV-TR notes that individuals with ASD might have unusual fear reactions, and it is also not uncommon for there to be a general tendency toward anxiety for many individuals with ASD. It is perhaps for this reason that the DSM-IV-TR excludes the diagnoses of social phobia and generalized anxiety disorder in the course of a pervasive developmental disorder. In practice, this guideline is often ignored and the comorbid diagnoses are in fact made, given that the concerns warrant specific treatment.

There are many aspects of having an ASD that may lead to this increased risk for anxiety, to the degree that some consider anxiety and the social impairment in ASD to have a bidirectional relationship (White et al., 2009). The characteristics of ASD that may contribute to an increased predisposition to anxiety are endless, but a few examples include:

- decreased understanding or acceptance of change,
- limited coping skills,
- limited independence skills,
- difficulty processing complex information,
- heightened sensitivity to environmental stimuli,
- decreased understanding of other's perspectives,
- sometimes acute awareness of being "different" or not fitting in, etc.

An increase in self-awareness is considered a risk factor for higher anxiety; therefore, anxiety is typically thought of as more common among individuals with ASD who have higher intellectual abilities, and older children, adolescents, and adults. Age patterns for anxiety in ASD may be disorder-specific and mirror patterns in non-ASD populations, such as higher rates of specific phobias in children and higher rates of social phobia and OCD in adolescents and adults (White et al., 2009).

There are many overt signs of anxiety that can be monitored in individuals with ASD, regardless of the individual's level of language ability. In addition to typical manifestations of anxiety, increases in the symptoms in Table 3.6 may also signify underlying anxiety in ASD.

In the sections below, additional special considerations for the different types of anxiety disorders are noted, which are again modifications incorporated in the Autism Comorbidity Interview (J. Lainhart, personal communication). Anxiety symptoms are likely to manifest differently in different environments, so gathering information from multiple reporters would be the ideal, particularly for younger children (White et al., 2009).

- **Separation anxiety disorder**
  A key distinguishing consideration for separation anxiety disorder diagnoses in ASD is whether the anxiety that appears related to separation from a caregiver is due to interpersonal attachment (the general concept

Table 3.6 – Anxiety Presentation in ASD

Increases in the following symptoms may be evidence of anxiety in individuals with ASD:

Repetitive questions or statements

Activity, hyperactivity, or restlessness

Temper tantrums

Crying

Withdrawal from or avoidance or situations

Aggression

Self-injurious behavior

Stereotypes, repetitive movements or behaviors

Note: The above concepts are from the Autism Comorbidity Interview (ACI; J. Lainhart, personal communication).

underlying separation anxiety disorder), or to reasons that should not be attributed to separation anxiety, such as: "1) anxiety, fear, or upset about change in routine; and 2) avoidance of situations for reasons having nothing to do with interpersonal attachment to the main caregiver" (ACI, J. Lainhart, personal communication). For example, the motivation for a child with ASD to react negatively to going to school in the morning may be to avoid stressors at school, such as being teased, too much noise, being forced into others' routines, etc. (e.g., reasons not having to do with the separation itself, but rather with aspects of the environment where the child is going after the separation occurs). This is different than a child who does not want to go to school primarily because going to school means leaving the caregiver. The involvement of interpersonal attachment should receive special consideration when probing anxiety surrounding calamitous events in particular; many children with ASD have preoccupations with calamitous events that are not worries per se, or they may worry about the non-separation aspect of these events.

● **Panic disorder**

The diagnosis of panic disorder is challenging due to the difficulty of discerning what is causing the panic in an individual with ASD. The underlying principle is that panic attacks are unexpected and without any precipitating stimuli. One strategy to differentiate causes is to consider whether or not a parent or other caregiver can *predict* their occurrence, in which case they should not be considered panic attacks. Otherwise typical panic attack symptoms should be considered, in addition to the manifestations of anxiety in ASD that may be slightly different in ASD, as summarized in Table 3.4 above.

● **Generalized anxiety disorder**

Given that generalized anxiety disorder embodies the idea of excessive worry, the key concern is determining whether the individual with ASD is in fact worrying or anxious about multiple things. This is obviously difficult to determine for nonverbal individuals, but this is also a challenge with higher-functioning individuals due to a common difficulty in expressing such feelings. In addition, some higher-functioning individuals with ASD lack the social inclination to report their worries to others, even if they have them. Worrying in ASD may commonly take the form of even more repetitive questions and statements than usual. Repetitive questions that should be considered indicative of anxiety would typically stop once the stressful thing in question is over. Repetitive questions focused on gaining more knowledge or facts regarding a special interest generally should not be attributed to anxiety.

Once the presence of worrying *has* been established, the next complication is determining the level of interference that the worrying presents. Since it may not be possible to determine how difficult the child or adult with ASD finds it to control worries or compulsive behaviors, clinicians can ask parents or caregivers how difficult it is for them to control these problems in their child.

● **Social phobia**

The main complication in the diagnosis of social phobia is determining the reason behind the social avoidance. To accurately diagnose social phobia, it is important to first establish if the individual understands and has demonstrated the concepts of feeling embarrassed or humiliated. It is also important for the individual to demonstrate that they have been afraid of doing or saying something for these reasons, and more broadly to have shown some indication of being concerned what others think of their behavior. Otherwise the diagnosis of social phobia may not be relevant or may not be an accurate reflection of the underlying behavior.

● **Specific phobia**

Specific phobias may manifest in much the same way in individuals with ASD as they do for typically developing populations. The one thing to keep in mind is that the fear should be developmentally inappropriate, and developmental age may be different from chronological age. To consider the fear a true phobia, it should be impairing in some way and take a great deal of effort for either the individual or caregivers to control.

● **Obsessive-compulsive disorder**

There have been many debates about OCD in ASD and how to differentiate repetitive behaviors from obsessive and compulsive behaviors (see Matson & Dempsey, 2009, for review). It is difficult to assess obsessions in individuals with ASD, both in those who are nonverbal and in those who are verbal enough to report the thought but have trouble communicating how intrusive or inappropriate it is. "Obsessions" that are better described as part of the ASD may be less well organized and complex than in true OCD. Furthermore, "random, non-persistent thoughts and talk, which may be repetitive in a given moment, need to be distinguished from obsessions, which, by definition, are persistent" (ACI; J. Lainhart, personal communication).

There are also many repetitive behaviors in ASD that are done repeatedly, but lack the driven quality inherent in compulsions. Circumscribed interests or preoccupations in ASD are different from compulsions, in that individuals with ASD typically get great joy from their circumscribed interests.

As noted in the Autism Comorbidity Interview, the following indicators may help determine if a behavior is a compulsion:

- The individual seems under pressure to perform the behavior
- The individual seems to have an irresistible urge to perform the behavior
- The individual is significantly preoccupied with performing the behavior
- The individual is preoccupied with the object on which the behavior is performed (e.g., on guard to perform the behavior)
- It is difficult for the subject to not perform the behavior or for the parent/caregiver to stop the individual from performing the behavior

Attention-Deficit/Hyperactivity Disorder (ADHD)

ADHD is another disorder that is considered extremely common in ASD (see Gillberg et al., 2009, for review of conceptual issues related to ADHD in ASD). This is to the degree that, like mood disorders, ADHD is often the first diagnosis before the ASD is identified for many individuals on the spectrum (Ghaziuddin, 2005). However, having an ASD is an exclusionary criterion for ADHD based on strict DSM-IV-TR guidelines (awaiting DSM-5 changes). Again, in practice, ADHD is frequently diagnosed and treatment for inattention, hyperactivity, and impulsivity is often needed.

There are several important differential diagnosis considerations regarding ADHD in ASD:

- It is important to consider the individual's mental age when making an ADHD diagnosis or deciding to treat, given that ADHD symptoms should be conceptualized regarding the degree of developmental inappropriateness.
- It is important to differentiate inattention concerns from lack of understanding, hearing impairment, transient behavioral reactions, or inattention better accounted for by anxiety, mood, or oppositional behavior (ACI; J Lainhart, personal communication).
- Individuals with ADHD may appear distracted, but it has a different quality if the "distraction" is based on being drawn to or seeking sensation from different stimuli.
- In some cases, distractibility is internal and due more to the underlying ASD symptoms (e.g., preoccupation with a special interest).

Oppositional Defiant Disorder

The diagnosis of oppositional defiant disorder should be conservatively applied in ASD. The incorrect use of an ODD diagnosis in ASD can lead to misunderstandings about where symptoms are coming from. The most common problem this leads to is viewing behaviors as purposeful or manipulative when they in fact stem from a skill deficit, which conclusion in turn could lead to an inefficient intervention approach (most likely a behavioral modification program as opposed to a focus on skill-building). Patterns of ODD presentation across various age groups in higher-functioning children with ASD also raise questions regarding whether the nature of the problem leading to the ODD is perhaps different from true ODD. Specifically, whereas ODD typically decreases with age or changes into conduct disorder among typical populations, rates of ODD are more consistent across age ranges (without decreasing and without becoming conduct disorder) among individuals with Asperger's disorder or high-functioning autism (Mattila et al., 2010).

Below are some key concepts to keep in mind when considering whether an individual with ASD has enough symptoms of ODD to warrant a comorbid diagnosis:

- Flat facial expressions are often part of having an ASD. It is important to consider one's overall range of affect before assuming lack of responsiveness to adult directives is an act of defiance.
- Insistence on sameness and difficulty with change are common symptoms of an ASD. These behaviors should not typically be considered a behavior done to exert control over others.
- Children with ASD often do things that annoy others. The relevant point for ODD is whether they are *purposefully* doing things to annoy others. Therefore, it is imperative to first ascertain whether they can recognize when others are annoyed, before considering this a relevant potential symptom.
- Symptoms of ODD such as blaming others/taking responsibility, resentment, and getting back at or hating others involve a high level of social understanding about nuances of interpersonal relationships. In each case, it is important to consider the child with ASD's baseline understanding of these concepts before applying any of these symptoms of ODD as present.

Summary

Psychiatric comorbidity is a significant and critical problem that all providers who work with individuals with ASD should be aware of, due to both its high rate of occurrence and its negative impact on functioning. However, the assessment of psychiatric comorbidity is quite complicated. There are few measures designed specifically to detect psychiatric comorbidity in ASD, and those that have been developed are in their infancy and require significantly more research to determine their validity and reliability. We summarized some of the available questionnaires and interviews, which can be used as a guide in the detection of comorbid diagnoses or risks. But, in all cases, providers must use their best clinical judgment and try to gather information from multiple sources in order to arrive at final diagnoses. There are many disorder-specific considerations, as noted above. Although each diagnostic decision warrants very careful consideration of all concepts discussed, what might be considered the key differential diagnostic concept for each disorder described is summarized in the Key Fact Box 3.2.

Clinicians should carefully consider underlying baseline functioning, how symptoms may overlap or stem from the ASD itself versus a separate disorder, and potential differences in the presentation of psychiatric concerns in ASD when completing the differential diagnosis process.

Key Fact Box 3.2 – Primary Differential Diagnosis Considerations by Disorder

Disorder	Key Concept or Question to Remember
Mood Disorders (Depression and Bipolar)	Individuals with ASD may be at heightened risk for depression. At the same time, it is important to remember that emotion dysregulation is often part and parcel of the ASD (i.e., you must establish a clear change from baseline for a mood disorder diagnosis!)
Separation Anxiety	Is the anxiety when separating from a caregiver due to interpersonal attachment (separation anxiety) or some other more idiosyncratic or ASD-related factor (i.e., resistance to change or to avoid social stressors)?
Panic Disorder	Panic attacks are, by definition, without any precipitants. Therefore, if parents can *predict* their occurrence, it is probably not panic disorder.
Generalized Anxiety Disorder	Do the individual's actions suggest worrying may be present, even if he or she does not explicitly describe feeling worried? If so, is it hard for others to control the worrying?
Social Phobia	Does the individual take notice of others' evaluation of his/her behavior and feel embarrassed or concerned?
Specific Phobia	Is the fear *developmentally* (not age-) inappropriate, and how hard is it to control the individual's fear reaction?
Obsessive-Compulsive Disorder (OCD)	Many of the preoccupations in ASD are enjoyable and preferred activities for the individual. Are the obsessions organized, intrusive, and distressing to the individual? Are the repetitive behaviors driven in quality?
Attention Deficit Hyperactivity Disorder (ADHD)	Is the "inattention" better accounted for by young developmental age, lack of understanding, hearing problems, a behavioral response, or other psychiatric concern?
Oppositional Defiant Disorder (ODD)	Is the defiant behavior truly purposeful and manipulative?

Further Reading

1. Baird, G., Pickles, A., Simonoff, E., et al. (2008). Measles vaccination and antibody response in Autism Spectrum Disorder. *Archives of Disease in Childhood, 93*(10), 832–837.

2. Bererjot, S., & Wetterberg, L. (2008). Autism Spectrum Disorder and psychiatric comorbidity in adolescents and adults. *Clinical Neuropsychiatry, 5,* 3–8.

3. Dhossche, D. M., & Wachtel, L. E. (2010). Catatonia is hidden in plain sight among different pediatric disorders: A review article. *Pediatric Neurology, 43,* 307–315.

4. Ghaziuddin, M. (2005). *Mental health aspects of autism and Asperger syndrome.* Philadelphia, PA: Jessica Kingsley Publishers.

5. Ghaziuddin, M., Ghaziuddin, N., & Greden, J. (2002). Depression in persons with autism: Implications for research and clinical care. *Journal of Autism and Developmental Disorders, 32,* 299–306.

6. Gillberg, C., Santosh, P. J., & Brown, T. E. (2009). ADHD with Autism Spectrum Disorder. In T. E. Brown (Ed.), *ADHD Comorbidities: Handbook for ADHD complications in children and adults* (pp. 265–278). Arlington, VA: American Psychiatric Publishing.

7. Johnson, C. P., Myers, S. M., & Council on Children with Disabilities–American Academy of Pediatrics (2007). Identification and evaluation of children with Autism Spectrum Disorder. *Pediatrics, 120*(5), 1183–1215.

8. Kakooza-Mwesige, A., Wachtel, L. E., Dhossche, D. M. (2008). Catatonia in autism: Implications across the life span. *European Journal of Child and Adolescent Psychiatry,* 17, 327–335.

9. Editors of Lancet (2010). Retraction: Ileal-lymphoid-nodular hyperplasia, non-specific colitis, and pervasive developmental disorder in children. *Lancet, 375*(9713), 445.

10. Leyfer, O. T., Folstein, S. T., Bacalman, S., Davis, N. O., Dinh, E., Morgan, J., et al. (2006). Comorbid psychiatric disorders in children with autism: Interview development and rates of disorders. *Journal of Autism and Developmental Disorders, 36,* 849–861.

11. LoVullo, S. V., & Matson, J. L. (2009). Comorbid psychopathology in adults with Autism Spectrum Disorder and intellectual disabilities. *Research in Developmental Disabilities, 30,* 1288–1296.

12. Manning, M., & Hudgins, L. (2010). Array-based technology and recommendation for utilization in medical genetics practice for detection of chromosomal abnormalities. *ACMG Practice Guidelines. Genetics in Medicine, 12*(11), 85–92.

13. Mattila, M. L., Hurtig, T., Haapsamo, H., Jussila, K., Kuusikko-Gauffin, S., Kielinen, M., et al. (2010). Comorbid psychiatric disorders associated with Asperger syndrome/high-functioning autism: A community- and clinic-based study. *Journal of Autism and Developmental Disorders,* DOI 10.1007/s10803-010-0958-2.

14. Matson, J. L., & Dempsey, T. (2009). The nature and treatment of compulsions, obsessions, and rituals in people with developmental disabilities. *Research in Developmental Disabilities, 30,* 603–611.

15. Matson, J. L., & Nebel-Schwalm, M. S. (2007). Comorbid psychopathology with autism spectrum disorder in children: An overview. *Research in Developmental Disabilities, 28,* 341–352.

16. Mazefsky, C. A., Anderson, R., Conner, C. M., & Minshew, N. J. (2010). Child Behavior Checklist scores for school-aged children with autism: Preliminary evidence of patterns suggesting the need for referral. *Journal of Psychopathology and Behavioral Assessment.* DOI: 10.1007/s10862-010-9198-1.

17. Mazefsky, C. A., Pelphrey, K. A., & Dahl, R. (under review). Using an emotional regulation framework to make conceptual advances in autism.

18. Mazefsky, C. A., Folstein, S. E., & Lainhart, J. E. (2008). Brief report: Overrepresentation of mood and anxiety disorders in adults with autism and their first degree relatives: What does it mean? *Autism Research, 1,* 193–197.

19. Mazefsky, C. A., Kao, J., & Oswald, D. P. (2011). Preliminary evidence suggesting caution in the use of psychiatric self-report measures with adolescents with high-functioning Autism Spectrum Disorder. *Research in Autism Spectrum Disorder, 5,* 164–174. DOI information: 10.1016/j.rasd.2010.03.006.

20. Miles, J. H., McCathren, R. B., Stichter, J., & Shinawi, M. In: R. A. Pagon, T. C. Bird, C. R. Dolan, & K. Stephens (Eds.), GeneReviews [Internet]. Seattle, WA: University of Washington, Seattle; 1993–2003 Aug 27 [updated 2010 Apr 13].

21. Price, C. S., Thompson, W. W., et al. (2010). Prenatal and infant exposure to thimerosal from vaccines and immunoglobulins and risk of autism. *Pediatrics,* 126, 656–664.

22. Schaefer, G. B., Mendelsohn, N. J., & Professional Practice, Guidelines Committee (2008). *Genetics in Medicine, 10*(4), 301–305.

23. Shen, Y., et al. (2010). Clinical genetic testing for patients with Autism Spectrum Disorder. *Pediatrics, 125*(4), 727–735.
24. Stewart, M. E., Barnard, L., Pearson, J., Hasan, R., & O'Brien, G. (2006). Presentation of depression in autism and Asperger syndrome: A review. *Autism, 10,* 103–116.
25. Volkmar, F. R., & Wiesner, L. A. (2004). *Healthcare for Children on the Autism Spectrum.* Bethesda, MD: Woodbine House, Inc.
26. Wakefield, A. J., Murch, S. H., Anthony, A., et al. (1998). Ileal-lymphoid-nodular hyperplasia, non-specific colitis, and pervasive developmental disorder in children. Lancet, 351(9103), 637–641.
27. White, S. W., Oswald, D., Ollendick, T., & Scahill, L. (2009). Anxiety in children with Autism Spectrum Disorder. *Clinical Psychology Review, 29,* 216–229.

Questions

1. Which of the following are *true* about medical workup in ASD?
   a. Seizures may affect up to one third of individuals with ASD.
   b. Regression in speech can be a sign of Landau-Kleffner syndrome.
   c. If motor and vocal tics last more than one year, then symptoms meet Tourette syndrome diagnosis.
   d. Muscle weakness or significant hypotonia can be a sign of a metabolic disorder.
   e. All of the above

2. A higher percentage of patients with which syndromes may have an ASD?
   a. Fragile X syndrome
   b. Tuberous sclerosis
   c. 15q duplication
   d. Angelman/Prader Willi syndrome
   e. All of the above

3. All of these are true about differences between repetitive behaviors in ASD and OCD *except* which one?
   a. Many repetitive behaviors in ASD lack the driven quality inherent in compulsions.
   b. Circumscribed interests in ASD are different from compulsions, in that individuals with ASD typically get joy from their circumscribed interests.
   c. A compulsion in OCD brings joy to the individual.
   d. A behavior is a compulsion if the individual seems to have an irresistible urge to perform the behavior.

4. Increases in which of the following symptoms may be evidence of anxiety in individuals with ASD?
   a. Repetitive questions or statements
   b. Crying and temper tantrums
   c. Avoidance of situations
   d. Aggression or self-injurious behavior
   e. All of the above

5. Which of the following statements are *true* about psychiatric diagnosis in individuals with ASD?
   a. Individuals with ASD may have heightened risk for depression, but emotion dysregulation is often part of ASD (e.g., must establish a clear change from baseline for a mood disorder diagnosis).
   b. Many of the preoccupations in ASD are enjoyable and preferred activities for the individual.
   c. The "inattention" may be better accounted for by young developmental age, lack of understanding, or hearing problems, rather than a true diagnosis of ADHD.
   d. The defiant behavior may not be truly purposeful and manipulative, and therefore not meet criteria for ODD.
   e. All of the above

Answers

1. e. All of the above
2. e. All of the above
3. c. NOT true
4. e. All of the above
5. e. All of the above

Neurobiology of Autism Spectrum Disorder

Kathryn McFadden, Nancy J. Minshew, and K. Suzanne Scherf

Autism: Lack of Reliability and Validity to Severity-Based Diagnostic "Subtypes" 88

Earliest Manifestations of Autism: Longitudinal Studies of Infants at Risk 90

The Profile of Cognitive and Neurological Functioning in Autism at Older Ages 92

Neurobiology and Pathophysiology of Autism 94

Functional MRI (fMRI) and fMRI Connectivity (fc-MRI) 98

Genetics of Autism 100

Syndromic Autism 102

Non-Syndromic (Idiopathic) Autism 104

Genetic Models 106

Conclusions 110

Further Reading 111

Questions 112

Answers 113

Over the past 15 years, dramatic advances in the genetic and neurobiological characterization of autism have resulted from the exponential growth in research technologies. These advances include a new understanding of:

- The early and probably prenatal, developmental neurobiological events that lead to subsequent brain developmental abnormalities, including alterations in forebrain connectivity
- How these early developmental neurobiological events are instantiated in molecular and microscopic pathophysiology
- How 15%–20% of cases of ASD are now linked to genetic or chromosomal abnormalities

In the near future, it is likely that ASD will be characterized, not by clinical nomenclature, but by the disturbance in developmental neurobiological mechanisms, such as axonal outgrowth or axonal pathfinding, and then by genotype (Zikopoulos & Barbas, 2010). Such characterizations will become increasingly more specific and precise with the continued growth in technology. The shift in focus to genetic- and neurobiologically based definitions of ASD highlights the inextricable link between biological mechanisms and treatment advances.

In this chapter, we provide an overview of:

- Invalid past diagnostic distinctions made on the basis of clinical severity
- Implications of infant and toddler manifestations of ASD in "at risk" siblings for the origin of the ASD syndrome
- Evidence that autism may be conceptualized as a disorder of complex information processing resulting from disordered development of the connectivity of cortical systems (e.g., failure of cortical systems specialization)

Importantly, we integrate this information with what is known about the genetic and developmental neurobiological aspects of ASD to constrain potential explanations about the "cause" of autism.

In order to understand potential causal factors leading to autism, it is critical to understand that *cause* has many different meanings, particularly in terms of the ultimate and proximal causes. From a medical perspective, causal factors refer both to the initiating or trigger factors (etiology) and to the resulting pathophysiology or sequence of events that "operationalize" the etiology. In contrast, when clinicians evaluate specific instances of behavior, as in "what caused the individual to act like that yesterday?" they are asking about a more proximal cause concerning the interplay between the current status of an individual and the demands of the circumstances; "cause" is then investigated by engaging in a functional analysis of behavior.

Autism: Lack of Reliability and Validity to Severity-Based Diagnostic "Subtypes"

ASD is defined and diagnosed differently in the community than in research settings. In clinical settings, each clinician operationalizes the diagnostic criteria according to their own knowledge and practices. Clinical populations often reflect a broader application of the ASD diagnosis and disregard the enormous variability among individuals with the same diagnosis. In research settings, the goal is to understand the causal mechanisms that lead to the disorder, in hopes of identifying specific mechanisms to guide development of more specific treatment approaches. Thus, *a research diagnosis considers the variability between individuals with ASD as a potential clue to the underlying pathophysiology and etiology of the disorder.*

Initial attempts to understand the cause of ASD were based on various clinical distinctions among cases, primarily related to variability in severity:

- "Low-" and "high-" functioning individuals with ASD based on overall severity
- Autism, Asperger's disorder, and pervasive developmental disorder–not otherwise specified (PDDNOS) based on variations in sociability measures, cognitive measures, structural brain imaging status, and family history indices have also been subject to intense investigation

Although this research documented the presence of unexplained heterogeneity among individuals with ASD and supported the notion that, in general, more severe abnormalities on these indices are associated with greater clinical severity, it failed to find support for the idea that these delineations distinguish valid or reliable subgroups. Furthermore, studies of incidence among family members revealed a high co-occurrence of autism, Asperger's disorder, and PDDNOS among siblings, including identical twins, and among affected members in extended families.

As a result of findings such as this and the lack of reliability in the community in making distinctions among the ASDs, the Fifth Edition of the Diagnostic and Statistical Manual (DSM-5) proposes to collapse all of these clinical syndromes into a single diagnosis of "autism spectrum disorder." Although this revision is appropriate for community diagnosis, and thus the allocation of clinical and support services, research studies will continue to rely on research diagnostic instruments like the Autism Diagnostic Interview (ADI) and the Autism Diagnostic Observation Schedule (ADOS) to make categorical distinctions between "autism and not autism" and "autism and autism spectrum disorder" (which includes Asperger's disorder and PDDNOS). These distinctions have played a vital role in advancing our understanding of the behavioral and neural profile of ASD over the past two decades, and are likely to continue to be used in research studies to establish consistency of group assignment across research sites. In order to compare results across studies, it is therefore important to be aware of what criteria and methods were used to define subject groups. Currently, the ASD designation may refer to autism, PDDNOS, and Asperger's disorder, or to high-functioning autism and Asperger's disorder. In addition, although clinical diagnosis may not distinguish between cases with an identified underlying cause such as tuberous sclerosis, Fragile X, or Rett's syndrome and those without such identified causes, these are important distinctions in studies investigating genetic and pathophysiological mechanisms.

> Variations in clinical severity among ASD cases are not valid indices of differences in pathophysiology or etiology.

Earliest Manifestations of Autism: Longitudinal Studies of Infants at Risk

As mentioned previously, autism is highly heritable, and approximately 15%–20% of infants with an older sibling diagnosed with autism will ultimately be diagnosable with ASD by three to four years of age.

Longitudinal research studies of these "at risk" infant siblings are defining the earliest signs or symptoms of autism both for improving early diagnosis and for implications regarding neurobiological mechanisms. The preliminary findings of these "infant sibs" studies were eloquently described and discussed by Rogers (2009). The key overall findings included:

- No developmental differences were detected at six months of age between "at risk" infants who go on to develop autism and those who do not.
- The earliest identifiable manifestations of autism were not in the form of a primary social impairment, as some behavioral theories had long predicted, but instead in the form of unusual responses to sensory stimuli, motor movements, and visual regard of objects.
- Developmental differences were first evident on standardized measures at 12 months.
- Social and language impairments, long hypothesized to be the *causative* features of autism, emerge later: between 12 and 24 months. Also, between 12 and 24 months, there appears to be a progressive widening of the performance gap between affected and unaffected infants.
- Very importantly, "associated symptoms," such as intellectual disability, irritability (temperament changes), poor affect regulation, reactivity to sensory stimuli and to change, activity level, and poor motor development were also integral parts of the clinical presentation at this early age.

Rogers eloquently summarized the conclusion of the findings when she wrote: "These findings do not support the view that autism is primarily a social-communicative disorder and instead suggest that autism disrupts multiple aspects of development rather simultaneously." "Children's developmental rates are decelerating markedly in a 12-month period, with IQs dropping from average (100) to below 50 for some children." This finding refutes the common mistaken belief that general intellectual disability (previously termed "mental retardation") in ASD reflects the co-occurrence of a separate disorder (i.e., a comorbid condition). Similarly, hyperactivity, attention deficit, emotion dysregulation (mood lability), sensory disturbances, and motor delays are also clearly part and parcel of the same pathophysiology that produces all the other manifestations.

These findings about the pattern of emergence of clinical manifestations in infants later diagnosed with autism are consistent with well-known principles about how neurological disorders of brain development present in childhood.

- Neurodevelopmental disorders present with a constellation of signs and symptoms that collectively reflect the impact of the underlying pathophysiological mechanism on the brain. Research in ASD indicates that the underlying developmental neurobiological mechanisms in ASD affect the development of the cortex and its connections and involve disturbances in neuronal organization and migration mechanisms.

- Signs and symptoms of a neurodevelopmental disorder are expressed in a developmentally appropriate time window (i.e., when corresponding skills are developing). Hence, the earliest abnormalities of ASD in infant siblings involving odd hand and arm movements, atypical reactions to sensory stimuli, and a visual preoccupation with unusual objects are consistent with the events of brain development that occur in the first year of life. In the second year of life, more elaborate brain connectivity develops to support the emergence of more advanced skills across all domains of function.

> As a result, ASD is manifested in the second year of life as an *expanding profile of disturbances in higher-order abilities that involve both conscious and non-conscious or automatic processing abilities vital to the governance of human behavior.*

- The presentation of ASD documented by the longitudinal infant sibling studies is typical of developmental neurobiological disorders of neuronal organization or migration (see Volpe [2008] for a discussion of clinical syndromes corresponding to neurodevelopmental disorders). These events are responsible for the intricate or specialized development of cortical connectivity that produces the specialized functions and abilities unique to humans.
- The distinctions that have been made between "core symptoms," "associated symptoms," and "comorbid" conditions are invalid at the neurobiological and genetic level.

The 8% of extremely premature infants (born before 28 weeks gestation) who are later diagnosed with cerebral palsy and ASD at outcome are the result of the impact of stroke (periventricular leukomalacia) on the proliferation and migration of neurons in this zone. The watershed region of vascular perfusion at this gestational age is periventricular and impacts the site of neuronal proliferation and migration path to the cortex. Ischemic events in the term or near-term infant produce a cortical pattern that is typically associated with hip and shoulder weakness, learning disability, and visuospatial difficulties.

The Profile of Cognitive and Neurological Functioning in Autism at Older Ages

The profile of impairments was previously investigated in children, adolescents, and adults with autism to ascertain common features among deficits and intact abilities that might reflect their neurological bases. Studies of children, adolescents, and adults with high-functioning autism had also revealed a broad but selective profile of altered cognitive and neurological abilities.

- In testable high-functioning adults and children with autism, there is a complex pattern of *deficits* in higher cortical sensory perception, skilled motor movements (praxis), cognitive memory, emergent language skills, concept formation aspects of abstract reasoning (Minshew et al., 1997; Williams et al., 2006). These are accompanied by *intact and sometimes enhanced skills* in attention, elementary sensory perception, elementary motor movements, associative memory, formal language skills, and rule-based aspects of abstract thinking.
- When both elementary and higher-order abilities in many domains are assessed, it becomes evident that deficits exist in several domains not considered to be integral parts of the autism syndrome, including aspects of the sensory-perceptual, motor, and memory domains. Furthermore, there are enhanced skills and impaired abilities within the same domains as deficits (e.g., memory, language, abstraction).

These findings led to several important conclusions.

- Domains with the most prominent clinical symptoms (concept formation, thematic and idiomatic language, social cognition) have the highest information-processing demands.
- Preserved abilities rely on elementary information-processing demands, particularly visual perception (see: Minshew et al., 2006, for detailed explanation).
- Causal explanations for ASD must account for the comprehensive pattern of both deficits and intact aspects of the disorder both within and across multiple domains.

- There is *no single primary deficit or triad of deficits*, brain regions, or neural systems causing autism.
- Rather, *autism broadly affects many abilities at the same time and systematically from its earliest presentation and throughout life.*
- This pattern could be characterized overall as reflecting a *disorder of complex or integrative information* processing, which results from altered development of cerebral cortical connectivity in ASD.
- Other investigators have characterized this profile in terms of "central coherence" and variations of local processing.

Just as the infant sibling studies have clearly demonstrated, studies of children and adults with autism have also demonstrated a broad but selective profile of deficits and intact or enhanced abilities that all reflect a relationship to information-processing demands. These findings also demonstrate that all of the manifestations are equally integral parts of the same syndrome. These patterns are known in child neurology to be the result of disturbances in the aspects of brain development referred to as "neuronal organizational events" and, in more severe cases with seizures, "neuronal migrational events."

Given this characterization of the behavioral syndrome of ASD, we now turn to review the state-of-the art science of the neurobiology, pathophysiology, and genetics of autism, which converges with the behavioral and neuropsychological evidence to indicate that ASD is a developmental neurobiological disorder. In particular, this work suggests that it is likely that genes affecting signaling pathways that regulate *neuronal organization* are strongly implicated in the etiology of autism.

Neurobiology and Pathophysiology of Autism

> ASD is now conceptualized as a developmental neurobiological disorder affecting elaboration of the forebrain circuitry that underlies the abilities most unique to human beings.

Neural circuitry may be considered at a number of different levels ranging from a few interconnected neurons to complex networks of interconnected brain regions. The development of this circuitry depends on the coordinated interactions of numerous genetic/molecular cascades and environmental/experiential exposures (see Tau and Peterson, 2010, for an excellent review of the normal development of brain circuits).

At the basic level, the physical substrate of neural circuitry is provided by neurons, their neuritic processes, and their synapses on neighboring or distant neurons. While this anatomical model of connectivity differs from that of functional connectivity, it is obvious that there is a relationship between the two, with the former underlying the latter in some manner. Wiring the brain requires that neurons proliferate, acquire the correct identities, migrate to the appropriate locations, extend axons, and make guidance decisions with a high degree of spatial and temporal fidelity. Converging evidence indicates that more than one of these processes may be altered in various combinations to produce the heterogeneous phenotypes observed in ASD.

Numerous morphometric studies have implicated perturbations in the processes of neocortical growth and organization in the development of ASD (reviewed in Lainhart, 2006). Studies examining head circumference (HC) and brain volume (BV) in individuals with ASD have demonstrated *altered brain growth trajectories across the lifespan.*

- Head circumference (HC) and brain volume (BV) were not significantly different from that of controls at birth.
- Up to 70% of infants with ASD exhibit abnormally accelerated brain growth in the first year of life. Approximately 20% to 25% of infants in this subset actually meet formal criteria for macrocephaly (i.e., HC of 2.0 standard deviations above the mean) in the first year.
- BV is significantly larger by two to four years of life, and some children meet criteria for megalencephaly (i.e., BV 2.5 S.D. above mean).
- The first two years of life are usually a period of rapid brain growth in infants as neurons undergo significant postnatal growth in cell size and elaboration (actually overproduction) of axons, synapses, and dendrites. It is possible that this process is exaggerated somehow in at least a subset of ASD.
- Whatever the neurobiological basis, abnormal growth rates in ASD tend to decline significantly after the initial acceleration, causing an *apparent "normalization"* of BV by adolescence or early adulthood.

> The functional significance of this is unknown, as up to one third of individuals with ASD may clinically deteriorate during this period while others may make significant gains in functioning. Mean HC remains somewhat elevated into adulthood, and rates of macrocephaly, although lower, remain increased overall.

Studies examining regional differences in brain growth note a rostral-caudal gradient in these altered growth trajectories. At the time of maximal brain growth in very early childhood, cerebral gray matter (GM) and white matter (WM) are both increased (by 18% and 38% respectively). The frontal cortical GM and WM show the most enlargement, followed by the temporal lobe GM and WM and the parietal GM. The occipital GM and WM and parietal GM tend not to vary significantly from normal. Within the frontal lobes, the GM areas most affected are the dorsolateral and mesial prefrontal cortex. Similarly, the WM most involved appears to be the radiate compartment and U-fibers immediately underlying these cortical areas and representing the intrahemispheric, cortico-cortical connections originating from cortical layers II and III.

After childhood, WM is no longer increased relative to typically developing controls, although GM volumes remain elevated. It is therefore thought that *"normalization" of BV is due to a decrease in WM relative to GM, a complete reversal of the age-dependent cortical thinning that typically occurs during this period*. Cerebral GM thinning is thought to be a sign of increasing maturity and is generally attributed to the concurrent processes of synaptic pruning and myelination. Excess (presumably weaker or imprecise) connections are eliminated during this period as both axon collaterals and terminal arbors are pruned through retraction or degeneration. This is necessary to develop precise functional connections and provide a substrate for neural plasticity. Again, this process may be aberrant in ASD, although this has not been demonstrated.

It must be noted that the above pattern of head and brain growth does not hold true for all individuals with ASD. Many show typical rates of head and brain growth, and a small subset even meet criteria for microcephaly, although this is more common in the setting of syndromic ASD. Therefore, *ASD as a whole may be best characterized as having greatly heterogeneous brain growth patterns relative to the non-affected population*. This variability is reflected at the microscopic level as well, and neuropathological studies have yielded equally heterogeneous results. This is due in part to the likely etiological/genetic variability underlying ASD, but also to the small sample sizes and frequent comorbidities (e.g., seizures), which typically complicate the interpretation of the findings of these studies. Fortunately, this has improved in recent years as more detailed studies of larger, clinically well-characterized samples are being carried out.

The first postmortem report of a non-syndromic case of ASD was reported in 1985 by Bauman and Kemper. After completing 10 additional cases over the next decade (Bauman & Kemper, 1998), three common findings emerged: 1) increased brain weight in children and decreased brain weight in adults, 2) increased packing densities of smaller-sized neurons (with underdeveloped dendritic arbors) in select forebrain limbic structures such as the anterior cingulate gyrus, and 3) decreased numbers of Purkinje neurons in the cerebellum. Bailey et al. (1998) similarly found increased brain weight as well as various cortical dysgenetic lesions in four out of six individuals with ASD. In a recent large-scale study, Weigel et al. (2010) reported a wide variety of heterotopias and dysplasic lesions in multiple cortical, hippocampal, and cerebellar regions in 12 out of 13 (92%) of ASD subjects analyzed. While somewhat inconsistent in particular details, these findings collectively point to dysregulation of neurogenesis, neuronal migration, and maturation in ASD.

Recent studies have also found subtle but pervasive microstructural abnormalities in cortical architecture, even in the absence of dysgenic lesions. Cassanova and colleagues (multiple studies) report increased numbers of minicolumns containing higher densities of smaller neurons in the cerebral cortices of ASD brains. This trend appears to be most pronounced in the frontal lobe, particularly the dorsolateral prefrontal cortex, and is not seen in more posterior regions such as the visual cortex. *Minicolumns* are the vertical cell columns created by sequential waves of migrating neurons travelling along radial glial fibers during early corticogenesis. Increased numbers of such arrays probably reflect excess early divisions of radial glial cells immediately prior to the onset of neurogenesis and migration.

In support of this, recent studies have found increased cortical gyration in the frontal lobes of ASD subjects, suggesting increased surface area (a function of the numbers of radial arrays). Furthermore, the distribution of minicolumn abnormalities correlates with patterns of accelerated growth in the early postnatal period (i.e., frontal > posterior). While probably not detectable at birth, the presence of even a small proportion of excess neurons could conceivably cause rapid postnatal growth in frontal regions. Cortical neurons are typically small in the perinatal period but, as previously mentioned, undergo exponential expansion in somatic and neuritic cytoplasmic volumes in the first two years of life. Also, as the neuronal proliferative cell cycle is tightly linked to cell fate specification, timing of migration, and ultimate laminar positioning, the frequent occurrence of cortical dysgenic lesions is not surprising. And, because neuronal identity and laminar position are two prime determinants of how a particular neuron integrates itself within wider brain circuitry (i.e., where it sends its processes and which neurons it contacts), final connectivity could easily be affected.

It is likely, however, that *altered proliferation is only one of many ways that neural circuitry may be perturbed and may be an underlying pathogenic process in only a small subset of ASD*. In fact, accumulating genetic evidence reviewed previously implicates a number of molecular pathways that serve as cross-regulatory factors that intertwine the above developmental processes contributing to neural circuitry. However, part of the difficulty in linking the genetic, neurobiological, and behavioral components of ASD is the large phenotype-genotype variability.

Until further specification of the molecular events has been accomplished, the concept of the ASD syndrome is that there are *commonalities across genes in the overall disturbances in cortical connectivity that produce the major features that define the syndrome(s) of ASD*. Differences in the specific mechanisms, superimposed on differences in familial inheritance, lead to the heterogeneity.

Functional MRI (fMRI) and fMRI Connectivity (fc-MRI)

This model of disturbances in cortical connectivity is also informed by findings from state-of-the-art neuroimaging techniques that evaluated the integrity of functional and structural connections among cortical and sub-cortical regions. The availability of functional neuroimaging methodologies for detecting localized increases in blood flow or blood oxygenation resulting from synaptic activity, including positron emission tomography (PET) and functional magnetic resonance imaging (fMRI), has provided an unparalleled opportunity for defining brain–behavior relationships in typically developing humans and in those with autism. These studies steadily defined neural systems abnormalities in ASD related to all of the defining features of autism, including the motor system, by identifying regional patterns of hypo- and hyper-activation related to specific perceptual, cognitive, social, and motor tasks (see Brambilla et al., 2004, for a review of the early studies, and Di Martino et al., 2009, for a recent meta-analysis).

The more elaborate ensembles of connections were sometimes called "the brain within the brain," such as the "social brain" and the "emotional brain." Other neuroimaging studies in ASD identified altered neural systems related to face-processing, formal language, executive functioning, cognitive inhibition, comprehension of idioms, metaphors, humor, prosodic processing, and even motor tasks. More recent studies have delineated new networks and cortical specializations in typical individuals that are also altered in ASD individuals. These networks include the biological motion-processing system, the gaze-processing system, the fronto-striatal reward systems, and a "default mode" system that is active when the mind is at rest and engaged in spontaneous or internally directed thought. Well-designed neuroimaging studies will continue to provide growing specification about the affected cortical networks and the mechanisms underlying the various manifestations of autism.

> Functional neuroimaging methods not only provided information about patterns of task-related activation abnormalities across networks, but also allowed the assessment of the temporal synchronization of activation among regions, or *functional connectivity*, within these networks during a specific activity.

By examining the cross-correlation of the time-series of activity, these studies demonstrated that alterations in activation were also associated with reduced functional connectivity in ASD, implying reduced communication, or coordination of activation modulation, among distant cortical regions (see Schipul et al., 2010, for a review of this work).

> Thus far, studies have identified *underconnectivity* with the frontal cortex as a specific characteristic of the altered connectivity in autism, and this characteristic is present across the same wide range of domains of complex information processing that are affected in the disorder, including social, language, executive, and motor processes.

Underconnectivity is also present when there is no experimenter-defined task, in the resting state. The most commonly replicated imaging pattern involves underdevelopment of connectivity with the frontal cortex and increased local activation posteriorly in the visual, parietal, or temporal cortices. This fMRI pattern has provided a neurobiological explanation for the cognitive profile of enhanced visual perception and impaired higher-order processing. In addition, measures of functional connectivity between specific areas have been shown to reliably predict the degree of impairment in specific domains among those diagnosed with autism. For instance, individuals with poorer social functioning measured by the ADI-R show lower functional connectivity between frontal and parietal cortices. These findings gave rise to the *underconnectivity theory* in autism, which now has sufficient support that it is accepted as a central feature of the pathophysiology of autism (reviewed in: Schipul, Keller, & Just, in press).

> Results from these studies are consistent with the notion that autism is a disorder of distributed neural systems (e.g., the connections between structures rather than the structures themselves).

More recently, advances in diffusion MRI have added to support the notion that alterations in brain structure underlie the disturbance in functional connectivity (also reviewed by Schipul et al., 2010). Diffusion-weighted imaging measures the direction and speed of microscopic water movement in the brain, allowing inferences about the microstructure of the tissue that constrains such movement. These studies have consistently found reduced structural integrity of white matter in adults with ASD, indicating reduced anatomical connectivity (although among very young children this pattern may be reversed, suggestive of early white matter overgrowth and supported by morphometric studies discussed below). In addition, like measures of functional connectivity, measures of anatomical connectivity derived from diffusion imaging have been shown to reliably predict symptom severity among individuals with autism. Diffusion imaging also allows for in vivo tracing of major white matter tracts (diffusion tractography), and studies relating the structural and geometric properties of specific tracts to the severity of specific symptoms are beginning to appear. For example, the structural properties of a tract connecting the right fusiform face area to the right hippocampus differ significantly among individuals with autism who have high or low face-recognition ability, but a similar relationship does not exist among typical individuals. Diffusion imaging and tractography technology is rapidly moving toward ultra–high resolution exploration of the entire "connectome," a complete map of all white matter connections among all cortical and subcortical gray matter regions.

Once this is accomplished, specific brain–behavior correlations can be investigated to ascertain the basis of ADHD, anxiety disorder, emotion dysregulation, and occasionally, obsessive compulsive disorder in ASD. A separate but interrelated focus is on efforts to define the development of brain organization from local neighborhoods to widely connected systems. Eventually, neural circuitry will be defined that is responsible for automatic processing, which may involve the majority of brain activity and functions that enable the human experience and life. This research will identify critical differences in neural systems for automatic processing between those with autism and typical peers that will explain some of the uniqueness of the ASD syndrome.

Genetics of Autism

In thinking about the genetic basis of autism, it is important to contrast *syndromic* (or *complex*) and *non-syndromic* (or *idiopathic/essential*) ASD. [This distinction is not necessarily accurate or precise in all instances. An excellent discussion of this concept is provided in Abramson & Geschwind (2008) and Miles et al. (2005)].

Syndromic ASD includes identifiable autism syndromes with known genetic causes, such as tuberous sclerosis complex, Fragile- X syndrome, Rett syndrome, and Smith-Magenis syndrome.
- Syndromic ASD is associated with a relatively higher propensity for dysmorphic features (including anatomical brain abnormalities), intellectual disability (ID), seizures, and female sex (sex ratios are almost equal).
- Syndromic ASD is also associated with a higher frequency of chromosomal abnormalities in general, many of which have been identified as part of the genome-wide microarray studies discussed below. However, it is not yet clear for many of these syndromes which features are typical of autism and which are unique.

Non-syndromic ASD is also called *idiopathic autism* and consists of cases with and without identifiable micro-deletions or duplications to the DNA.
- Some of these microgenetic alterations are present within the abnormal chromosomal regions in syndromic ASD cases, thus providing a link.
- Individuals with idiopathic ASD are more likely to be male, with sex ratios approximately 1:4 (F:M) but approaching 1:7 in milder cases.

The syndromic/non-syndromic ASD distinction remains a clinically valuable approach to the evaluation of patients at this time, and should serve to remind *all* involved with the care of individuals with ASD to examine every case for signs of tuberous sclerosis, Fragile-X syndrome, and the many other syndromes.

In research, the distinction between syndromic and non-syndromic cases is beginning to blur, in that genes involved in non-syndromic cases are being found to lie within abnormal chromosomes or chromosomal regions that result in syndromic cases. The identification of ASD-relevant genes and copy number variation or CNV has demonstrated that they are distributed across the genome, which has explained why ASD has long been associated with a variety of chromosomal syndromes ("nonspecifically") rather than with a few chromosomes consistently.

Syndromic Autism

Overall, approximately 10% of children being evaluated for ASD are found to have an identified medical condition with a known genetic lesion such as Fragile X or tuberous sclerosis. An additional 10% or more have an identifiable chromosomal structural abnormality or copy number variation associated with ASD.

See Table 4.1 from Abrahams and Geschwind (2008) article: "ASD-related syndromes."

Table 4.1 – ASD-Related Syndromes

Syndrome	Gene(s) associated with the syndrome	Proportion of patients with the syndrome that have an ASD	Proportion of patients with an ASD that have the syndrome
15q duplication—Angelman syndrome	*UBE3A* (and others)	>40%	1–2%
16p11 deletion	Unknown	High	~1%
22q deletion	*SHANK3*	High	~1%
Cortical dysplasia-focal epilepsy syndrome	*CNTNAP2*	~70%	Rare
Fragile X syndrome	*FMR1*	25% of males; 6% of females	1%–2%
Joubert syndrome	Several loci	25%	Rare
Potocki-Lupski syndrome	Chromosome position 17p11	~90%	Unknown
Smith-Lemli-Optiz syndrome	*DHCR7*	50%	Rare
Rett syndrome	*MECP2*	All individuals have Rett syndrome	~0.5%
Timothy syndrome	*CACNA1C*	60%–80%	Unknown

Table 4.1 – ASD-Related Syndromes *(Continued)*

Syndrome	Gene(s) associated with the syndrome	Proportion of patients with the syndrome that have an ASD	Proportion of patients with an ASD that have the syndrome
Tuberous sclerosis	*TSC1* and *TSC2*	20%	~1%

The rates quoted in the table depend on the population that is being evaluated. For example, rates are higher in individuals from simplex families compared with multiplex families, and are higher in dysmorphic and mental retardation populations compared with idiopathic populations. "High" is used for syndromes in which no good estimates exist (that is, only a handful of individuals with the syndrome in question have been identified). It should also be noted that none of the studies cited here indicates that assessment for the autism spectrum disorder was performed blind to a patient's primary diagnosis. An expanded version of the table with additional variables can be found in *Supplementary information S1 – reference in* Source *below* (table). **KEY**: *CACNA1C*, calcium channel voltage-dependent L type alpha 1C subunit; *CNTNAP2*, contactin associated protein-like 2; *DHCR7*, 7-dehydrocholesterol reductase; *FMR1*, Fragile X mental retardation 1; *MECP2*, methyl CpG binding protein 2; *SHANK3*, SH3 and multiple ankyrin repeat domains 3; *TSC1*, tuberous sclerosis 1; *TSC2*, tuberous sclerosis 2; *UBE3A*, ubiquitin protein ligase E3A.

Source: Abrahams, B. S., & Geschwind, D. H. (2008). Advances in autism genetics: On the threshold of a new neurobiology. *Nature Reviews, Genetics, 9*(5), 344. Permission granted for use by Nature Publishing Group.

Recent genome-wide scans using microarray technology have demonstrated a substantial role for small chromosomal deletions or duplications (i.e., copy number variation or CNV) in the etiology of ASD. Sebat and colleagues (2007) showed that at least 10% of sporadic and 2% of familial ASD may be caused by de novo CNVs. Subsequent studies found this frequency to approach 25% in complex ASD. Recurrent CNVs have also been identified; in particular, duplications of 15q11-13, deletions and duplications of 16p11, and deletions of 22q11-13. Confirmed by multiple studies, these alterations account for approximately 0.5 to 1.0% of cases in large series. Many ASD-associated CNVs are located in areas previously associated with intellectual disability or chromosomal syndromes with a substantial ASD phenotype e.g. Phelan-McDermid Syndrome (22q13), Prader-Willi (15q11-13), and velocardiofacial syndrome (22q11). The list of known ASD-associated CNVs will probably increase as higher-resolution microarray technology evolves.

Non-Syndromic (Idiopathic) Autism

There is considerable debate concerning the genetic architecture underlying the remaining cases (i.e., the majority of idiopathic autism). Arguments can be made for either the effects of single, but rare Mendelian causes (for which documented CNVs are presumably the tip of the iceberg) or the interaction of numerous common, but low-risk alleles. Genetic linkage and association studies have been traditionally employed to address the latter model, but have failed to consistently identify susceptibility loci. This has been partially due to inadequate study sample sizes.

The formation of multi-institutional groups such as the Autism Genome Project (AGP) Consortium and the International Molecular Genetic Study of Autism Consortium (IMGSAC), as well as the establishment of shared resource banks such as the Autism Genetic Resource Exchange (AGRE) Consortium, have gone a long way toward ameliorating this problem. Using microarray technology to perform whole genome scans on samples numbering in the hundreds or thousands, these collaborative efforts have identified and replicated susceptibility loci on chromosomes 7q22-32, 17q21, and more recently on chromosome 5p14.1. While promising, the paucity of consistent results underscores the significant genetic variability involved, as well as the need for even larger sample sizes in order to identify potential common risk alleles.

Obviously the competing "common variants" and "rare variants" models are not mutually exclusive, as complex diseases most likely result from the actions of functional mutations on a background of normal genetic variation. Still, the majority of the more than 25 candidate loci currently under investigation are rare Mendelian mutations, CNVs, and genes/chromosomal regions associated with syndromic ASD. Not surprisingly, a number of models have been generated to organize this growing list in terms of common molecular signaling pathways, common functions, or common developmental pathways in an attempt to both identify a common, underlying ASD pathophysiology as well as point to new potential candidate genes.

Genetic Models

ERK/PI3K Pathway Model

Many of the known syndromic disorders with a significant ASD phenotype have indicated a common set of molecular targets that participate in a well-characterized *molecular cascade* (reviewed in Levitt & Campbell, 2009). Specifically, the genes involved in these disorders, such as tuberous sclerosis complex (TSC1/2), Fragile X syndrome (FMR1), neurofibromatosis, type 1 (NF1), and Rett's syndrome (MECP2), all impinge on or are directly involved in the ERK/PI3K intracellular signaling pathway.

In response to upstream tyrosine kinase signaling, ERK and PI3K activate mammalian target of rapamycin (mTOR) which, via further kinase signaling, serves to increase mRNA translation of multiple downstream genes responsible for a number of cellular functions, particularly proliferation, growth, survival, fate decisions, and motility. NF1 and TSC1/2 are direct participants in this *signaling pathway*. Disruptions in their function all have the result of increasing mTOR signaling. Others have more indirect effects. For instance, MECP2 encodes a protein that regulates the transcription of downstream genes involved either directly in the ERK/PI3K pathway or the upstream MET RTK pathway. Again, the effect is to increase mTOR signaling.

While the consequences of altered ERK/PI3K signaling are consistent with many of the anatomical and neuropathological findings in ASD, it must be noted that this pathway is common to most organs. Genetic lesions in key members produce conditions with more severe and widespread clinical manifestations than is generally seen in non-syndromic ASD. It is therefore more likely that potential ERK/PI3K-related genetic lesions causing non-syndromic ASD occur further upstream and impart a more subtle and brain region–specific orientation to the downstream effects. The MET gene is one such upstream activator of the ERK/PI3K pathway. Located in the 7q31 candidate region, MET is important in forebrain development, particularly interneuron proliferation and motility. A common promoter variant that affects MET function in vitro, as well as a number of MET mutations, has been found to be associated with a small subset of ASD cases.

Synaptic CAM Model

A second model for the pathogenesis of ASD, focusing on abnormal formation and/or maintenance of synaptic connections, has been suggested by the identification of NLGN3, NLGN4X, NRXN1, and SHANK3 in candidate loci. These are all synaptic cell adhesion molecules (or CAMs), which are crucial for the initial contact between pre- and postsynaptic neurons and serve to maintain cell adhesion and assemble/anchor synaptic scaffolding proteins (reviewed by Betancur et al., 2009).

The neuroligins are postsynaptic CAMs involved in the maturation and function of synaptic connections. Various mutations and splice isoforms have been identified in NLGN3 and NLGN4X, the two X-linked genes in the neuroligin family. Alterations of NLGN4X are not restricted to ASD, having been reported in Tourette syndrome, ADHD, anxiety, and depression, as well as in healthy carriers.

The neurexins are the pre- and postsynaptic binding partners of the neuroligins. Rare NRXN1 deletions, chromosomal abnormalities and sequence variants in NRXN1 have been identified not only in individuals with ASD, but healthy carriers and individuals with schizophrenia. Mouse models of a number of neurexin and neuroligin mutations have variably shown abnormalities in communication and social behavior. These findings have not been consistent and appear somewhat dependent upon genetic background of the mouse strain.

SHANK3 is a postsynaptic density scaffolding protein involved in dendritic spine morphogenesis and synaptic function and plasticity. SHANK3 is now known to be the gene responsible for the ASD and intellectual disability phenotypes in 22q13.3 deletion syndrome. Numerous large- and small-scale genetic lesions involving SHANK3 have been reported in association with ASD, and taken together, comprise an estimated prevalence approaching 0.5% of cases.

Numerous other synaptic CAMs and scaffolding proteins are also under investigation as ASD susceptibility genes. These include various cadherins and protocadherins, members of the Ig CAM superfamily (e.g. L1CAM), and the contactins. The contactins are a subfamily of the Ig CAM superfamily of genes and are involved in axonal pathfinding and synapse formation. CNTN4 is the gene responsible for ID and ASD-like features in 3p deletion syndrome and is highly expressed developmentally during the period of synaptogenesis. Alterations of CNTN4 have been found in a number of ASD probands. However these are of uncertain significance as they are most frequently inherited from unaffected parents. Also implicated in ASD are the contactin-associated proteins. These are structurally similar to the neurexins, but their exact function is not known. Homozygous alterations of CNTNAP2, a gene highly expressed in the frontal and anterior temporal lobes, are associated with cortical dysplasia, epilepsy, ID, and ASD-like features. Heterozygous alterations have been found in ID, language delay, obsessive compulsive disorder, and a small proportion of non-syndromic ASD cases.

Overall, with the possible exception of SHANK3, alterations in most candidate CAM genes do *not* appear to account for an appreciable proportion of ASD individually and are as likely to be found in association with other conditions or unaffected individuals alike. Additionally, single-gene mouse models of synaptic candidates usually have no discernable behavioral phenotype, although this alone does not exclude any candidate gene as potentially contributing to risk for ASD in humans.

Axonal Pathfinding/Positional Information Model

A third model for the pathogenesis of ASD focuses on the developmental neurobiological processes of neuronal axon outgrowth and targeting. This is suggested by the identification, not only of the aforementioned synaptic CAMS, but also of several members of the Leucine rich repeat (LRR) family, as well as multiple mediators of axonal microtubule stabilization as potential candidate genes. When wiring the brain, neurons must not only proliferate and migrate to the appropriate locations, they must also extend axons and make guidance decisions with a high degree of spatial and temporal fidelity. The growing end of the axon must travel toward its cortical or subcortical target, often over large distances, in response to numerous attractive and repellent guidance cues. Target cells are then specifically recognized through cell adhesion molecules on the surfaces of both axon and target, and, once initial contact is made, synapse formation commences. Perturbation in any or all of these developmental processes would be expected to impact anatomical connectivity.

From work in rodents and primates, it has been increasingly recognized that many of the molecular cascades underlying neurogenesis and layer specification play a key role in the later process of axon guidance, and they interact, directly and indirectly, with the "classic" axon guidance molecules (netrins, Slits, semaphorins, ephrins and growth factors). The molecular pathways controlling cell migration are also "recycled" in this manner, as is evidenced by the extracellular protein reelin. Reelin has been implicated in the etiology of a small proportion of ASD by genome-wide association, and neuropathological and expression data. While long known to control the positioning of migrating cortical neurons, recent studies show reelin also promotes the development of dendritic processes in the forebrain and affects synaptic transmission. Therefore, alterations of reelin signaling would clearly be expected to have multiple effects on developing neural circuitry.

In reverse fashion, additional roles for the classic axonal guidance molecules have also been discovered. For example, the LRR-containing secreted Slit proteins, established mediators of axonal branching and guidance, have been recently found to influence the proliferation, differentiation, and migration of cortical interneurons. The Slit genes have been implicated in the etiology of ASD based on recent genome-wide association studies, and again, could be predicted to have various effects on developing neural circuitry if perturbed.

These findings suggest that many of these proteins can be thought of more generally as providing positional information, cues that may be variously interpreted by responding cells as division, fate specification, migration, or neuritic sprouting/pathfinding signals. In other words, they are recycled for various developmental processes mechanistically requiring positional information. Therefore, genetic alterations involving members of these pathways would be expected to have pleiotrophic phenotypic effects and would be very capable of producing the varying abnormalities of architecture and connectivity observed in ASD brains.

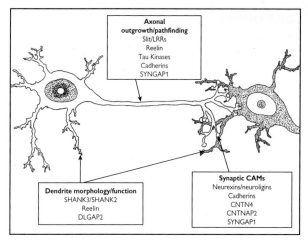

Figure 4.1. Functional impact of global rare copy number variation in autism spectrum disorder. Used with permission *Nature*, June 9, 2010 (Epub, ahead of print).

Syndromic ASD—ASD associated with evidence of disruption of early morphogenesis as evidenced by one or more dysmorphic features; e.g., microcephaly.

Non-syndromic ASD—ASD without significant dysmorphology.

Copy Number Variations (CNVs)—are gains or losses of large segments of DNA sequence (ranging from one kilobase to several megabases in size) and caused by deletions, duplications, inversions, or translocations.

Conclusions

- Across all domains impacted by autism, the common thread is the preservation of elementary skills, with greatest impairments in the abilities that require the most on-line integration of information.
- State-of-the-art science of the genetics, neuropathology, behavioral, and brain basis of autism indicates that this pattern results from selective disturbances in cortical connectivity.
- Recent genetic advances have identified a multitude of abnormal and mutated genes for ASD that all share a role in the development of neuronal connections and share common molecular signaling pathways.
- A little is known about the molecular pathophysiology of ASD, but far from enough to explain the specific connection of these genes to the impact ASD has on cortical circuitry.
- These findings have produced a convergent developmental neurobiological model of autism as a disorder of neuronal organization and in some cases neuronal migration, not one caused by social-information processing deficits or by environmental factors like vaccinations.

This work was supported by award numbers HD060601 (P. I. Mazefsky) and HD055748 (P. I. Minshew) from the Eunice Kennedy Shriver National Institute of Child Health & Human Development, and SAP# 4100047816 (P. I. Minshew) from the Pennsylvania Department of Health. The content is solely the responsibility of the authors and does not necessarily represent the official views of the National Institutes of Health or the Pennsylvania Department of Health.

Further Reading

1. Abrahams, B. S., & Geschwind, D. H. (2008). Advances in autism genetics: On the threshold of a new neurobiology. *Nature Reviews, Genetics, 9(5)*, 341–355.
2. Bailey, A., Giunta, B., & Obregon, D. (1998). A clinicopathological study of autism. *Brain, 121,* 889–905.
3. Bauman, M., & Kemper, T. (1985). Histoanatomic observations of the brain in early infantile autism. *Neurology, 35,* 866–867.
4. Bauman, M., & Kemper, T. (1998). Neuropathology of early infantile autism. *Journal of Neuropathology and Experimental Neurology, 57,* 645–652.
5. Betancur, C., Sakurai, T., & Buxbaum, J. (2009). The emerging role of synaptic cell-adhesion pathways in the pathogenesis of Autism Spectrum Disorder. *Trends in Neuroscience, 32,* 402–412.
6. Brambilla, P., Hardan, A. Y., di Nemi, S. U., et al. (2004). The functional neuroanatomy of autism. *Functional Neurology, 19,* 9–17.
7. Di Martino, A., Ross, K., Uddin, L. Q., Sklar, A. B., Castellanos, F. X., & Milham, M. P. (2009). Functional brain correlates of social and nonsocial processes in Autism Spectrum Disorder: An activation likelihood estimation meta-analysis. *Biological Psychiatry, 65,* 63–74.
8. Lainhart, J. (2006). Advances in autism neuroimaging research for the clinician and geneticist. *American Journal of Medical Genetics, Part C (Semin. Med. Genet.)* 142C, 33–39.
9. Levitt, P., & Campbell, D. (2009). The genetic and neurobiologic compass points toward common signaling dysfunctions in Autism Spectrum Disorder. *Journal of Clinical Investigations, 119,* 747–754.
10. Miles, J., Takahashi, T., Bagby, S., et al. (2005). Essential versus complex autism: Definition of fundamental prognostic subtypes. *American Journal of Medical Genetics, 135A,* 171–180.
11. Minshew, N. J., Goldstein, G., & Siegel, D. J. (1997). Neuropsychologic functioning in autism: Profile of a complex information processing disorder. *Journal of the International Neuropsychological Society, 3,* 303–316.
12. Rogers, S. J.(2009). What are infant siblings teaching us about autism in infancy. *Autism Research, 2,* 125–137.
13. Schipul, S. E., Keller, T. A., & Just, M. A. (2011). Inter-regional brain communication and its disturbance in autism. *Frontiers in Systems Neuroscience, 5(10)*.
14. Schipul, S. E., Keller, T. A., & Just, M. A.(In Press). Disturbances in frontal-posterior brain connectivity in autism. *Frontiers in Systems Neuroscience.*
15. Sebat, J., Lakshmi, B., Malhotra, D., et al. (2007). Strong association of de novo copy number mutation with autism. *Science, 316,* 445–449.
16. Tau, G. Z., & Peterson, B. S. (2010). Normal development of brain circuits. *Neuropsychopharmacology, 35,* 147–168.
17. Wegiel, J., Kuchna, I., Nowicki, K., et al. (2010). The neuropathology of autism: Defects of neurogenesis and neuronal migration, and dysplastic changes. *Acta Neuropathologica, 119(6),* 755–757.
18. Williams, D. L., Goldstein, G., & Minshew, N. J. (2006). The profile of memory function in children with autism. *Neuropsychology, 20(1),* 21–29.
19. Zikopoulos, B., Barbas, H. (2010). Changes in prefrontal axons may disrupt the network in autism. *Journal of Neuroscience,* Nov 3; *30(44),* 14595–14609.

Questions

1. Which of the following are *true* about early infant studies in ASD as reported by Rogers?
   a. Studies find no developmental differences at six months of age between "at risk" infants who go on to develop autism and those who do not.
   b. Developmental differences were first evident on standardized measures at 12 months, when all "core" symptoms of ASD were present, including deficits in joint attention, repetitive behaviors, and language delays.
   c. The earliest identifiable manifestations of autism were not in the form of a primary social impairment, but instead in the form of unusual responses to sensory stimuli, motor movements, and visual regard for objects.
   d. These longitudinal studies indicate that social and language impairments, long considered the causative features of autism, emerge later: between 12 and 24 months. Also, between 12 and 24 months, there appears to be a progressive widening of the achievement gap between affected and unaffected infants.
   e. All of the above

2. Which of the following is *not* true about "Syndromic ASD"?
   a. Includes autism syndromes with known genetic causes, such as tuberous sclerosis complex, Fragile- X syndrome, Rett syndrome, and Smith-Magenis syndrome.
   b. It is associated with a relatively higher propensity for dysmorphic features (including anatomical brain abnormalities), intellectual disability, seizures, and female sex (sex ratios are almost equal).
   c. It is associated with a higher frequency of chromosomal abnormalities in general.
   d. It is of unknown genetic origin and more likely to be male, with sex ratios approximately 1:4 (F:M) but approaching 1:7 in milder cases.

3. Studies examining head circumference (HC) and brain volume (BV) in individuals with ASD have demonstrated all of the following *except*:
   a. Not significantly different from controls at birth.
   b. Up to 70% of infants with ASD exhibit abnormally accelerated brain growth in the first year of life. Approximately 20% to 25% of infants in this subset actually meet formal criteria for macrocephaly in the first year.
   c. BV is significantly larger by two to four years of life, and some children meet criteria for megalencephaly.
   d. Apparent "normalization" of BV by adolescence/early adulthood.
   e. The first two years of life are usually not a period of rapid brain growth in typically developing infants.

4. Which of the following are *true*?
   a. Fifteen to 20% of cases of ASD are now linked to genetic or chromosomal abnormalities (15%–20% of infants with an older

sibling diagnosed with autism will ultimately be diagnosable with ASD by three to four years of age).

b. There are commonalities across genes in the overall disturbances in cortical connectivity that produce the major features that define the syndrome of ASD.

c. Functional neuroimaging methods not only provided information on patterns of task-related activation abnormalities across networks, but also allowed the assessment of the temporal synchronization of activation among regions, or *functional connectivity*, within these networks during a specific activity.

d. *Underconnectivity*, with frontal cortex as a specific characteristic of the altered connectivity in autism, is present across the wide range of domains of complex information processing that are affected in ASD, including social, language, executive, and motor processes.

e. All of the above.

5. Which of the following are *true* of genetic models of ASD?

a. Many of the known syndromic disorders with a significant ASD phenotype have indicated a common set of molecular targets that participate in a well-characterized molecular cascade.

b. The genes involved in these disorders—tuberous sclerosis complex (TSC1/2), Fragile X syndrome (FMR1), neurofibromatosis, type 1 (NF1), and Rett's syndrome (MECP2)—all impinge on or are directly involved in the ERK/PI3K intracellular signaling pathway.

c. Synaptic cell adhesion molecules (or CAMs) are crucial for the initial contact between pre- and postsynaptic neurons and serve to maintain cell adhesion and assemble/anchor synaptic scaffolding (i.e., abnormal formation and/or maintenance of synaptic connections has been suggested by the identification of NLGN3, NLGN4X, NRXN1, and SHANK3 in candidate loci).

d. When wiring the brain, neurons must not only proliferate and migrate to the appropriate locations, they must also extend axons and make guidance decisions with a high degree of spatial and temporal fidelity (i.e., abnormalities in developmental neurobiological processes of neuronal axon outgrowth and targeting).

e. All of the above.

Answers

1. e. All of the above

2. d. This is true of Non-Syndromic (Idiopathic) ASD: it is of unknown genetic origin and more likely to be male with sex ratios approximately 1:4 (M:F) but approaching 1:7 in milder cases.

3. e. This is false. It is correct to state that the first two years of life is usually a period of rapid brain growth in normal development of infants.

4. e. All of the above.

5. e. All of the above.

Functional Behavioral Assessment (FBA)

Jennifer B. Alfieri, Rebecca Burkley, and
John J. McGonigle

Description of the Functional Behavioral Assessment (FBA) *117*

How a Functional Behavioral Assessment (FBA) Is
    Conducted *118*

The Purpose of Conducting a Functional Behavioral
    Assessment *120*

Where a Functional Behavioral Assessment Occurs and
    How to Conduct the FBA *124*

Who is Qualified to Conduct a Functional Behavioral
    Assessment? *131*

Summary *131*

Further Reading *132*

Questions *132*

Answers *133*

The previous chapters have focused on recognition and diagnosis of autism spectrum disorder, medical and psychiatric evaluation, neurobiology, and genetics. This chapter will cover behavioral assessment and methodology used broadly for any challenging behaviors, and specifically in ASD and developmental disorders. It is a prelude to the next set of chapters on interventions, including several types of behavioral treatments. Much of the behavioral assessment is completed by professionals other than physicians, who are trained and supervised in this method. It is the integration and synthesis of the work by a multidisciplinary team that builds the comprehensive assessment and intervention plan for individuals with ASD. This chapter will explain the Functional Behavioral Assessment (FBA) that is required in schools and by most psychological and behavioral health service providers. It is based upon Applied Behavior Analysis (ABA) theory and methodology. Child and adolescent psychiatrists, other physicians, educators, health care providers, and behavioral health clinicians should understand the concepts, approach, and utility of FBA and ABA in working with individuals with ASD.

Description of the Functional Behavioral Assessment (FBA)

The term *functional behavioral assessment* comes from what is called a "functional assessment" or "functional analysis" in the field of applied behavior analysis (O'Neill et al., 1997).

Functional behavioral assessment is a systematic process in which challenging behaviors are analyzed to help determine the purpose behind them before developing an intervention. It is a problem-solving approach in which a clinician works with an individual and each of his or her support staff to identify variables that may influence the presence of a specific behavior or behaviors.

An FBA is an individualized assessment, but it requires a team effort. It is considered to be evidence-based and is the current gold standard of approaching challenging behaviors for individuals with ASD. FBA links with positive behavior support practices to ensure that interventions are individualized and are based on the hypothesized etiology/cause (function) of a behavior. A comprehensive FBA exists within the larger context of "positive behavior support" (PBS).

Positive behavior support is a proactive, respectful, and supportive approach to identifying, prioritizing, assessing, hypothesizing, intervening in, and monitoring behaviors that interfere with skill acquisition and socialization.

A behavior or behaviors that an individual, caregiver, or support staff (e.g., parent, teacher, therapist, etc.) desires to change is initially identified. In individuals with ASD, there may be several behaviors that interfere with a variety of life domains that could be selected for change. Therefore, identifying and prioritizing which behaviors to target first is imperative (see goals of positive behavior support in Key Fact Box 5.1).

Key Fact Box 5.1—Goals of Positive Behavior Support

- Increased achievement
- Improved quality of life
- Access to reinforcers
- Access to integrated environments
- Access to social situations
- Future employment
- Observed enjoyment of lifestyle

How a Functional Behavioral Assessment (FBA) Is Conducted

The number of behaviors identified for intervention in a treatment plan is individualized and will vary according to rates and severity of the identified behavior[s].

- Behaviors that are destructive (e.g., physical aggression, self injury/self-mutilation, etc.) and pose a safety risk to the child, other individuals, or property should be considered first.
- Disruptive behaviors (e.g., tantrums, screaming, off-task behaviors, etc.) are often the next group of behaviors to be treated due to their interference with social and academic inclusion, acceptance by the community, and one's general quality of life.
- Challenging behaviors that are disturbing may be treated after the first two categories show improvement.

Once one or more challenging behaviors are identified and prioritized, the Functional Behavioral Assessment (FBA) process can begin. FBA consists of three main steps:

1. Informal data collection
2. Direct observation
3. Analysis of the information that was obtained

Step 1. Informal data collection may include:

- Review of the child's record, such as previous evaluations and/or progress notes from past providers.
- Obtaining indirect interviews, which can be optimized by using rating scales, checklists, and formal and semiformal interviews.
- Obtaining information from a variety of sources in several settings.
- Interviews with parents or caregivers, siblings, extended family and friends, early childcare providers and teachers, and therapists.
- Discussion with the individual, whenever possible in the FBA, although the age and functioning level of the child will help determine his or her type of involvement.

Broad information is gathered, including main areas of concern, preferences and strengths of the child, current routines of the child and family, medical and physical determinants, history of interventions and their outcomes, and dynamics of the family (including community supports). Specific questions are also posed that allow for (1) detailed description of the behavior (e.g., form, frequency, duration, intensity); (2) the presence of ecological variables (e.g., medications, medical issues, sleep patterns, nutrition); (3) daily demands of the day (e.g., existence of a schedule at home, early education center, community); (4) events or situations that predict the occurrence of the behavior (e.g., time, setting, presence of others, triggers, situations in which the behavior always or never occurs); (5) potential functions or reasons that the behavior may occur, efficiency of the challenging behavior; (6) the ability of the child to communicate wants and needs to others; and (7) other events in the environment that either support or hinder the child.

Step 2. Direct observation is a key feature of FBA and allows for the team to collect objective data regarding the behavior. Information is gathered as the challenging behavior occurs through a descriptive or sequence analysis:

- **A**ntecedents - the events that precede the behavior
- **B**ehavior - thorough details of the behavioral response)
- **C**onsequences - the events that follow the behavior

The "ABCs" of behavior provide the FBA team with pertinent information about events that may reliably predict as well as maintain the challenging behavior. In addition, thorough details of the actual response are recorded and assist in operationally defining the target behavior. During the direct observation periods, data can be collected on relevant dimensions of behavior, including its frequency, duration, and intensity.

Step 3. The analysis of information gathered both directly and indirect occurs during the last step of the FBA. A clinician from the team will typically summarize and graph the data to:

- determine the interaction of the individual with his or her environment
- identify variables common to antecedent and consequent events
- identify patterns that relate to various dimensions of behavior, such as frequency, duration, and intensity

The goal of an FBA is to prioritize (rank) and define problem behavior, to identify reliable triggers as well as any maintaining variables, to develop a hypothesis about the function of the behavior, and to link assessment to intervention by designing a comprehensive behavior support plan (see FBA 6 step process in Key Fact Box 5.2).

Key Fact Box 5.2–The Functional Behavioral Assessment Is Part of a 6-Step Process:

Step 1. Specifically define the behavior of concern (topography).
Step 2. Choose an accurate data system and collect data.
Step 3. Analyze the data.
Step 4. Develop a hypothesis based on the data analysis.
Step 5. Develop a positive behavior support plan tailored to the person and based on the etiology of the behavior of concern.
Step 6. Evaluate the effectiveness of the support plan.

The Purpose of Conducting a Functional Behavioral Assessment

Failure to base the intervention on the specific cause (*function*) of a behavior may result in increased rates of the identified challenging behaviors, increased frustration and stress for the person, family, caregiver and support staff; ineffective and unnecessarily restrictive procedures; loss of placement; and referral to more restrictive placement.

For example, consider the case of a young child who has learned that screaming is an effective way of avoiding or escaping unpleasant tasks. Using "timeout" in this situation would provide the child with exactly what he wants (avoiding the task) and is likely to make the problem worse, not better. Without an adequate functional behavioral assessment, we would not know the true function of the young child's screaming and therefore may select an inappropriate intervention.

In order to increase the likelihood that an intervention will result in success for an individual, it is reasonable to assume that one must correctly identify the "maintaining variable" (function) of the challenging behavior and replace it with an alternative and appropriate behavior that serves the same function. Taking the time to conduct an FBA ensures clinical responsibility and increases the likelihood that the team will design an intervention that correctly addresses the underlying reason for the behavior. Not only is an FBA considered to be evidenced-based and a best-practice approach to addressing challenging behaviors, but for children and adolescents in school, it is also mandated by law for Individualized Education Plans (IEPs) per the 1997 and 2004 reauthorizations of Individuals with Disabilities Education Act IDEA). Also, in most states, an FBA is a requirement under mental health policy as a part of the behavior plan to treat behavior problems.

> A core assumption of an FBA is that all behavior is purposeful in that it serves a function, albeit not always consciously, for the person engaging in it. The objective of the FBA is to not only define and eliminate the behavior of concern, but to thoroughly understand how the behavior functions and the variables that maintain the behavior in order to prompt, teach, and increase acceptable alternative repertoires. By looking at the larger contingencies of the behavior, one can be more active in creating supportive environments and contacting natural reinforcers to ensure that the challenging behavior is irrelevant, ineffective, or inefficient.

When it is necessary to conduct a functional behavioral assessment

Functional behavioral assessments have been used extensively for individuals with developmental delays, including ASD, who exhibit challenging behavior. FBAs should be considered when the person's challenging behavior interferes with skill acquisition, when the behavior interferes with socialization and social reciprocity, when the behavior interferes with activities of daily living (ADLs such as maintaining hygiene, accessing the community, keeping medical appointments, etc.), or when identified behaviors of concern interfere with general health and well-being (e.g., medical issues, sleep problems, self-destructive behavior).

When a functional behavioral assessment should be completed

Once an FBA is completed, the reason for the behavior has been identified, and a comprehensive PBS plan is consistently and effectively implemented, the ongoing monitoring of the response to the treatment will provide guidance for future specific interventions. The response to treatment is continually monitored by an individualized data system that is sensitive to behavioral change. The data are reviewed and compared to a baseline measure to determine if a behavior has responded to the intervention. Changes in the behavior support plan or extending the functional behavior assessment may need to occur because of a limited, partial, or lack of response or if side effects of the intervention are observed.

The areas to consider regarding motivations for challenging or interfering behaviors

All behaviors serve a function, which is an act on the social environment. The challenging or interfering behavior can serve a variety of functions for individuals with ASD. Areas to consider when completing a functional behavior assessment are listed in Key Fact Box 5.3.

Key Fact Box 5.3–Possible Functions of Behavior

The function of a behavior is to:

Obtain Something	*Avoid/Escape Something*
Attention/Social Interaction	Attention/Social Interaction
Materials/Tangible/Activity	Materials/Tangible/Activity
Sensory Stimulation	Sensory Stimulation

The following are possible *motivating factors* that can interfere with the person's ability to be successful in completing a task, activity, or assignment and function within the daily environment:

- Biological (genetics—behavioral phenotypes (Fragile X syndrome, Angelman syndrome, tuberous sclerosis)
- Physiological (hunger, thirst, pain)
- Medical (dental, seizures, apnea, hypoglycemia, cluster headaches)
- Psychiatric/emotional/behavioral
- Medication (side effects)
- Trauma
- Environment (including caregiver interactions)
- Cognitive, executive functioning deficits (processing/joint attention)
- Communication (expressive/receptive)
- Social skill deficits
- Attention (gaining access to preferred items, people)
- Escape or avoidance (from unpleasant situations/experiences/people/ demands)

- Sensory (self stimulation: can involve anything for the individual that involves tactile, auditory, visual, proprioceptive, and oral stimulation)
- Access to tangibles: the individual seeks a desired object (tangible item)/ activity

In many cases it is possible to rule out some of the motivating factors that interfere with the child's behavior. However, if there are biological or medical issues impacting the challenging behaviors, then it is important to address the medical concerns first, before the behaviors can be addressed effectively and efficiently through behavioral methods. When it is determined that the individual's behavior interferes with skill acquisition, socialization, daily functioning, or overall health and well-being, then it is important to conduct a functional behavioral assessment.

Where a Functional Behavioral Assessment Occurs and How to Conduct the FBA

An FBA should be conducted in each setting in which the child spends a portion of his or her daily life. Although it may seem reasonable to only conduct an FBA in the setting or settings in which challenging behavior occurs, it can be equally valuable to observe the person and gather data in an environment in which challenging responses are absent. Identifying antecedent conditions that elicit more desirable behaviors, or observing consequences that diminish or stop the behavior of concern, can be very beneficial and can assist a treatment team in altering environmental conditions.

After gathering information via indirect measures, the clinician can prioritize which environments (including location, time of day, presence of people, etc.) to observe and collect data first. Key steps during the preparation period of data collection can be pivotal to its effectiveness and efficiency. Prior to recording data, it is important to identify the purpose behind the data collection, to prioritize and operationally define the behavior of concern, to decide in which environments and how often data will be recorded, to determine who will record data, to design a user friendly system, and to ensure that data will be graphically displayed for analysis.

> Data should be collected from a variety of settings, times, and days. Following sufficient data collection, the FBA team should look for consistency across sources of information as well as patterns of antecedents and consequences.

Upon graphing data, three main characteristics can be used to analyze the data: level (quantity of the behavior), slope (trend), and variability. Information about predictable antecedents and maintaining consequences often emerges from the data and is instrumental in developing a hypothesis regarding the function that the behavior serves for the person. If those data suggest no clear patterns or trends, the team typically returns to the data collection process and refines the data collection procedures. The FBA can also manipulate the behavior of concern to test the accuracy of a hypothesis by adding or eliminating a variable and looking at its impact on behavior (see example of hypothesis statement in Key Fact Box 5.4).

The formulation of a hypothesis statement allows for the linkage of assessment to intervention via the development of a positive behavior support plan. The team will summarize and integrate the results of the FBA

> **Key Fact Box 5.4–Hypothesis Statement**
>
> "When (antecedents), child will (behavior of concern), in order to (perceived function of the behavior of concern)."
> *Example: When given a direction from the teacher, Karlee jumps out of her seat in order to get the attention of her teacher.*

to move forward with developing a comprehensive treatment plan for the individual. Problem behavior[s] will be prioritized and defined operationally. Typically, one to three behaviors are targeted for intervention at a time. The team determines which behavior or behaviors to address first. Behaviors that are destructive (danger to self, others, or property) are the highest priority and are treated before merely disruptive or disturbing repertoires are targeted. Aspects of the FBA, including identification of all environmental factors that may trigger or maintain the behavior, are identified and become the basis for the behavior support plan (see FBA summary in Table 5.1).

A competing behavioral model approach (O'Neill et al., 1997) is used to lessen slow- and fast-acting triggers to the problem behavior, to replace the behavior of concern with a short- and long-term appropriate behaviors that serve the same function, and to ensure that immediate and eventual natural contingencies are in place to promote alternative options and foster durable results over time. The positive behavior support plan considers the overriding dynamics of the behavior and includes proactive antecedent-based strategies and replacement-skills training, as well as consequence-based interventions and lifestyle supports.

How the cause or function of a behavior is determined

There are three main ways of determining the function (cause) of the behavior:

- Interviews and rating scales (indirect)
- Direct and systematic observation of the person's behavior (direct)
- Manipulating different environmental events to see how behavior changes

The first two are generally referred to as functional *assessments* whereas the third is generally referred to as a functional *analysis*. Several different interviews and rating scales have been developed to try to identify the functions (cause) of behaviors. However, the reliability of the available scales is usually poor, and these should be used *only as a starting point* for systematic and direct observation of the person's behavior. The best way to determine the cause or function of the challenging behavior is through gaining information from a variety of sources and methods.

Table 5.1 – Functional Behavioral Assessment (FBA) Summary Chart

Antecedent/ Setting Event Interventions	Alternative Skills Instruction	Consequence Interventions for Problem Behavior and Alternative Skills	Long-term Supports
Modify or eliminate Introduce	Teach replacement behavior Teach coping/ tolerance Teach general skills	Reduce outcomes Provide instructive feedback Develop crisis-management plan	Make lifestyle changes Strategies to sustain support

- **Interviews and Rating Scales (indirect functional assessment)**

Gathering information from others through an interview is important because it allows significant others (parents, siblings, teachers, therapists, etc.) who know the child to identify the behavior in simple terms and to help identify possible causes or triggers of the behavior. The interviewer is able to ask detailed questions (e.g., what, when, and how questions) and to better understand various conditions that might affect the appearance of the challenging behavior. The interviewer will also be able to assist in developing behavioral interventions once she or he has finished talking to significant others in the individual's life. It would be in the best interest of the interviewer to speak with the child, if the child is able to communicate effectively with the interviewer. Many times, when someone outside of the child's immediate environment asks questions regarding the challenging behaviors, the youngster will explain why they are behaving in a certain way. However, if this is not an option, it is best to interview the family, caregivers, and support staff in the person's life, as discussed above.

There is a variety of rating scales available to assist in identifying the function, etiology, or cause of the challenging behavior. Therefore, it will be necessary to identify one or two behavior-assessment scales that will best fit the child's clinical needs. (See the attached list of available scales in Table 5.2.) However, these instruments are not diagnostic and should only be used as a starting point for systematic and direct observation of the person's behavior, since reliability of these scales is usually poor. Relying solely on interviews and rating scales should never be considered an adequate functional assessment.

One of the most reliable methods for accurately assessing behavior involves direct observation the individual's behavior in her or his natural environment and analyzing the behavior's antecedents (environmental events that immediately preceded the problem behavior) and consequences (environmental events that immediately followed the problem behavior). Observations are specific to conditions that set the behavior in motion as well as the conditions that maintain the identified challenging behavior.

- **Direct and Systematic Observations (direct functional assessment)**

Observing the individual's behavior in their natural environment over a period of time is the preferred method of direct observation. Direct observation of the behavior usually occurs after the functional behavioral interview process is completed. This will help the clinician identify which behaviors to look for in the natural environment. The clinician should observe the behavior in several different settings (home, school, community) so that he or she will have an accurate understanding of the child and of the behaviors.

Antecedent-Behavior-Consequence Data Chart (ABC)

During the ABC recording, the observer must give full attention to the person she or he is observing and document or score every occurrence of the behavior. Observation periods can vary and are based on the setting, type, frequency, and duration of the behavior in question. In the majority of cases, a 20- to 30-minute observation will yield sufficient data to formulate an initial hypothesis. The ABC recording allows the clinician or observer to record a descriptive account of all of the behaviors, antecedents (what occurred before the behavior), and consequences (what occurred after the

Table 5.2 – Frequently Used Functional Behavioral Assessment (FBA) Instruments

Rating Scales	Developed by	Targets
Functional Assessment Interview	R. E. O'Neill, R. H. Horner	What is the problem of concern? Describe positive social behaviors? Setting events related to the problem behavior? Many more questions
Kansas FBA Interview	Adapted from O'Neill, Horner, R. W. Albin, J. R. Sprague, K. Storey, & J. S. Newton	Outlines specific questions for the clinician to ask significant others: problem behavior of concern, positive social behavior, setting events that impact behaviors, consequences for problem behaviors, effort to engage in problem behavior, functional alternative behaviors known, reinforcers, history of problem behaviors, and hypothesis for problem behaviors
Student-Assisted Functional Assessment Interview	L. Kern, G. Dunlap, S. Clarke, & K. Childs	Provides perspective from the student's point of view, which will allow the clinician to determine the environmental factors that affect the student's behavior
Motivation Assessment Scale (MAS)	V. Mark Durand & Daniel B. Crimmins	Assists professionals in understanding problem behaviors in individuals. The MAS is research-based and is easy to administer in a variety of different locations (home, school, community) and for all ages of individuals from young children to adults. This scale allows clinicians to understand the function of the behavior and then develop a positive behavior support plan or intervention for the individual.
The Problem Behavior Questionnaire	Lewis, Scott, & Sugai, 1994	Asks a series of 16 questions with a specific target behavior in mind and rates the occurrence of behavior on a percentage from 10% to 90% or "Never to Always" occurring. This questionnaire allows the professional to identify the function (escape or attention) of the behavior.

(continued)

Table 5.2 – Frequently Used Functional Behavioral Assessment (FBA) Instruments (continued)

Rating Scales	Developed by	Targets
Behavior Rating Scales: -Connors Rating Scales -Child Behavior CheckList -Behavior Assessment System for Children	Connors CBCL - Achenbach BASC - Reynolds & Kamphaus	There are multiple scales for parents, teachers, and children of various ages:questionnaires that address inattention and hyperactivity, and detects internalizing and externalizing problems.

behavior) that surrounded each instance of the target behavior. This anecdotal data collection allows the observer to identify potential triggers to the behavior and develop interventions.

Ecological Assessment

This assessment is an expansion of the ABC data collection in that it gathers additional information on the environment in which the person lives, works, goes to school, etc. Physiological conditions, physical components of the environment, interactions with others, the home environment, and past reinforcers all play a part in an individual's behavior, which may need to be assessed more thoroughly if the challenging behaviors become too complex (Cooper et al, 2004).

Scatter Plots

Designed to record specific behaviors at the exact point in time that they occur allows one to identify possible patterns of behavior. On a scatter plot, the chart is divided into specific times of day (e.g., 30-minute intervals) and typically includes data over an interval of a week or longer. After several days, the observer often is able to identify specific times of the day when the target behavior is most likely to occur. This allows the clinician to develop an intervention plan based on the time of the day and the activity or demand that typically occurs at that time.

Functional Observation Assessment Form (FOAF)

Developed by O'Neill and his colleagues (1997), the FOAF combines the essentials of an ABC chart and a scatter plot. This form tracks the antecedents, behavior, perceived function, setting event, and consequences of a behavior. It allows a clinician to view the behavior over a period of time. Problem behavior typically falls into one or more of three general categories:
1) behavior that produces attention and other desired events (e.g., access to tangibles, desired activities)
2) behavior that allows the person to avoid or escape demands or other undesired events/activities

3) behavior that occurs because of internal or sensory consequences (relieves pain, feels good, etc.)

The antecedents and consequences of the target behavior are analyzed to determine which function[s] the behavior fulfills. Problem behavior can also serve more than one function, which can make developing an appropriate treatment plan more challenging (see examples of direct observation data forms in Table 5.3).

Table 5.3 – Examples of Direct Observation Data Forms

Forms	Developed by	Records
Antecedent, Behavior, Consequence (ABC) Chart		The ABC recording allows the clinician or observer to record a descriptive account of all of the behaviors, antecedents (what occurred before the behavior), and consequences (what occurred after the behavior) that occurred in the individual's natural environment.
Ecological Assessment		An expansion of the ABC data collection to gather additional information on the environment of the person's home, work, and school, and the physical components of their life
Scatter Plot		Records specific behaviors and determines at what points the behavior occurs more often than it does at other times. On a scatter plot, the chart is divided into specific times of days (30 minutes) and over several days.
Functional Assessment Observation Form	R. E. O'Neill, R. H. Horner, R. Albin, K. Storey, & J. R. Sprague (1990)	The FOAF combines the essentials of an ABC chart and a scatter plot. This form tracks the antecedents, behavior, perceived function, setting event, and consequences of a behavior.

- **Manipulating Different Environmental Events (functional analysis)**

In some cases, direct observation does not provide a clear picture of a behavior's function. When this occurs, systematically manipulating various environmental events becomes necessary. The most common way of systematically manipulating the environment is to put the person in several different situations and carefully observe how their behavior changes. This is called *functional experimental analysis*.

Hypothesis testing is becoming more frequent and standard in clinical settings. Functional (experimental) analysis may be conducted when a trend or pattern is not present in the data collected from a thorough FBA, or it can be used to confirm or reject suspected functions of behavior via the scientific method. The antecedents to and the consequences of the behavior of concern are systematically altered to indicate their influence on that behavior.

The separate manipulation of antecedents and consequences is often performed in an analogous condition if the experimental analysis is not conducted in a naturally occurring situation. A functional analysis typically has four conditions (three test conditions and one control) and includes *contingent attention*, *contingent escape*, *alone*, and a *control condition* (Iwata et al., 1994). The use of a functional analysis warrants thorough consideration, however, due to potential ethical issues.

For example, to determine the function of screaming, one could arrange for attention to be given to the child each time she screams and measure how frequently her screaming occurs. One could also make demands on the child, terminating them each time she screams, and measure how frequently this occurs. In addition, one could leave the child alone and measure how often her screaming occurs. If screaming is more frequent when attention is given, it would be hypothesized that screaming occurs to gain attention. If screaming is more frequent when demands are made on her, one could conclude that screaming has served to let the person escape or avoid demands. Finally, if screaming is more frequent when she is left alone, it can be assumed that the behavior is occurring because of its sensory consequences.

Who is Qualified to Conduct a Functional Behavioral Assessment?

Direct observation should be carried out only by a person who is experienced in applied behavior analysis and who has been thoroughly trained in collecting data about and analyzing human behavior. Directly manipulating environment events should be conducted only by a well-trained behavior analyst or a clinician with a high degree of training and experience. One must use caution in manipulating variables that elicit behavioral responses because of possible unwanted behavioral side effects that can pose a danger to the person and clinician if not monitored correctly.

Although it is recommended that clinicians who are leading an FBA have had extensive graduate level coursework, supervised experience, and/or relevant certifications or licensures (e.g., board-certified behavior analyst, licensed psychologist, etc.), it can be expected that the practitioner of an FBA should be knowledgeable in the basic tenets of applied behavior analysis, have participated in a comprehensive and systematic training in the process of functional behavior assessment, demonstrated competence in the conceptual application of an FBA, and have clinical supervision accessible when needed. Someone knowledgeable about behavior must be in the classroom family home, directly observing and measuring the behavior. Although this takes time, it is usually time well spent, because the intervention is more likely to be effective than one developed without careful consideration of the behavior's function[s].

A team effort is recommended for an FBA, due to the time that it requires. The team is often multidisciplinary (teachers, psychologist, therapist, occupational therapist, speech and language therapist, parents, caseworkers, etc.) and is involved in the indirect and direct gathering of data. If an actual behavior analysis is conducted, the FBA team should be directly supervised by a credentialed BCBA to ensure that ethical considerations and potential risks and benefits are identified and weighed during the experimental manipulations of variables that elicit or maintain the challenging behavior.

Summary

It is imperative that a proper assessment be conducted prior to developing and implementing a behavior support plan. The use of functional behavioral assessment and functional analysis offers the most valid methods for determining the function of a behavior. Such an assessment includes examination of prior records; interviews with teachers, staff, and family; as well as direct observation of the child. The use of FBA technology requires experienced clinicians who have training in assessment, and ideally, applied behavior analysis. Once the results of the assessment have been analyzed, a more informed and effective treatment plan can be developed.

Further Reading

1. Cooper, J. O., Herron, T. E., & Heward, W. L. (2007). *Applied behavior analysis* (2nd ed.). Upper Saddle River, NJ: Pearson.

2. Durand, V. M., & Crimmins, D. (1992). *Motivation assessment scale.* Topeka, KS: Monaco & Assoc.

3. Horner, R. H., Sugai, G., Todd, A. W., & Lewis-Palmer, T. (2005). School-wide positive behavior support: An alternative approach to discipline in schools. In L. Bambara & L. Kern (Eds.), *Positive behavior support.* New York: Guilford Press.

4. Iwata, B. A., Dorsey, M., Slifer, K., Bauman, K., & Richman, G. (1994). Toward a functional analysis of self-injury. *Journal of Applied Behavior Analysis, 27,* 197–209. (Reprinted from *Analysis and Intervention in Developmental Disabilities, 2,* 3–20, 1982).

5. O'Neill, R. E., Horner, R. H., Albin, R. W., Sprague, J. R., Storey, K., & Newton, J. S. (1997). *Functional assessment and program development for problem behavior: A practical handbook.* Pacific Grove, CA: Brooks/Cole.

6. Tobin, T. J. (1994). *Behavior challenges: A teacher's guide to functional assessment.* Eugene, OR: University of Oregon, College of Education, Behavior Disorders Program.

Questions

1. What are the A-B-Cs of a functional behavioral assessment?
   a. Anecdotal, Behavioral, Consequence
   b. Antecedent, Behavior, Consequence
   c. Assessment, Behavior, Consistency
   d. None of the above

2. Name two effective ways to determine the reason or function of a challenging behavior.
   a. Just observe the behavior and draw a conclusion regarding the function of the behavior.
   b. Conduct a direct observation and interview with those who know the child.
   c. Conduct a functional behavior assessment.
   d. Both b and c

3. What is the role of data collection in the FBA and positive behavior support plan?
   a. Assist in supporting your hypothesis of the function of the behavior.
   b. Allows the team to develop a plan to address the behavior in specific goals and interventions.
   c. Record data only after choosing an agreed-upon intervention.
   d. Helps to determine the function of the behavior.
   e. a, b, and d

4. When should a functional behavior assessment be completed?
   a. When the behavior interferes with skill acquisition.
   b. When the behavior interferes with socialization and social reciprocity.
   c. When the behavior interferes with activities of daily living.
   d. All of the above

5. Challenging behavior can best be classified under what two broad functions?

a. To obtain and to escape/avoid.
b. To change the outcome of a caregiver's response and to delay an event.
c. To communicate frustration and to label emotion.
d. To seek attention from another person and to demonstrate stress.

Answers

1. b. Antecedent, Behavior, Consequence
2. d. both b & c
   - Conduct a direct observation and interview with those who know the child
   - Conduct a functional behavioral assessment
3. e. a, b, & d
   - Assist in supporting your hypothesis of the function of the behavior.
   - Allows the team to develop a plan to address the behavior in specific goals and interventions.
   - Helps to determine the function of the behavior.
4. d. All of the above
   - When the behavior interferes with skill acquisition.
   - When the behavior interferes with socialization and social reciprocity.
   - When the behavior interferes with activities of daily living.
5. a. To obtain and to escape/avoid.

Introduction to Treatment Chapters: Treatment Overview

Benjamin L. Handen, Johanna Taylor,
Kylan Turner, and Martin J. Lubetsky

Evidence-Based Practice for Children with ASD *138*
Complementary and Alternative Treatments *140*
Helping Caregivers Access Evidence-Based Treatments *142*
How ASD Treatments Are Implemented in the Community *144*
Summary *145*
Further Reading *146*

Up to this point, the chapters have covered diagnostic assessment, medical and psychiatric evaluation, neurobiology, and behavioral assessment. This chapter will provide an overview of the remainder of the book, which is focused on treatment. The goal of the following chapters is to provide a summary of current knowledge of best practices and evidence-based treatment, when possible. These chapters will cover early intervention and educational and adult services, as well as psychosocial treatments and psychopharmacology. The primary focus will be on practices where there is ample research support.

In autism spectrum disorder (ASD), much of the intervention occurs in the school. For young children, that may be in the home or in preschool. For transition-age and adults, that might occur in the vocational training setting. Additional treatment may occur in the clinic in individual, group, or family work; in the home; or in social groups and activities.

The past 40 years have seen significant changes in the diagnosis of ASD (see Chap. 1, "DSM Diagnostic Criteria") and in the development of best treatment practices. Many of the current practices in the field have been affected by both court cases and changes in federal law. There has been an extensive amount of research on the neurodevelopmental and genetic underpinnings of ASD (see Chap. 4, "Neurobiology") as well as the development of a wide range of psychosocial and pharmacological interventions (see subsequent chapters). In the 1960s, behavioral psychologists first began to treat children with ASD and other developmental disorders in institutional settings. Court cases, such as *Wyatt vs. Stickney* (1971), led to changes in policy regarding the right to treatment of individuals in institutions at around the same time that the deinstitutionalization movement began to take hold in the United States. Public Law 94-142 was adopted in 1975, further strengthening the concepts of normalization and least-restrictive environment. The requirement for early intervention and early comprehensive educational services was made into law in 1986 (PL 99-457). Finally, the Individuals with Disabilities Education Act (IDEA), which was first passed in 1990, and amended in 2004, emphasized the inclusion of children with disabilities in classrooms of typically developing peers (see Chap. 10, "Educational Issues").

With this transformation in educational practices for children with ASD and other developmental disabilities came significant changes in psychosocial treatment as well. For example, in the early 1970s, the use of the TEACCH (Treatment and Education of Autistic and Communication–related handicapped CHildren) model was introduced in the state of North Carolina. By the 1980s, behavioral psychologists, utilizing the applied behavior analysis (ABA) approach, had begun a move from the use of more consequence-based to an antecedent- and reinforcement-based treatment model. The use of functional behavioral analysis and functional behavioral assessment gradually became a recognized and important aspect of the assessment of behavioral concerns prior to initiating treatment. The succeeding decades saw the development of interventions such as discrete-trial training, incidental teaching, pivotal response training, verbal learning, and the PECS (Picture Exchange Communication System), to name but a few. Model preschool programs were also established, including the LEAP (Learning Experiences: an Alternative Program for preschoolers and parents—started in Pittsburgh, Pennsylvania), the Denver Model, and the Walden Program (in Atlanta).

There have also been significant changes in the psychopharmacological treatment of individuals with ASD. Early studies of haloperidol in the 1970s (Campbell et al., 1978) have been followed by research examining a wide range of symptoms, including overactivity, anxiety, irritability and aggression, self-injury, and repetitive behaviors in ASD. While no medication has yet been identified that is capable of treating the core features of ASD, two medications have recently been approved by the FDA specifically to target symptoms of irritability and agitation (see Chap. 14, "Medications").

Finally, the last 40 years have seen the growth of complementary and alternative treatments in ASD. This field has grown to the point that 33% to 50% of families with a child with ASD report having used some form of complementary treatment (see Levy & Hyman, 2003). Most popular is the casein-free/gluten-free diet. However, families also have frequently used nutritional supplements and vitamins. Some treatments, such as secretin (a peptide hormone that helps to regulate release of digestive fluids) and facilitated communication, have been proven to be ineffective following a number of well-controlled trials. However, the vast majority of interventions that fall under the category of complementary or alternative treatments have not been well studied. Some, such as the use of chelation therapy described in recent reports, in fact can be quite dangerous.

Evidence-Based Practice for Children with ASD

There has been considerable emphasis in recent years on the use of evidence-based practices in many fields. This has been especially so in medicine and education. As discussed previously, there are numerous available treatments for ASD—some with a strong theoretical basis and research support, and others with only meager documentation as to their efficacy. In 2009, The National Autism Center (NAC) and Maine's Department of Health and Human Services (DHHS), with the Maine Department of Education, conducted projects to examine the effectiveness of available treatments for children with ASD. Both designed rating scales that utilized a combination of assessment measures to categorize the interventions.

The NAC's National Standards Project constructed a "Scientific Merit Rating Scale" to judge the efficacy of each treatment, while Maine used an already existing tool, the "Evaluative Method for Determining Evidence Practice" in autism (Reichow, Volkmar, & Cicchetti, 2008). This method rated each study based on primary (necessary for validity ratings) and secondary (i.e., level of evidence) indicators. The NAC (2009) assessed the experimental design (e.g., randomized control trial vs. single-subject), variable measurements (e.g., types of data collected, treatment fidelity, reliability), diagnosis of participants (e.g., confirmed diagnosis, instruments utilized), and generalization of target skills (e.g., maintenance of skills, data collected). Interventions were then placed into one of four categories (Established, Emerging, Unestablished, Ineffective/Harmful), which placement was determined by the level of supporting evidence available in the literature, their scientific merit, and reported treatment effects. The Maine DHHS report categorized interventions in six levels (Established Evidence, Promising Evidence, Preliminary Evidence, Studied and No Evidence of Effect, Insufficiently Studied, Evidence of Harm). The specific findings of the NAC and Maine DHHS reports are summarized in Chapter 12.

> Two reports (National Autism Center's National Standards Project and Maine's Department of Health and Human Services with the Maine Department of Education, 2009) offer updated information to both parents and professionals and provide a standardized method with which to judge and compare treatments in the field of ASD.

Complementary and Alternative Treatments

Similar to the National Standards Project, the chapters that follow examine treatments that are commonly implemented by parents and professionals to address the core and associated symptoms of ASD. No clear etiology has been identified for ASD, which allows for a wide range of treatments to exist. Although interventions utilizing a behavioral approach were strongly supported by the NAC treatment reviews and Maine's DHHS, as indicated previously, many families often turn to complementary and alternative approaches that currently lack empirical validity, or are not yet proven by rigorous scientific research trials.

Commonly used unconventional interventions are often defined in the literature as "complementary and alternative medicine (CAM)." Reports of the efficacy of CAM treatments are based predominantly on anecdotal reports from families and tend to lack scientific validation through large randomized controlled trials. Parents of children with ASD often report that they selected a CAM treatment for ASD because they believed the treatment was natural, safe, and had limited adverse side effects. Over 50% of parents surveyed used CAM because they hoped one or more alternative treatments would cure their child of ASD (Hanson et al., 2007; Wong & Smith, 2006; Levy, 2008). Table 6.1 provides a list of some of the most commonly used CAM interventions in ASD, most of which are not covered in this manual. None has been identified as "established" in the NAC and Maine DHHS reports.

It is important to be aware of all of the bio-integrative approaches being used by parents. This requires that the clinician specifically ask about them during evaluation and ongoing treatment. The physician and health care provider should have knowledge of all aspects of care and all interventions, in order to provide optimal oversight and recommendations to parents.

Table 6.1 – Complementary and Alternative Medicine (CAM) Interventions

Vitamins (e.g., B6 & Magnesium, Melatonin, DMG)
Dietary Supplements
Casein-Free/Gluten-Free Diet
Live Stem Cell and Stem Cell Therapy
Antifungal Treatment (i.e., candida, yeast)
Immunoglobulin Therapy
Hyperbaric Oxygen Treatment (HBOT)
Vision Therapy
Auditory Integration Training
Chinese Medicine and Acupuncture
Somatic Therapy
Craniofacial Therapy
Animal Therapy
Sensory Integration Training
Massage Therapy
Deep Pressure/Squeeze Machine
Sensory Diet
Music Therapy
Options/Son-Rise Therapy
Holding Therapy
Secretin
Chelation Treatment

(Hanson et al., 2007; Wong & Smith, 2006; Levy, 2008)

Helping Caregivers Access Evidence-Based Treatments

In addition to special education services and outpatient treatments (e.g., speech, occupational, or physical therapy, etc.), intensive services for children with ASD are often delivered in the child's home. These services typically include comprehensive treatment packages, such as intensive behavioral interventions and social skills training, and are delivered in environments where the child typically functions. This delivery method is not simply recommended due to the obvious convenience of meeting the high intensity of required hours of therapy, but is intended as a means to implement generalization of target behaviors taught in other environments. Additionally, in acknowledging parents and caregivers as the most salient and permanent figures on a child's therapeutic team, the notion of educating parents about how to determine which interventions contain an appropriate evidence base may assist in improving the child's functional outcome over time. There are only so many hours in the day, and devoting limited resources and time to therapies that are of questionable value can have a long-term impact.

In an effort to ensure that caregivers develop an awareness of developments in the evidence base for therapies for children with ASD, it is crucial that they be actively and explicitly taught critical skills to become good consumers of therapy and strong advocates on behalf of their children. Caregivers have a wide range of resources for information, including the Internet, books, parent support groups, and professionals. Once a child has been diagnosed with ASD, the parents will need to rapidly become educated about available services in their area. This process typically starts with the professional who makes the initial diagnosis (which may be a child and adolescent psychiatrist or psychologist). Families are often provided with a list of referrals to local service providers, including the local education system (which has legal responsibility to provide services after a child turns three years of age). Many support and advocacy groups specifically serve families of children with ASD and can often provide additional information about local available services. Many diagnostic clinics continue to follow families during this initial post-diagnostic period to insure that appropriate educational and mental health services have been obtained.

Some parents may find it difficult to decide among various treatment or programmatic options and have little basis upon which to make an informed decision. It is recommended that *parents compile a list of questions* that they would like to ask a provider regarding a possible treatment for their child. Exkorn (2005) developed the following list of questions that can serve as a guide:

- What is this treatment, and what does it intend to do?
- What is the intensity of the treatment?
- Is there real science to support this treatment?
- Will this treatment complement the rest of my child's treatments?
- How am I involved in supporting my child's treatments?
- How will my child's progress be measured?
- What is the cost of the treatment?

In addition to judging possible treatment alternatives for their child, families will also eventually need to make a decision regarding school placement. Ekkorn (2005) has provided another set of criteria to help parents and professionals *assess the appropriateness of various school options*:

- Evaluate the environment, staff credentials, scheduling, and mission of the program.
- Determine how long the school or program has been in existence.
- Determine whether the school's philosophy is consistent with parent or family values.
- Determine whether the school's program has been consistent in its use and application of certain well-established treatments for children with ASD.

How ASD Treatments Are Implemented in the Community

Many interventions for children with ASD are provided in the community rather than via a traditional outpatient model. The majority of children and adolescents with ASD have individual education plans (IEPs) with their school districts. Depending upon the needs of the child, educational services can range from a small, intensive classroom that specializes in working with children with ASD, to providing only limited support services (e.g., a weekly social skills group) within a regular education program. Young, preschool-age children may receive intensive in-home services or attend developmental preschool programs. Ancillary services, such as speech and language therapy, occupational therapy (OT), and physical therapy (PT), are also obtained privately or as part of a child's IEP at school. Some states also provide in-home and community-based mental health services until an individual turns 18 years of age. In general, in-home services are more often provided during the toddler and preschool years, with services increasingly provided in schools and outpatient programs once a child reaches school age. The clinician working with a child or adolescent with ASD is likely to need to interface with a range of other professionals who also are working with the patient or his family. Consequently, it will be important to have a general knowledge of what types of services are offered by these specialists.

An important role of the child and adolescent psychiatrist/pediatrician/neurologist/psychologist is to help the family to insure that all educational and psychosocial services are optimized for the child.

- For the preschooler, this means that at least 25 hours per week of services need to be provided (National Research Council, 2001).
- For the school-age child, the child's IEP needs to address learning, behavioral, and social skills needs.
- As adolescence approaches, new issues arise, such as transition planning for vocational training or post-secondary education.

Often, the child's treatment team works closely with the child and adolescent psychiatrist to address the child's behavioral needs. There are also times when a family will consider a complementary and alternative intervention for their child. It is important to maintain a positive and open relationship with families so that they will feel comfortable sharing such information. Unless a complementary treatment is clearly dangerous (e.g., chelation) or there is strong research evidence against it (e.g., secretin), it may be best to explore with the family how to assess its effectiveness. In addition, it may be helpful to talk about how long a proposed treatment should be in effect before improvement can be noted (so that it can be given a fair assessment).

Summary

This book will focus upon a review of the more promising treatments, both psychosocial and psychopharmacological. As part of a larger treatment team, the effectiveness of a professional working in the field will be significantly enhanced by possessing knowledge of the entire range of treatment options available to the individual with ASD. The next few chapters will discuss early childhood interventions both in-home and in-preschool; speech and language interventions; and specialized recommendations for feeding, sleep, and toileting treatment. The remaining chapters will focus on school-age, transition-age, and adult issues, behavioral/psychotherapeutic interventions including social skills training, and pharmacological treatment.

- The child and adolescent psychiatrist/pediatrician/neurologist/ psychologist is part of a larger multidisciplinary treatment team that includes: teacher, speech therapist, occupational therapist, physical therapist, behavioral specialist, mental health clinicians, other medical specialists, individual with ASD, and parents.
- There have been recent efforts to identify best practices (evidence-based treatments) for the treatment of children with ASD that have documented a number of established and possibly emerging interventions.

Further Reading

1. Beaulieu, A., Tweed, L.,& Connolly, N. (Eds.) (2009, October). Interventions for Autism Spectrum Disorder: State of the evidence. (A collaboration of the Maine Department of Health and Human Services & the Maine Department of Education). Augusta: Muskie School of Public Service and the Maine Department of Health and Humans Services.

2. Campbell, M., Anderson, L. T., Meier, M., et al. (1978). A comparison of haloperidol and behavior therapy and their interaction in autistic children. *Journal of the American Academy of Child and Adolescent Psychiatry, 17*, 640–655.

3. Hanson, E., Kalish, L. A., Bunce, E., Curtis, C., McDaniel, S., Ware, J., & Petry, J. (2007). Use of complementary and alternative medicine among children diagnosed with autism spectrum disorder. *Journal of Autism and Developmental Disorders, 37*(4), 628–636.

4. Howard, H. A., Ladew, P., & Pollack, E. G. (Eds.) (2009) *The National Autism Center's National Standards Project "Findings and Conclusions".* Randolph: National Autism Center.

5. Levy, S. E., & Hyman, S. L. (2003). Use of complementary and alternative treatments for children with autistic spectrum disorders is increasing. *Pediatrics Annals, 32*,685–691.

6. Levy, S., & Hyman, S. (2008). Complementary and alternative medicine treatments for children with Autism Spectrum Disorder. *Child and Adolescent Psychiatric Clinics of North America, 17*(4), 803–820.

7. Lord, C., McGee, J.P. (Eds.) (2001). National Research Council, Division of Behavioral and Social Sciences and Education. Educating children with autism. Committee on Educational Interventions for Children with Autism. Washington, D.C.: National Academy Press.

8. Wong, H. H. L., & Smith, R. G. (2006). Patterns of complementary and alternative medical therapy use in children diagnosed with Autism Spectrum Disorder. *Journal of Autism and Developmental Disorders, 36*, 901–909.

Early Childhood Interventions

Louise A. Kaczmarek, Kylan Turner, and Jennifer B. Alfieri

Defining Dimensions of Early Childhood Interventions 150
Additional Considerations in Early Childhood Interventions 153
Early Intensive Applied Behavior Analysis Approaches 154
Other Intensive ABA Approaches 160
Other Intensive Naturalistic Approaches 167
Summary 168
Further Reading 169
Questions 170
Answers 171

This chapter will review the basic dimensions of early childhood interventions and provide an overview of (1) two comprehensive intensive applied behavior analysis (ABA) approaches: discrete trial training (DTT) and applied verbal behavior (AVB): and (2) three naturalistic approaches also grounded in applied behavior analysis. In addition, this chapter will summarize other intensive and naturalistic behavioral approaches (see Chapter 2 for early identification and diagnosis, and Chapter 5 for the basics of a functional behavioral assessment).

The average age at which children with ASD are being diagnosed has decreased in recent years due to research advances in early identification. In addition, research has demonstrated that children who receive intervention earlier have better outcomes. Consequently, early childhood interventions—that is, those designed for children under five years of age—can have long-reaching effects on the quality of children's lives and those of their families.

Over the years there have been many interventions developed for young children with ASD. Thus far, research has not demonstrated that any particular intervention approach is better than the others. Rather, interventions are selected and individualized based on the characteristics of the child and the preferences of the family. Most early childhood interventions have focused on preschool children (ages three to five years). However, many of these are now being used with increasingly younger children, and some, like the Early Start Denver Model described below, are being developed specifically for children who are diagnosed before the age of three, who may not be diagnosed but are showing early signs of the disorder, or who are considered at high risk because they have an older sibling with ASD. The American Academy of Pediatrics recommends that if a child is showing signs of ASD, the pediatrician should refer the child to early intervention services so that intervention can commence on the basis of a delay even before a diagnosis of ASD is made, especially since there are often long delays in many communities in scheduling diagnostic evaluations for ASD.

Key Fact Box 7.1–Early Childhood Intervention Programs for Children with ASD

- Children with autism are being diagnosed at increasingly younger ages due to increased knowledge about the nature of autism and better screening and assessment measures.
- Research has shown that children with autism who receive early intensive intervention have better outcomes.
- Early childhood interventions have been developed for increasingly younger children, including children as young as 12 months of age.
- Thus far, research has not demonstrated that any particular intervention approach is successful with all children with autism and universally appropriate for all families.
- The American Academy of Pediatrics recommends that young children who are showing signs of autism should be referred to early intervention services in their local communities.
- The American Academy of Pediatrics recommends that young children with autism receive at least 25 hours of intervention per week, 12 months of the year.

Defining Dimensions of Early Childhood Interventions

Early childhood interventions differ along a number of critical dimensions, which include:

- theoretical approach
- degree of comprehensiveness
- intensity
- location
- the identity of the interventionist[s]
- structure
- supportive materials

Theoretical approaches. Most interventions are based on behavioral or developmental psychological theories. Behavioral interventions generally utilize the principles of applied behavior analysis, with underpinnings in learning theory, specifically those of B. F. Skinner. Developmental approaches are generally rooted in the developmental psychology literature and draw loosely from such multiple developmental theories as those of Piaget, Vygotsky, Ainsworth, Bruner, and others. A relationship-based approach is generally considered a type of developmental approach that is based on social-emotional theories of development and the corresponding empirical literature. Some interventions, especially those that are comprehensive, may combine more than one theoretical approach.

Degree of comprehensiveness. Many early childhood interventions that have been developed are comprehensive in nature; that is, they are designed not only to address specific autistic deficits but also to affect a child's functioning in multiple aspects of life. They offer a greater magnitude of service and are typically broader in scope and more intense. More focused interventions may be directed specifically to social skills, language and communication skills, or specific behavioral issues such as sensory sensitivities, behavioral excesses, or self-injurious behaviors. Many comprehensive approaches are composed of multiple focused interventions that are theoretically unified and packaged together. Some comprehensive approaches may have a primary focus on one of the areas of autistic symptoms but have an intervention framework that addresses those and other deficits in multiple areas of a child's life.

Intensity. The intensity of the intervention is considered to be the number of hours per week of intervention. Although considerable research is still needed, there is some convincing research that has suggested that children engaged in higher intensity interventions (20–40 hours per week) have more positive outcomes than those in lower intensity interventions (10 hours per week or less). Interventions that take between 20 and 40 hours per week are often referred to as "intensive." *The American Academy of Pediatrics recommends that children be engaged actively in intervention for at least 25 hours per week, 12 months of the year.*

Location. Early childhood interventions may be delivered in a child's home, clinic, or classroom. Classroom configurations can vary from specialized settings (exclusively children with ASD, or children with ASD and other types of disabilities) to inclusive settings that also include typically developing children. Interventions in clinics and children's homes tend to be exclusively one-to-one therapeutic sessions; i.e., one therapist or teacher and one child. Classrooms may include group activities, often based in traditional preschool curricula, but may also include one-to-one therapeutic sessions. Home-based programs may be structured like one-to-one therapeutic clinic sessions in a specific part of the house, or interventions may be delivered within the normal routines, activities, and contexts of the family. Interventions that occur during typical routines and activities in children's homes or preschool classrooms are called "naturalistic interventions." Many programs may include a combination of locations and intervention delivery modes.

Interventionists. Most interventions are designed to be delivered by trained professionals and/or supervised by them, but many also include parents and other family members. Depending on the approach, parents may be considered the primary intervention agents, partners with the professional interventionists, or agents for maintaining and generalizing acquired skills established through professional interventions. Some approaches, especially historically, may not offer or may even prohibit parent participation.

Parent education and training. Approaches differ as to the degree of training parents receive and nature of the training. Programs may feature sessions with groups of parents, individualized sessions focused on one child and family, or have no parental component at all. Individualized parent training may take place in a clinic setting or in the child's home. Individualized sessions may also include the child and opportunities for the trainer or educator to model intervention techniques, observe parents delivering the intervention, and provide feedback on intervention delivery. Some programs take a didactic approach in which parents not only learn the intervention strategies as they apply to their child, but also are provided with readings, paper and pencil exercises, and occasionally "tests" on what they have learned.

Structure. The structure of the intervention may vary with the adult-imposed direction. Some approaches require children to respond specifically to the treatment agenda of the therapist in very tightly controlled conditions. In such approaches a child typically sits at a table across from the therapist, who follows a specific curriculum or treatment regimen based upon the child's assessment results. Discrete trial training is an example of one such approach. At the opposite end of the spectrum are child-centered approaches in which the therapist follows the child's lead, and the prescribed treatment is delivered within the context of child-selected activities and interests. The more naturalistic approaches are usually delivered within the routines and activities of the child's home or inclusive classroom. Others may be delivered in playroom-type clinical settings. Comprehensive interventions may combine several different structures.

Supportive materials. The materials that are available to support early childhood treatment approaches vary with the approach. Some approaches come with developed materials, such as assessment tools, curricula, treatment manuals, or training videos that can be readily used by interventionists, including parents.

Key Fact Box 7.2–Dimensions of Early Childhood Programs for Young Children with ASD

- Comprehensive early childhood interventions are those that are designed to address a child's development and functioning in all domains, and typically include motor skills and self-care in addition to language, social interaction, play, and other areas of characteristic of autism such as joint attention, imitation, and behavior.
- Most early childhood interventions are based either in behavioral or in developmental psychology. Many utilize a combination of these theoretical approaches.
- Intensive interventions are those in which a child is engaged from 20 to 40 hours per week.
- Depending on the approach, interventions may be delivered in highly structured, adult-directed settings in preschools, clinics, or children's homes, or within the context of natural routines and activities in these same settings, such as mealtimes, playtimes, and community excursions.
- Interventions may be delivered by trained professionals from a variety of disciplines (e.g., psychology, special education, occupational therapy), paraprofessionals who are supervised by trained professionals, or parents and other family members.
- Many approaches offer varying degrees of training and support to parents, who may be considered primary therapists, co-therapists, or agents for extending an intervention to the home setting.

Additional Considerations in Early Childhood Interventions

Several other issues arise in understanding early childhood interventions for the treatment of autism. These include:

- Payment for services
- Intervention development and research
- Empirical support

Payment for services. Who pays for services and which services are covered differs by state. All states provide early intervention services to children with autism. Typically, early intervention services are provided in the home for infants and toddlers (until age three) and in classrooms for children between the ages of three and five years. However, early intervention services in many states do not generally cover the level of intensity of services that is being recommended for young children with autism. Some states may pay for these more intensive services under other legislation and in other departments (e.g., mental health services). Public and private insurance plans may also finance some or all of these services. Unfortunately, in many states intensive services are paid for out-of-pocket by parents.

Intervention development and research. Many interventions have been developed within institutions of higher education, especially within university-based research and treatment institutes that seek government and foundation grants to support their activities. Others have been developed by individuals or groups of individuals who establish private clinics and centers.

Empirical support. The amount of empirical support for different treatment approaches varies significantly. However, in general, more empirical support is needed for all approaches, and studies comparing the efficacy and effectiveness of different approaches are sorely lacking.

Early Intensive Applied Behavior Analysis Approaches

Early intensive applied behavior analysis approaches, often referred to as *early intensive behavioral interventions* (EIBI), represent the systematic application of the principles of applied behavior analysis. Interventions, which are typically adult-directed, occur in highly structured learning environments in the child's home, school, or clinic, and are typically implemented by highly trained therapists or teachers. Two early intensive behavioral interventions, which are described below, are discrete trial training (DTT) and applied verbal behavior (AVB).

Discrete Trial Training

Defining features of DTT. "Discrete trial training" is a systematic teaching methodology rooted in learning theory and based on the principles of applied behavior analysis. DTT can be a primary approach when teaching young children on the autism spectrum or used in combination with other interventions. When DTT is the primary intervention, teaching interactions typically occur when the child and trainer are positioned face-to-face at a table. This therapy, which usually takes place over 25 to 40 hours per week, is both comprehensive and intensive. Trained therapists who deliver the one-to-one therapy may be provided by an agency or privately hired by the family, depending upon the child's state of residence. Parents may also deliver a portion of the DTT hours.

DTT is characterized by *breaking down skills to the smallest level that a child needs*, a process that is referred to as *task analysis*, and teaching a skill using a *five-step teaching unit known as a "discrete trial."* A discrete trial consists of:

- the general antecedent condition, known as a "motivative operation" (MO), whose presence is intended to motivate the child to attend and respond;
- a change in the environment called a "discriminative stimulus," like a question, command, or instruction that is intended to cue the expected child behavior;
- the behavior of the child;
- the consequence that reinforces the child's behavior if it was performed correctly, or if it was not, additional feedback to assist the child to perform the behavior correctly;
- an inter-trial interval, usually one or two seconds of time before the process is repeated.

To assist the child in learning the skill/behavior, discrete trials are presented repeatedly and consistently. If the child is having trouble displaying the expected behavior, systematic prompts that help the child perform the behavior are provided in addition to the discriminative stimulus. Prompts will vary depending upon the nature of the behavior being taught and can be in the form of physical assistance, additional instructions, models of the correct behavior, gestures, or additional visual information. Like all aspects of a discrete trial, prompts are presented consistently and systematically. Performance of the expected behaviors or approximations to the behaviors are then followed by high levels of reinforcement to ensure that the child will display the behavior again. If the child displays the behavior incorrectly, then prompts may also occur as corrections in order that the child will display the desired response. The therapist will deliver the most valuable reinforcer when the child emits his or her best response. If the response is appropriate, but not the child's best effort, a less preferred reward is provided. Prompted responses are reinforced highly during initial training trials to let the child know what is expected.

Such trials are presented repeatedly within a session (referred to as "massed trials") and as necessary across sessions until a child is responding independently and the single skill has been mastered. As part of the discrete trial program, children will often have 15 to 20 different skills or behaviors that they are learning at the same time. Work on each of these skills will occur during a given session, which can last from two to four hours. Sessions are often broken up into shorter sittings. One or more sessions may be scheduled on a given day. Therapists are trained to deliver a discrete trial in exactly the same manner each time, as this improves the chances that the child will learn the behavior.

Skills that are taught using DTT may not be easily transferred and used by the child outside of the teaching setting. Consequently, learned skills are often subject to explicit programming for generalization to more natural environments and settings, other people, and different materials. This typically occurs through more informal teaching opportunities that are interspersed between DTT sittings.

History and empirical research base for DTT. Although clinical researchers and practitioners have used discrete trial training since the mid-1960s, it became more widespread with children with autism following the publication of Ivar Lovaas's seminal 1987 study. In the 1987 study, nine of the 19 children (47%) who received an average of 40 hours of one-to-one DTT for an average of three years entered regular first-grade classrooms unassisted. Only one (2%) of the children in the control group who received an eclectic model of standard special education completed first grade successfully. A follow-up study (McEachin et al., 1993) found that eight of the nine children remained in regular education at the average age of 13, and continued to be indistinguishable from their peers on a variety of standardized measures. Much controversy followed, criticizing the study for lack of random assignment, disparity in the subjects, and questions of internal validity. Since the seminal 1987 study, the Lovaas Institute for Early Intervention (LIFE) and several of its direct and indirect affiliates have been conducting research to replicate or expand the initial study. In 2005, Sallows and Graupner published a long-term outcome study that resulted in 48% of the subjects' reaching best-outcome status as children who were indistinguishable from their peers in regular first-grade education. Nearly a dozen long-term outcome studies have since been published by peer-reviewed journals, and they consistently show that sustainable and clinically significant gains can be made by comprehensive and well supervised EIBI programs whose primary teaching methodology consists of DTT.

Prerequisites for DTT. Nearly all children on the autism spectrum can benefit from discrete trial training in some circumstances. Breaking skills down to the individual level of where a child is experiencing difficulty and teaching skills within the discrete trial format often result in faster acquisition.

Intensive behavioral intervention programs whose primary approach includes DTT and a comprehensive behavioral curriculum are particularly helpful for young toddlers and preschoolers who demonstrate marked delays in imitation, cooperation, attention to task, and receptive and expressive language skills. DTT can be of significant benefit for a child who matches this type of learning profile due to the breakdown of skills, use of repetitive trials, consistency of teaching formats, systematic use of prompts, and high level of reinforcement. Young children who do not yet learn efficiently through observational learning and naturalistic teaching are excellent candidates for an early intensive behavioral treatment program that is centered on DTT methodologies.

Curriculum and transition in DTT. Initial therapy sessions focus on developing rapport with the early learner, and teaching cooperation, imitation, functional communication, and early toy manipulation. As the trainer begins to successfully teach the child how to learn specific skills, a wide range of preschool learning domains are targeted such as receptive and expressive language, and pre-academic repertoires such as matching, functional play skills, fine and gross motor skills, self-help, early quantitative concepts, and beginning joint attention repertoires. Most DTT curriculums are organized into learning domains and progress through more complicated levels or phases. There is no one set curriculum. Different authors have produced different curricula.

In general, intermediate learners progress to early abstract language concepts and focus more heavily on conversation and pretend play. More advanced learners may concentrate on programming that addresses social awareness, observational learning, rolling conversation, cooperative play, and expressive reasoning skills.

Comprehensive, high-quality behavioral intervention programs that are intensive in nature and aimed at the young toddler or preschooler with ASD are becoming more available across the country. The Lovaas Institute for Early Intervention, Autism Partnership, and The Center for Autism and Related Disorders (CARD) are three well-established, national programs that have clinical sites and consultation services throughout the United States and abroad.

Typically, when a child is learning the majority of new, adaptive behaviors through observational learning and more naturalistic methods, transferring skills with ease to other settings and people, and retaining what he or she has learned without difficulty, a transition away from discrete trial teaching is encouraged. At this time, the trainer shifts focus and serves primarily in the role of behavioral shadowing as the child begins to attend preschool, play dates, and more age-appropriate community-based activities.

The ultimate goal of DTT is to move toward generalization of skills to other settings, materials, and people, and to shift to other styles of learning as soon as possible. By the time the child is in a full-day educational placement, the intensity of one-to-one hours reduces dramatically, and the team begins to plan for transition to a treatment modality whose primary teaching interaction is not DTT.

Parental role in DTT. A high level of participation by parents and primary childcare providers is vital to the success of DTT. Depending on the geographical area in which a child resides, parents may need to take the primary role of organizing, training, monitoring, and often paying for a team of trainers to provide DTT to their child. Although many states have resources available, access to highly trained program consultants, one-to-one therapists, and sufficient funding can vary widely across regions. Typically, DTT therapists are hired by parents privately, or are provided through professional agencies and deliver the majority of the child's therapy hours. Parents may conduct DTT sessions as well, or assume the responsibility of generalizing and transferring skills during naturally occurring daily life. It is crucial to consider the amount of time and resources that a parent may have at their disposal when considering DTT as a viable treatment option for one's client.

Regardless of what role a parent takes in the therapy, treatment is optimized by family engagement, practice and transfer of skills beyond training sessions, and capitalizing on teaching opportunities throughout the child's day. A proactive clinical team will help to build capacity with the child's family and support parents in becoming the child's lifelong teacher.

Applied Verbal Behavior

Defining features of AVB. Applied verbal behavior (AVB) is a systematic teaching methodology, based on the principles of applied behavior analysis and B. F. Skinner's conceptual analysis of verbal behavior, which focuses on increasing language skills in children with ASD.

Verbal behavior refers to the *behavior of a speaker that is mediated by another person's behavior* (the listener). Asking for a cup of coffee is an example of verbal behavior, as it is mediated by another individual. Deciding to get a cup of coffee by oneself is a non-verbal behavior and is not mediated by another person.

The classification of language based on Skinner's functional analysis of language demonstrates one of the key features of AVB. New terms for function-based language repertoires were coined by Skinner and describe communicative processes from a behavioral perspective. Examples of verbal behavior that are the core operants and are heavily targeted in an AVB program include:

- Mand—derived from *demand* or *command*, is essentially a request for an item, activity, attention, assistance, or information.
- Tact—consists of commenting about an item that is present and is perceived from one's sense of sight, touch, hearing, smell, or taste.
- Mimetic—an imitative response of either gross, fine, or oral motor movements.
- Echoic—mimetic in nature and describes verbal imitation.
- Intraverbal—a conversational response to a stimulus that is not present, and relies on recalling information or an experience.

A comprehensive AVB program aims to promote language skills in children with ASD by capturing and contriving hundreds of learning trials each day. Motivation is initially assessed and optimized through rapport-building procedures in which therapists pair themselves, the teaching environment, and learning materials with reinforcement. As a child begins to approach the adult to gain reinforcers, demands are gradually introduced. Learning occurs via systematic mand training (requesting), natural environment teaching (capturing and contriving learning opportunities that occur incidentally), and intensive teaching trials that typically occur between the therapist and the child at a youth table. The use of discrete trials is standard; however, the delivery of prompts, the rate at which a child is reinforced, the interspersing of different types of tasks during teaching sessions, and the expectation of fast, fluent responses differ markedly from discrete trial training. Although vocal responding is emphasized, non-vocal learners may be taught to use sign language as a response form at the inception of treatment.

History and empirical research base for AVB. Skinner's 1957 publication, *Verbal Behavior*, introduced the idea of how typically developing individuals acquire language and how behavior principles and procedures could account for this process. In addition, in 1982, Jack Michael, who worked closely with Skinner for many years, re-conceptualized the role that motivation plays in learning. During the late 1990s, a larger number of behavior analysts began to combine and apply both of these conceptual frameworks to the development of specific verbal behavior teaching methodologies for young children on the autism spectrum.

Applied verbal behavior relies on the same behavioral literature as discrete trial training. There are dozens of peer-reviewed studies to support well-established procedures (errorless teaching, schedules of reinforcement, interspersal training, fluency, etc.) that are primarily utilized during AVB sessions. Over the past decade, other single-case-design studies have been conducted to buttress AVB as a new development in the field of ABA. Although AVB is currently a primary treatment model within early intensive behavior intervention, no long-term outcome studies have been published to date based specifically on the approach that has become known as applied verbal behavior.

Prerequisites for AVB. The ideal candidate for AVB shares many similarities with the candidate for DTT. A young child who is struggling to communicate his or her basic needs or wants effectively could benefit from an initial focus on mand training in which the child is taught to request. If a child has had a negative experience with past therapy situations, the implementation of reinforcement-pairing procedures that typically are in place as therapy begins may also be helpful in teaching a child that good things (reinforcers) are associated with the presence of a trainer. Because teaching a wide variety of targets and operants across the verbal behavior repertoire is encouraged, the practitioner should be mindful of how successfully a child can shift attention and discriminate across multiple stimuli. The use of massed trials (repetition of the same instruction) is discouraged in AVB, so it is important to consider the whether a child can learn when a variety of demands are interspersed during a single teaching session.

Curriculum and transition in AVB. Most AVB programs are guided by both an assessment and a curriculum that analyzes and teaches a repertoire of verbal behavior. In 1998, Sundberg and Partington published the Assessment of Basic Language and Learning Skills (ABLLS) and its corresponding curriculum, which outlines hundreds of skills within basic and more expanded operants. The ABLLS–Revised (Partington, 2006) is now widely available, and Sundberg has recently expanded upon his early work through the Verbal Behavior Milestones Assessment and Placement Program (VB MAPP; Sundberg, & Michael, 2001). Both of these tools analyze a wide range of verbal behavior and pivotal learning-readiness skills and assist in identifying a child's strengths as well as potential learning objectives. As a child reaches the upper end of their ABLLS or VB MAPP, the clinical team begins to plan for a child's transition to less-intensive teaching modalities and school-age instruction.

Parental role and involvement in AVB. Active parental participation when using an analysis of verbal behavior is pivotal to a child's progress. Because the AVB approach emphasizes mand training and natural environment teaching, parents have the opportunity to contrive and capture hundreds of learning interactions throughout the day in an environment other than one-to-one intensive teaching. The likelihood that a child will be able to generalize skills taught in formal AVB sessions and transfer skills is significantly increased when the family follows through with intervention recommendations consistently.

Other Intensive ABA Approaches

Although the two approaches described above are probably the most widely used intensive applied behavior analysis approaches, there are at least two additional approaches that should be mentioned. **Precision teaching**, initially developed by Ogden Lindsley, refers to a method for making educational decisions that are based on systematically monitoring a child's performance. **Fluency training**, whose origins lie in precision teaching, focuses on increasing the accuracy and speed of a mastered behavior or skill. Although precision teaching and fluency training were developed independently from DTT, many of their principles are utilized within the DTT and AVB interventions described above.

Intensive Naturalistic Approaches

Intensive naturalistic approaches generally are more developmental in nature, and many, although not all such approaches, utilize the principles of applied behavior analysis to varying degrees. These approaches are implemented within the child's natural routines and activities of home, school, and community and almost always involve a strong focus on parental implementation of the interventions. Three examples of intensive naturalistic approaches that will be described in-depth are: pivotal response training (PRT), Learning Experiences: An Alternative Preschool (LEAP), and Early Start Denver Model (ESDM).

Pivotal Response Training

Defining Features of PRT. Pivotal response training is a comprehensive, intensive naturalistic intervention for children with ASD that utilizes the principles of both applied behavior analysis and a developmental approach. PRT addresses *specific pivotal behaviors* that, when learned within the child's daily routines and activities, result in *collateral changes in*

Key Fact Box 7.3–Early Intensive Behavioral Interventions (EIBI)

- **Discrete trial training (DTT)** is a systematic teaching methodology based on the principles of applied behavior analysis, which can be used as the primary approach to teaching young children with autism or in combination with other interventions.
- DTT is characterized by the breakdown of skills into smaller behavioral units and the presentation of learning tasks as five-step teaching units called "discrete trials."
- Lessons involve the repeated, consistent presentation of discrete trials that are followed by high levels of reinforcement specific to each child.
- DTT therapy sessions, when applied as the primary approach, usually take place over 25–40 hours per week by trained therapists in classrooms, clinics, or homes.
- **Applied verbal behavior (AVB)**, which uses B.F. Skinner's conceptual analysis of verbal behavior as its foundation, is an intensive, comprehensive intervention approach that applies many of the same teaching strategies as DTT, as well as additional strategies specific to verbal behavior.

language, socialization, and behavior that improve broad and generalized areas of functioning. Currently, there are five pivotal areas of focus within the PRT framework: motivation, responsiveness to multiple cues, self-management, self-initiations, and empathy. Parents are trained to be primary-intervention providers of PRT. However, PRT's efficacy is enhanced when a coordinated team approach is implemented across people, settings, and environments. The ultimate goal of this model is to alter the child's repertoire of functioning so that they approach a more typical developmental course across all areas of development.

History and empirical research base for PRT. The developers of PRT (R. L. Koegel, L. K. Koegel, and L. Schreibman) studied the efficacy of various interventions for specific behaviors seen to be problematic in the skill acquisition of children with ASD. Through attempts to understand which behaviors hold the greatest impediment, or might promote the most learning, the notion of *pivotal* behaviors emerged as an expansion of the "natural language paradigm." PRT is delivered in the child's natural environment in order to reap the greatest benefit of more frequent and genuine generalization opportunities with familiar caregivers in naturally occurring contexts and environments. The three primary goals of addressing pivotal behaviors include teaching responsively to multiple cues across learning environments, decreasing the necessity for constant involvement of intervention providers, and providing as many services in the natural environment as possible.

PRT has been evaluated in recent systematic reviews and has been consistently ranked as an intervention with a well-established evidence base. The National Autism Center (2009), in its systematic review of evidence-based practice in ASD, evaluated a series of 14 single-subject-design and group comparison studies on PRT. In this review, PRT was reported to be most effective for children (ranging in age from three to nine years) with autistic disorder in addressing the core deficits of the diagnosis. Specifically, PRT was found to demonstrate improvement in communicative, interpersonal, and play behaviors with children with ASD. Additional studies have investigated the efficacy of the parent-training paradigm within PRT and have also revealed positive results in the acquisition, generalization, and maintenance of parent skills in promoting natural language in their children (Koegel & Koegel, 2006). This information taken together provides compelling support for PRT as an intervention to address the core deficits of ASD, as well as evidence that these skills are generalized spontaneously and are maintained over time in both the children and their parents.

Prerequisites for PRT. The children who would most benefit from PRT are children who are relatively young (i.e., three to nine years of age). Additionally, children with parents who are eager to learn how to deliver the intervention to their child in their home and community would benefit from the service delivery model.

Curriculum and transition in PRT. Although an essential feature of PRT is the delivery of the intervention in homes by parents, the PRT model can also be used successfully in classrooms when teachers and therapists participate as members of the PRT team. In schools, the PRT model is intended to be utilized within a general comprehensive educational curriculum for typically developing children. Practitioners are meant to infuse PRT teaching opportunities into the program. It is simply advised that the curriculum serving as a framework be of sufficient quality for the child's developmental age and continue to present appropriate expectations as the child transitions through their education (e.g., preschool, elementary, and middle and high school).

Additionally, given the naturalistic delivery of the intervention, parents and other caregivers are trained to effectively implement the interventions to address pivotal behaviors in the home and community when opportunities naturally occur in the child's or family's routines. Clinicians as well as parents learn to identify and capture naturally occurring teaching opportunities, so that the child acquires the skills and generalizes them most naturally. Due to the role that parents assume as intervention providers, learning these skills and effectively implementing them over time consistently and across environments will produce the most optimum benefit for children within the PRT model.

Parental role in PRT. Parental involvement when utilizing the PRT model is critical to the delivery of the intervention in the natural environment. The design of the model places parents as the primary intervention providers; consequently, parents receive formal training in workshops facilitated by PRT therapist trainers (usually 25 hours over the course of five days), which includes doing activities and workshops available in the PRT training manuals (also available on the internet from the Koegel Autism Center at the University of California at Santa Barbara). Parents are also provided ongoing training and consultation from PRT clinicians on how to best implement the interventions in the natural environment and how to incorporate the pivotal behaviors as target behaviors within the interventions. Therefore, the efficacy of the intervention is largely dependent upon the involvement and ongoing training of the caregivers.

While much of the research on early and intensive interventions suggests that a high intensity of services be provided (20 to 40 hours per week), the guidelines for PRT suggest that the type of intervention being delivered is a variable to consider in determining the necessary intensity for a given child. Due to the parent-training model and the naturalistic delivery of services, the developers of PRT suggest that thoughtful, consistent delivery of interventions for the pivotal behaviors in the natural environment yields beneficial effects on par with the high number of hours recommended for other treatments deemed to be effective. Essentially, given the parent-education model of PRT, parents are intended to be providing this intervention during all of the child's waking hours and doing so in as seamless a manner as possible within the natural routine.

Learning Experiences: an Alternative Program for preschoolers and parents (LEAP)

Defining Features of LEAP. Learning Experiences: an Alternative Program for preschoolers and parents is a comprehensive and inclusive educational program designed for preschoolers with ASD. The inclusive preschool emphasizes a strong foundation of naturalistic teaching components and interdisciplinary collaboration between related therapy providers and educators. *Social interactions* between children with ASD and typically developing peers are targeted by employing strategies to *address behaviors/ skills across contexts within the classroom*. Generalization of skills is further targeted by embedding all treatment goals into the natural routine of the school day. In addition to the generalization-focus of the preschool environment, LEAP also facilitates a behavioral skill training program for parents and involves families to the fullest extent possible (i.e., in the school, home, and community). The LEAP model is also data-driven and tailored to the unique needs of each child.

History and empirical research base for LEAP. The LEAP model, which was developed by Dr. Philip Strain and colleagues at the University of Pittsburgh, created a comprehensive program that incorporated and integrated multiple interventions based on applied behavior analysis, such as peer-mediated interventions, incidental teaching, and prompting strategies. A primary goal was to create a service delivery mechanism that is intensive not simply in terms of the number of hours of direct intervention, but in the concentrated and coordinated efforts targeting various areas in the child's daily life.

Over 36 studies have investigated the outcomes of child and family participants in the LEAP model preschool. This research base demonstrates improvement in a broad array of developmental areas pertinent to the diagnosis. Several of these studies were longitudinal and evaluated the performance and functioning of children participating in LEAP compared to that of children who were not. A longitudinal outcome study (Strain & Hoyson, 2000) evaluated the progress of six initial LEAP participants on measures of autism classification, developmental functioning, parent–child interactions, social interaction, and school history. Results revealed improvement during two years in the program and continued maintenance for up to five years after exiting the program on all measures. Specifically, autism symptoms as rated by the Childhood Autism Rating Scale were reduced from an average of 35 to 22 following program participation. Changes in developmental functioning were evaluated using two different assessments (the Learning Accomplishment Profile and the Stanford-Binet). The children gained approximately 1.41 months in their development for each month of participation within the program. Improvement in social interaction behavior was also demonstrated across the LEAP participants, with a 21% increase in the mean level of social interactions, which closely approximated the mean level of social interactions of typically developing peers in the program. Finally, in an evaluation of school data associated with the six children following their participation in the LEAP program, five were noted to no longer require special education services in their school placements.

Prerequisites for LEAP. The prerequisites for children with ASD receiving interventions delivered through the LEAP model are consistent with those of the other early childhood interventions that have been discussed in this chapter. Primarily, children who are preschool age (i.e., three to five years old), and whose families are involved in the treatment process are most likely to receive the most optimal benefit from participating in the LEAP model.

Curriculum and transition in LEAP. The Quality Inclusion Curriculum was developed by Phillip Strain (2010) specifically for educational programming in the LEAP model. This teacher training curriculum contains multiple strategies, guidelines, and learning materials for teachers to use in inclusive classrooms. The training curriculum is based on a strong foundation of behavior-analytic principles, both in providing strategies to reduce challenging behavior and promote desirable behavior, and in the provision of natural, rather than contrived or arbitrary, reinforcement. Essential to the mission of this curriculum is a focus on the development of communication and social skills in the natural environment through peer-mediated techniques and environmental arrangement.

In the LEAP model, teachers, family service coordinators and the child's family create opportunities within the school day, the home, and the community to address target behaviors. Careful documentation of progress includes the collection of data in each of these environments to ensure that children are progressing toward target goals within each activity. The transition process is comprehensive and carefully planned. Typically, this transition process is meant to begin well before the child turns five in order to properly map the child's treatment goals for the long term.

Parental role and involvement in LEAP. Parents of LEAP participants are strongly encouraged to take an active role in assisting to implement the intervention process with their child in the home setting. Parents are invited to attend the skills training program delivered at the LEAP site offered for several hours each week. This training program intends to teach parents generalized (rather than task-specific) skills, focusing on behavior modification for their child in the home environment.

The longitudinal follow-up study mentioned earlier (Strain & Hoyson, 2000) evaluated changes in parent–child interactions. In this study, an interval-coding system was used to evaluate these interactions (in three 20-minute samples per parent–child dyad) and demonstrated that the six child participants improved in these interactions from a mean rating of 51% of appropriate behavior at program entry to 98% following two years in the program. In particular, marked decreases in noncompliant behaviors were demonstrated in all child participants during these interactions. This rating of appropriate behavior was approximately maintained (falling only to a mean of 97%) over the subsequent follow-up period. This suggests that parent–child interactions may improve through participation in the program.

Early Start Denver Model (ESDM)

Defining features of ESDM. The Early Start Denver Model is a comprehensive, intensive, naturalistic, social-developmental intervention model for the youngest children, ages 12 to 36 months of age, diagnosed with or at risk for autism. The model represents an *integration of applied behavior analysis, developmental, and relationship-based approaches* administered by parents and professionals in the home, preschool, community, and/or clinic. The model focuses on optimizing motivation within natural environment's routines and activities in order to: (1) increase the reward value of social engagement for the child; (2) develop coordinated, interactive social relations so that the child starts to learn through social experiences; and (3) facilitate play activities that include joint routines so the child will learn skills typically deficient in children with autism, such as imitation and flexible play with toys.

History and empirical research base for ESDM. The ESDM was developed by Sally Rogers, Geraldine Dawson, and colleagues at University of California–Davis and the University of Washington. It is based on the joint application of two previously developed comprehensive models for the treatment of young children with autism—the Denver Model and pivotal response training (PRT). The Denver Model, which was also developed by Sally Rogers for somewhat older children (24 to 60 months of age), contributes to the ESDM its approach to affective and relationship-based skills, play skills, and communication skills. PRT contributes its naturalistic application of the principles of applied behavior analysis to increase the child's motivation to learn new skills and to improve a child's response to multiple cues within a format that is similar to the way a typical child might learn. In addition, the instructional practices of the ESDM are based on the basic practices of effective teaching used in applied behavior analysis.

To date, there have been only been a few studies on the ESDM published in peer-reviewed journals. In addition to four earlier studies that demonstrate the efficacy of the earlier Denver Model, there have been four specifically related to the ESDM. The studies included a randomized controlled trial and several single-subject-design studies. The randomized, controlled trial (Dawson et al., 2009) featured interventions administered by both professionals and parents in the home environment to 24 children between the ages of 18 and 30 months over a two-year period. Children received an average of 15.2 hours per week of intervention delivered by trained professionals, 16.2 hours per week delivered by parents, and 5.2 hours per week of other therapies outside of the intervention. Parents received training during semi-monthly meetings. Children in the ESDM group demonstrated greater improvements in IQ, adaptive behavior, and autism diagnosis over the comparison group of 24 children who received an average of 9.1 hours per week of community-based therapies and 9.3 hours per week of community-based group interventions. Another study revealed that the ESDM resulted in improvements in social and communication behaviors when applied in the home setting exclusively by parents who attended a 12-week training program

Prerequisites for ESDM. The approach is intended for toddlers (i.e., children under age three) who are diagnosed with or considered at-risk for autism. The authors indicate that the approach is inappropriate for children under about nine months of age and children over 60 months. The delivery of the intervention requires no specific prerequisites on the part of the child. The approach requires parents who are willing to learn and apply the strategies in their homes during family routines and activities.

Curriculum and transition in ESDM. The ESDM offers a comprehensive sequence of developmental skills based on the following domains: receptive communication, expressive communication, joint attention, imitation, social skills, play skills, cognitive skills, fine motor skills, gross motor skills, and self-care skills. The skills are found in the criterion-referenced curriculum checklist (Rogers and Dawson, 2010), which consists of four levels that roughly cover the developmental periods of 12 to 18 months, 18 to 24 months, 24 to 36 months, and 36 to 48 months. The checklist is skewed to emphasize the delays and needs found in children with autism.

Children are assessed using the curriculum checklist. Based on the assessment results, two to three short-term objectives are written in each developmental area, with the expectation that they will be mastered within a 12-week period. After a 12-week period, additional objectives are added or old ones revised.

Interventions are carried out within the context of child-centered joint-play routines, with and without objects. In addition to being the context for learning, such routines are intended to create positive emotional states in children in order to recalibrate their social responsiveness. Challenging behaviors are addressed through positive behavioral approaches. Since developmental delays in autism seem to be related to decreased learning opportunities, the ESDM intervention must be implemented at least as intensively as the high level of social interactions underlying typical early development. Data collection and the use of data-based decision-making are also essential components.

Parental role in ESDM. In order to achieve the level of intensity of interaction needed to alter the developmental trajectory of autism, parental involvement is considered an essential part of the ESDM. Parents and family members as co-therapists are expected to embed the intervention techniques within natural family routines for at least one to two hours per day. Parents receive training and coaching on the intervention strategies and support in embedding the techniques into home routines.

> ## Key Fact Box 7.4–Early Intensive Naturalistic Behavioral Interventions
>
> - Intensive naturalistic approaches are based on child development, although many, but not all, such approaches utilize the principles of applied behavior analysis to varying degrees.
> - Naturalistic approaches almost always involve a high level implementation of interventions by teachers, therapists, or parents within the child's natural routines and activities of the home, school, and community.
> - **Pivotal response training (PRT)** is a naturalistic approach that focuses on teaching a child's parents and often the child's teachers to address pivotal behaviors that, when learned within the child's daily routines and activities, result in positive improvements in the core deficits areas of autism.
> - **Learning experiences: An Alternative Preschool (LEAP)** is a comprehensive, inclusive preschool program for children with autism that emphasizes naturalistic instruction within classroom activities and the facilitation of social interactions with typically developing children.
> - **Early Start Denver Model (ESDM)** is a naturalistic intervention model for children under three years of age that integrates a developmental and relationship-based approach with the principles of applied behavior analysis, including the training of parents as co-therapists.

Other Intensive Naturalistic Approaches

There have been several additional naturalistic developmental intervention approaches that have been developed for children with autism. Among them are the following.

- **Developmental, Individual difference, Relationship-based model (DIR)/Floortime**

  Conceived by Stanley Greenspan and Serena Wieder, DIR is a *comprehensive, play-based, problem-solving framework* for developing intervention programs that addresses the unique needs of individual children based on their natural interests and emotions to enhance their relationships with others and provide the fundamental foundation for development.

- **Relationship Development Intervention (RDI)**

  RDI, developed by Steven Gutstein, is a program developed for parents that addresses the core deficits of autism by *deconstructing and re-programming the fundamental relationships* that guide children in their development.

- **Responsive Teaching**

  Proposed by Gerald Mahoney and colleagues, this is a model designed to assist parents and other caregivers to maximize their interactions with their children within daily routines in order facilitate the cognitive, communication, and social-emotional development of children.

- **SCERTS Model**

  Developed by speech language pathologists Barry Prizant and Amy Wetherby, the SCERTS model provides a comprehensive system for teaching young children with autism to become competent social communicators, including skills related to emotional regulation (see further explanation in Chapter 8 on language interventions).

Summary

This chapter offers an in-depth review of five early childhood interventions for children with ASD. The interventions are described in their purest sense according to the materials that have been published in journals, books, and websites by the proponents of each model. Not all of these interventions are available in every community, and when offered in a given community, not all models will necessarily be implemented with the same rigor as by those who originally developed the approach. Hopefully, those proposing to follow a single model will also offer evidence that staff have been appropriately trained.

However, many community-based programs may offer eclectic approaches combining elements of various types of interventions within a single program. Although we are beginning to understand better the types of approaches that seem to be successful for young children with autism and their families, we really have no way of knowing the extent to which eclectic, community-based approaches are successful. For that information, probably it is best to examine the reputation of a program within its own community and to weigh the dimensions of a given program in terms of the extent to which it seems to meet the needs of any given family.

Further Reading

1. Carr, J. E., & Firth, A. M. (2005). The verbal behavior approach to early and intensive behavioral intervention for autism: A call for additional empirical support. *Journal of Early and Intensive Behavioral Intervention*, 2, 18–27.

2. Dawson, G., Rogers, S., Munson, J., Smith, M., Winter, J., Greenson, J., Donaldson, A., & Varley, J. (2009). Randomized, controlled trial of an intervention for toddlers with autism: The Early Start Denver Model. *Pediatrics*, 125, 17–23.

3. Koegel, R. L., & Koegel, L. K. (2006). *Pivotal response treatments for autism*. Baltimore, MD: Paul H. Brookes.

4. Lovaas, O. I. (1987). Behavioral treatment and normal educational and intellectual functioning in young autistic children. *Journal of Consulting and Clinical Psychology*, 55, 3–9.

5. McEachin, J. J., Smith, T., & Lovaas, O. I. (1993). Long-term outcome for children with autism who received early intensive behavioral treatment. *American Journal on Mental Retardation*, 97, 359–372.

6. National Autism Center (2009). *National standards report: Addressing the need for evidence-based practice guidelines for Autism Spectrum Disorder*. Randolph: National Autism Center (http://www.nationalautismcenter.org/pdf/NAC%20Standards%20Report.pdf), accessed on December 8, 2010.

7. Partington, J. W. (2006). *Assessment of basic language and learning–Revised*. Pleasant Hills, CA: Behavior Analysts, Inc.

8. Rogers, S., & Dawson, G. (2010). *Early Start Denver Model for young children with autism: Promoting language, learning, and engagement*. New York, NY: Guilford Press.

9. Sallows, G. O., & Graupner, T. D. (2005). Intensive behavioral treatment for children with autism: Four-year outcome and predictors. *American Journal on Mental Retardation*, 110, 417–438.

10. Strain, P. S. (2003). *The Quality Inclusion Curriculum: Proven results for children with Autism Spectrum Disorder and behavior and emotional issues!* Tualatin: Teacher's Toolbox (http://www.ttoolbox.com/quality.htm), accessed on December 8, 2010.

11. Strain, P. S. & Hoyson, M. (2000). The need for longitudinal, intensive social skill intervention: LEAP follow-up outcomes for children with autism. *Topics in Early Childhood Special Education*, 20(2), 116–122.

12. Sundberg, M (2008). *The Verbal Behavior Milestone Assessment and Placement Program (The VB-MAPP)*. Concord, CA: AVB Press.

13. Sundberg, M. L., & Michael, J. L. (2001). The benefits of Skinner's analysis of verbal behavior for children with autism. *Behavior Modification*, 25, 698–724.

Questions

1. The American Academy of Pediatrics recommends which of the following for young children with autism?
   a. Referral to early intervention if a young child is showing the signs of autism, even before a diagnosis of autism is made
   b. Intensive one-to-one behavioral intervention in a clinical setting
   c. Intensive intervention of at least 25 hours per week, 12 months of the year
   d. a & c

2. Who pays for early intensive autism services in most states?
   a. Early intervention services through the Individuals with Disabilities Education Act pays for at least 40 hours of intervention per week in most states
   b. Private health care plans supplemented by public health care plans cover these costs in most states
   c. Intensive services in most states must be paid out-of-pocket by the parents of the children with autism
   d. Medical assistance covers up to 30 hours of these expenses in most states

3. Pivotal Response Training (PRT) and the Early Start Denver Model (ESDM) are considered naturalistic interventions for which reason?
   a. Because parents are considered essential intervention agents
   b. Because they are delivered in the home, school, and community settings
   c. Because they focus on taking advantage of the child's natural motivations within daily activities and routines
   d. All of the above

4. Characteristics of the LEAP model include:
   a. Primarily one-to-one instruction in the preschool environment
   b. A comprehensive educational program delivered in an inclusive preschool environment
   c. Piecemeal delivery of therapeutic services (e.g., occupational, speech, and physical therapy) occurring at separate times of the day in different locations
   d. All of the above

5. Features of early intensive behavioral interventions such as discrete trial training (DTT) and applied verbal behavior (AVB) include which of the following:
   a. One-to-one instructional delivery by trained therapists in adult-structured learning environments focused on the breakdown of skills and the presentation of learning tasks in trials that are consistent and systematic
   b. One-to-one instructional delivery that is mainly administered by parents with a focus on pivotal behaviors in natural environments such as motivation, responsiveness to multiple cues, self-management, self-initiation, and empathy

   c. Group instructional delivery by teachers in inclusive classroom settings that focuses on the use of peer-mediated interventions, peer-tutoring, social skills training, and environmental arrangements

   d. All of the above

Answers

1. d. a & c
2. c. Intensive services in most states must be paid out-of-pocket by the parents of the children with autism
3. d. All of the above
4. b. A comprehensive educational program delivered in an inclusive preschool environment
5. a. One-to-one instructional delivery by trained therapists in adult-structured learning environments focused on the breakdown of skills and the presentation of learning tasks into trials that are consistent and systematic.

Language Interventions

Diane L. Williams and Lori J. Marra

Referrals to a Speech-Language Pathologist *175*

Speech and Language Assessments *176*

Assessment Related to Challenging Behaviors *177*

Models of Service Delivery for Speech-Language Therapy *178*

Speech-Language Interventions *180*

Developmental Pragmatics Approaches *186*

Pivotal Response Training *187*

Applied Verbal Behavior *188*

Traditional Speech-Language Therapy *188*

Summary *189*

Further Reading *190*

Questions *190*

Answers *191*

This chapter will review speech and language assessment and intervention in children with autism spectrum disorder. The evaluation and treatment is completed by a professional who has been trained as a speech and language specialist and has had experience working with individuals with ASD. The child and adolescent psychiatrist, pediatrician, neurologist, psychologist, other healthcare provider, and educator refers to the speech-language pathologist (SLP) for guidance in the multidisciplinary treatment team and planning. Services are often provided in the school as well as in a clinical setting.

Impairment in social communication is one of the diagnostic criteria for ASD; therefore, communication is universally affected in individuals with ASD. Social communication includes many nonverbal aspects such as eye gaze and facial expression. It also includes the use of spoken language to interact with others, which is referred to as *pragmatics,* or the functional use of communication. In addition, all individuals with ASD have some level of difficulty with comprehension of spoken language.

The degree of affectedness of spoken language can vary widely in individuals with ASD.

Sixty to 70% of individuals with ASD are low-verbal or nonverbal, with substantial difficulty with the understanding of spoken language and the ability to use it for functional communication (Fombonne, 2005). However, most children with ASD develop some spoken language skills.

In a study of a large sample of nine-year-olds with ASD, fewer than 15% were classified as nonverbal (defined as using fewer than five words per day) (Lord et al., 2006). Most children with ASD who acquire spoken language have extreme difficulty using it for spontaneous, flexible, and functional communication.

Children with ASD generally have large amounts of immediate or delayed echolalia in which they immediately imitate what someone else says or repetitively use language they have heard from sources such as television, movies, books, or videogames. For example, one young child with ASD would use the phrase "one fish, two fish, red fish, blue fish" (from a Dr. Seuss book) whenever he noticed something red. Echolalia is thought to result because children with ASD have an abnormally large "attentional window" for language, resulting in learning larger "chunks" of language. Multiple words are treated as if they were a single word.

Individuals with ASD may use what appear to be perseverative utterances; that is, repetitively saying the same sentence or phrase over and over. Some perseverative utterances are attempts at functional communication with a mismatch between the surface structure or literal meaning of the words and the intended meaning. For example, one little girl with ASD would use the phrase, "Go swimming?" to mean "What's the next activity?" Another boy would say, "Crispy chicken" at an increasingly high pitch to indicate that he was becoming over-stressed.

Thirty to 40% of individuals with ASD are verbal with the ability to use spoken sentences and connected discourse. These individuals typically have some difficulty with auditory comprehension (understanding what is said to them), reading comprehension, and pragmatics (the functional and social use of communication). Verbal individuals with ASD may also have more restricted meanings for words so that they easily understand that "bank" means "a place where money is kept" but may become confused when that same word is used to mean "the side of a river." Even high-functioning individuals with ASD may have difficulty with understanding the social use of language because they interpret words literally and have difficulty making inferences. Highly verbal individual with ASD may monopolize the conversation by going on and on about a topic that is interesting to them and failing to give their communication partner a turn to speak.

Language proficiency or verbal ability is consistently associated with positive outcomes in social and adaptive functioning for children and adults with ASD. Therefore, it is important that a child's communication and language skills be addressed as soon as developmental concerns appear.

Referrals to a Speech-Language Pathologist

Because of the universality of language and communication problems, all children with ASD should be seen by a speech-language pathologist as soon as possible after diagnosis for a complete evaluation. *An SLP is a state-licensed professional* who has a minimum of a master's degree and holds a Certificate of Clinical Competence in Speech-Language Pathology (CCC-SLP) from the American Speech-Language-Hearing Association (ASHA), the professional organization that oversees the practice of speech-language pathology. A SLP has specialized training in the assessment and diagnosis of communication and language disorders and the implementation of behavioral interventions for these disorders. SLPs are trained to work with individuals on communication development from birth, well before spoken language develops; therefore, even very young children who are suspected of having ASD should be referred for a speech and language evaluation. Also, it is important that the child's hearing be evaluated to rule out any unidentified hearing loss.

Speech and Language Assessments

Even though the name of the profession would seem to suggest that SLPs focus exclusively on spoken language, they actually embrace a broad view of communication in all of its forms. Therefore, an SLP will assess both nonverbal and verbal communication. The form of the assessment will vary depending on the age and ability level of the child or adult who has (or is suspected to have) ASD. Again, depending on the age and ability level of the individual with ASD; the assessment may include formal observations of communication; a sample of any spoken language; interviews with the primary caregivers, teachers, and other significant communication partners; and/or standardized testing.

Typical behaviors that are measured during the assessment process include:

- The initiation of spontaneous communication
- Communication of a range of communication functions including requesting objects and actions, refusing, protesting, commenting, and answering
- Reciprocity of both verbal and nonverbal communication
- Comprehension of spoken language
- Comprehension of nonverbal communication
- Comprehension of written words (reading)
- Productive use of communication using different modalities, including natural gestures, speech, manual signs, pointing to pictures, and writing words

Assessment Related to Challenging Behaviors

Many children and adults with ASD may exhibit challenging behaviors that interfere with their ability to interact with others, function well in their home environment, and learn in a school setting. Many of these behaviors may actually have a communicative intent that is not necessarily obvious to family members and school personnel. A program that focuses only on attenuating the behavior may ultimately be unsuccessful because the individual with ASD will simply develop a new behavior (which will then need to be ameliorated) so that he or she can communicate the underlying message. Teaching functional communication skills has been successfully used to replace challenging behaviors in children with ASD (see Chapter 5 on functional behavior assessment, and Chapter 7 on early childhood interventions).

The SLP can play an important role in managing these challenging behaviors.

- The first step will be to observe the occurrence of the behavior or to gathered detailed information about instances of the behavior from the family and teaching staff.
- Next, the SLP will try to determine what the antecedent events for the behavior are.
- Then the SLP will try to interpret the meaning of the challenging behavior.
- Finally, the SLP will develop a more socially acceptable means for the individual with ASD to communicate the intended message.

For example, when a child with ASD becomes cognitively "overloaded," he may stand suddenly and tip over a table. The program of intervention for this behavior would be to train parents and teaching personnel to recognize the beginning signs of "overload" and make downward adjustments in the demands of the task. A second objective of intervention would be to give the child a more socially acceptable way to communicate that the task is too hard or too much, such as saying, "I'm done" or by pointing to a red "stop" sign.

Models of Service Delivery for Speech-Language Therapy

Following the diagnostic assessment, the SLP will develop an appropriate treatment plan that meets the needs of the child and their family. Treatment may be provided through various models of service delivery, depending on the age of the child, the severity of the child's language and communication problems, and the needs of the child and family. Different models of service delivery are also important to achieve functional outcomes that will work in different environments (see Table 8.1). Due to the significant social communication impairment, family members, peers, and other communication partners may find it difficult to communicate with individuals with ASD. Therefore, an important component of any speech-language therapy program is to provide training to the significant communication partners of the individual with ASD.

- **Family-centered practices**

For children younger than three years of age, intervention is typically family-centered and may be delivered either in the home or in the child's daycare setting. The primary focus of intervention is parent education. Parents are taught to recognize and encourage their child's idiosyncratic attempts at communication, to help the child learn other means to communicate, and to help their child learn the representational and symbolic thinking that is necessary to develop spoken language. Past the age of three years, speech and language intervention becomes more child-centered. However, the family should continue to be centrally involved. Family priorities and concerns should be considered during intervention planning, and the family should participate in the process of intervention by helping the child use the skills developed in therapy or in the classroom during daily life.

- **Direct or pull-out therapy**

After the child reaches three years of age, speech and language intervention may be directly provided to the child. These services may occur one-on-one with the therapist or they may be provided to the child as part of a small group of children who have ASD or other developmental language disorders. Pull-out therapy is beneficial for helping the child develop new skills that require more direction or intensive practice.

Table 8.1 – Models of Service Delivery

Models of Service Delivery for Speech & Language Intervention for ASD

- Family-centered practices
- Direct, pull-out
  - Individual
  - Small group
- Collaborative services in natural environments
- Consultative
- Peer-mediation

However, if the child *only* receives pull-out therapy, these skills may not generalize to other settings. To maximize effectiveness, pull-out therapy should only be one component of a child's intervention services.

- **Collaborative services in natural settings**

 Additional focus on communication and language development will be provided to the child within the preschool or K–12 classroom setting. The SLP will work collaboratively with the teacher to teach her what to target and how to interact with the child to maximize the use of language and communication. At the same time, the teacher will help the SLP understand the language and academic demands of the curriculum so that the SLP can help the child develop the skills needed to meet these demands.

- **Consultative services**

 Some verbal, high-functioning children may not qualify for direct speech and language therapy services. To qualify for services in the school system, the child's communication and language problems must adversely affect his or her academic performance. Even if the child does not receive direct services, she or he may be eligible for consultative services based on the ASD diagnosis. In this case, the teacher consults with the SLP whenever aspects of the curriculum prove difficult for the child. For example, in math class, a child with ASD who is proficient at arithmetical calculations may experience difficulty in dealing with the language and abstract thinking of word problems. The SLP can provide assistance by developing an individualized educational approach for the child based on the child's understanding of language.

- **Peer-mediation**

 This is an approach that has been successfully used to increase the interaction and spontaneous communication skills of children with ASD. In this model of service delivery, the SLP provides training to the child's same-age typically developing peers on how to communicate and interact with the child. The therapist and teacher then encourage the children to use these skills in the classroom on a daily basis. The participation in a greater number of interactive experiences increases the social communication and language skills of the children with ASD; however, peers must continue to be prompted to continue to use the facilitative strategies.

Speech-Language Interventions

Intervention to promote communication and the speech and language abilities of individuals with ASD will be behavioral and includes a range of different approaches. Which approach is appropriate is determined by the SLP based on the age, verbal abilities, overall cognitive ability, and needs of each individual with autism (see Table 8.2). To have the greatest impact on the developmental process, language intervention should be initiated as soon as the child is identified as having a problem.

ASHA has developed guidelines that direct the practice of SLPs with respect to intervention with individuals with ASD (ASHA, 2006a). In addition to being initiated as early as possible, communication and language intervention should be integrated into any other type of intervention program that the child is receiving, such as applied behavioral analysis (ABA). Alternatively, programs of intervention have been developed that specifically target the development of social communication and language skills in children with ASD. Several of the commonly used interventions implemented for children with ASD by SLPs are described below.

As a profession, SLPs have become increasingly concerned about delivering *evidence-based practice*. There are as yet no large, randomly

Table 8.2 – Language Interventions for Children with ASD by Age and Level of Spoken Language

Level of Spoken Language	Age (at which the intervention is typically used)	Speech & Language Interventions for ASD
Newly diagnosed toddler	Under 3 years	Parent Education Models
Nonspeaking or low verbal	3 years and older	Augmentative and Alternative Communication (AAC)
Nonspeaking or low verbal	3 years and older	Total Communication (speech + manual sign)
Nonspeaking or low verbal	3 years and older	Picture Exchange Communication System (PECS)
Nonspeaking to fluent speech	Developmentally 8 months or older	Developmental Pragmatics Approaches (e.g., SCERTS®)
Nonspeaking to low verbal	3 to 13 years	Pivotal Response Training (PRT)
Nonspeaking to low verbal	3 years and older	Applied Verbal Behavior (AVB)
Imitative or fluent speech	≈ 3 years of age through adulthood	Traditional Speech-Language Therapy

assigned, matched control samples with sufficient sample sizes and adequate statistical power comparable to clinical efficacy trials for pharmacological interventions. Studies comparing the efficacy of one approach versus another are also not available. However, there is empirical support for a number of approaches for enhancing the communication skills of children with ASD. Determining which intervention approach is appropriate for a particular child is as much art as science. As is typical of most behavioral interventions, no intervention is equally effective for everyone, and not everyone benefits to the same degree.

- **Augmentative and Alternative Communication**

Augmentative and alternative communication (AAC) strategies are categorized as "unaided" or "aided." *Unaided* methods of communication rely on the user's body to convey messages. These methods could include vocalizations, gestures, sign language, head nods, and eye gaze. *Aided* communication methods require the use of tools or equipment in addition to the user's body. Aided communication methods include single photographs or pictures, picture books or boards, electronic devices with speech output, or laptop computers. Many parents are initially resistant to using AAC with their child, even when the child is nonverbal or low-verbal, because they fear that the child will become so reliant on this method of communication that he or she will not be motivated to communicate with spoken words. Contrary to this popular belief, AAC systems will NOT inhibit speech development. In fact, there is scientific evidence that indicates the *use of AAC promotes the development of spoken language* (ASHA, 2006a). Furthermore, even if the child does not develop fluent speech, the use of an AAC system will enhance his or her language development and give the child a means of communication, which will reduce her or his frustration and decrease the occurrence of challenging behaviors.

Because of these positive benefits, AAC should be initiated with any child who has failed to develop functional spoken language by age two, regardless of the child's level of cognitive function. The assumption that children with severe disabilities (i.e., Down syndrome, ASD, cerebral palsy) had to meet a specific cognitive level of function before they would be able to benefit from an AAC system has been shown to be unfounded (Romski et al., 2006). The keys to success with AAC intervention are a collaborative service-delivery model, instruction in a natural everyday environment, and a focus on both comprehension and production.

System for Augmenting Language

One specific AAC intervention method that has been used successfully with moderate to severely affected children with ASD is the System for Augmenting Language (SAL) approach (Romski et al., 2006). This approach is based on how typically developing children learn language, and it links AAC to both the input and output modes of communication. SAL has five integrated components:

1. *Selection of a portable Voice Output Communication Aid (VOCA)* that is appropriate for the child. A number of VOCAs are commercially available that can be used even with young or low-functioning children. Some examples are Hawk (Adam's Lab), CheapTalk (Enabling Devices), TechSpeak and TechTalk (AMDI), and Go Talk (Attainment Corp).

2. *Choosing visual-graphic symbols and lexicon that are functionally relevant for the child.* The child must be able to interpret the visually depicted information. Photographs may be needed for some children, whereas commercially available picture symbols may work for others. These pictorial symbols are used to create overlays that are placed on the VOCA.

3. *Teaching through natural, everyday environments with an emphasis on functional communication exchanges.* Instructing the child to use the communication technique when it is needed promotes generalization and increases spontaneous use.

4. *Instructing the communication partners to use the device.* During interactions with the child, the communication partner activates and uses device as a model. The partner shows the child how to be both a speaker and a listener.

5. *Monitoring ongoing use.* The SLP provides support to ensure that the SAL program continues to be implemented. Changes in the child's programming are also made in response to feedback from the child, the family, and other communication partners.

- **Total Communication**

  The primary unaided communication technique that is used with nonspeaking or low-verbal individuals with ASD is manual signing. The signing system that is used is typically an adaptation from American Sign Language (ASL) used in a format called Total Communication, in which speech is combined with sign. Early studies reported that children with ASD had increased initiation in communication after learning some manual signs (Goldstein, 2002). The use of manual signs is also associated with increases in vocalizations or spoken words in numerous studies. Other studies report limited productive use of manual signs by the children with ASD who were studied. Most of the studies do not report language progress beyond a few words using this approach; however, the Total Communication approach appears to be particularly effective with low-verbal children with ASD who have poor verbal imitation. Concern has also been raised regarding the effects of possible motor apraxia on the production of manual signs for some children with ASD. This body of research suggests that manual signing should be implemented as part of the communication intervention for nonspeaking or low-verbal children with ASD, but that it should not be considered as the primary or sole means of communication. It should be used in conjunction with other forms of AAC.

- **Picture Exchange Communication System**

  Picture Exchange Communication System (PECS) was developed in 1985 for use with preschool-aged children with ASD and other social communicative disorders who displayed no functional or socially acceptable speech. It was designed to help children approach others to communicate and to actively interact with others instead of only responding to a direct cue to do so. Currently, PECS is used with a wide variety of diagnoses or educational classifications (e.g., adults with developmental disabilities). PECS consists of three integrated components (Frost & Bondy, 2002):

1. *Functional objectives.* The focus is on the development of functional communication skills that are necessary for independence. The materials or vocabulary used are associated with everyday items (e.g., clothing, food, activities of daily living).

2. *Powerful reinforcement.* This should be as natural to the situation as possible (e.g., after naming the color and size of a toy car, the child gets to play with the car) and should be given in timely manner. The reinforcement should be explicit and known (e.g., visual representation of what the reinforcer or "deal" is).

3. *Communication and social skills.* The behaviors being developed are not rote picture identification but involve behavior directed to another person, who in turn provides related, direct, or social rewards.

The initial step in using the PECS system is to have the child give a picture of a desired item to a communication partner in exchange for that item. The clinician creates opportunities for communication within physical environments by doing the following:

- The adult identifies what the child may want within an activity (something highly reinforcing).
- The adult arranges for that item to "disappear" or to be somewhat out of reach, creating a need for the child to initiate communication.
- The child picks up picture and gives it to the adult.
- The adult gives the desired item to the child.
- The child plays with the item for 15 to 20 seconds.
- The adult takes the item back from the child, and the next trial begins.

PECS is designed to progress the child through six phases as described in Table 8.3.

Clinical studies indicate that PECS is successful in teaching children to communicate and, in some cases, to develop some spoken language skills. For example, out of 66 children who used PECS for more than one year, 39 (59%) acquired speech as their sole means of communication (Brunner & Seung, 2009).

Although the picture exchange format appears to be a highly successful one for young and low-functioning children with ASD, clinical experience suggests that the later stages of the PECS system may be confusing to some children, causing them to abandon use of the technique at this point. Specifically, Phase 4, in which the *"I want"* card is combined with the card of the desired item, can be challenging to teach. Functionally, the child has been communicating the message contained in *I want* by giving the adult the card of the desired item. The new requirement of adding the *"I want"* card may, therefore, be very confusing and frustrating to some children. They are being required to do an additional behavior with no related increase in communication. An alternative suggestion is to build the use of two picture symbols by following the model of semantic relationships development in typical children. By using this approach, the child is not simply increasing the length of the communication, but is communicating additional meaning. For example, two-word combinations can be created by adding a descriptor such as size or color to an object. *Big + ball* or *small + ball* signals a request for a *particular* ball. The meaning of the word *ball* is changed by the other concept that occurs with it, creating a request for a particular ball. Other typical combinations are *action + object* (*throw + ball*; *turn on + light*); *object + location* (*puzzle piece + in*; *string + out*), and *possessor + object* (*my + squish ball*).

Table 8.3 – Six Phases of PECS

Phase	Title	Content
1	Physical exchange	Child is taught to hand a picture card to a communication partner with item in sight.
2	Distance and persistence	Child is taught to go to the PECS board, get a picture card, seek out a communication partner, and to place the card in the partner's hand to receive reinforcement. The distance between the child, the board, and the partner is increased, and the setting is varied.
3	Discrimination of symbols; discrimination of requests	Child is taught to discriminate among multiple pictures on the PECS board.
4	Sentence structure	Child combines *I want* card and the card of the desired item, seeks out a communication partner, and gives the strip. The partner inserts a delay between the words "I want" and the item label, then provides social praise if the child independently provides the label. Addition of attributes encouraged.
5	Answering a question	Child is taught to respond to the question: "What do you want?"
6	Commenting in response to a question	Child is to respond to the question, "What do you see?" by selecting a card depicting the same object and combining it with an *I see* card to describe, then comment about, an aspect of the environment. Social reinforcement provided.

Developmental Pragmatics Approaches

Developmental pragmatics approaches have also been successful in developing communication and language skills in young children with ASD. The Social Communication, Emotional Regulation and Transactional Support (SCERTS) model (Prizant et al., 2006), the Developmental Individual Relationship Based Model (DIR), and the Hanen approach are examples of this type of treatment. A developmental pragmatics approach focuses on the establishment of a full range of functional communication behaviors (rather than only spoken language) during reciprocal communicative exchanges. The SCERTS Model, a developmental pragmatics approach in common use by SLPs, is described below.

- **SCERTS® Model**

Many SLPs are currently trained in implementation of the SCERTS Model, a developmental pragmatics approach that was developed by a multidisciplinary team of professionals trained in communication disorders, special education, occupational therapy, and developmental and behavioral psychology. SCERTS is based on 25 years of research and clinical and educational practice. Although the development of language and communication is a central objective of this approach, it extends beyond this to enhance socio-emotional abilities and provide support to families. The SCERTS model helps children with ASD *develop functional, social communication skills while regulating emotional behavior.* Specific guidelines and training are provided to families, educators, and therapists to coordinate the child's program and maximize the child's progress. All those who interact with the child are considered "potential developmental facilitators." Unlike other approaches that are adult-initiated, the SCERTS model promotes child-initiated communication in the course of everyday activities.

SCERTS is implemented as a team approach and includes assessment prior to the implementation of intervention. It is based on a family-centered philosophy, with the parents as active members of the team. The child is actively engaged in intensive instruction (25 hours per week, 12 months per year). Intervention is integrated into the child's everyday activities, and learning opportunities are identified across home, community, and school settings.

The primary elements of SCERTS are:

1. *Social communication (SC)*: Development of spontaneous, functional communication; emotional expression; and secure and trusting relationships with children and adults
2. *Emotional regulation (ER)*: Development of the ability to maintain a well-regulated emotional state to cope with everyday stress, and to be most available for learning and interacting
3. *Transactional support (TS)*: Development and implementation of supports to help partners respond to the child's needs and interests, modify and adapt the environment, and provide tools to enhance learning (e.g., picture communication, written schedules, and sensory supports)

SCERTS also provides educational and emotional support to families and fosters teamwork among professionals. The SCERTS model can be used with a wide variety of developmental disorders, across the child's lifespan, within different social settings (e.g., school, home, community) and with a variety of communication partners. One of the unique qualities of SCERTS is that it can incorporate practices from other approaches, including contemporary ABA (e.g., pivotal response treatment, LEAP), Treatment and Education of Autistic and Communication related handicapped Children (TEACCH), Floortime, Relationship Development Intervention (RDI), Hanen, and Social Stories®.

Pivotal Response Training

Another intervention approach that has been successful in teaching language to young children with ASD is pivotal response training (PRT) (Koegel et al., 1999). A "pivotal behavior" is thought to be one from which other behaviors develop. A behavior that is thought to be pivotal for communication and language to develop is motivation. A motivated child tries harder, which increases her or his interest in the educational situation, and the likelihood that she or he will apply the learned behaviors in other situations increases. PRT and other *naturalistic behavioral language* interventions use principles of ABA during interactive, discrete teaching episodes in the context of ongoing activities in which the child is interested. Naturalistic behavioral approaches have been successful in teaching prepositions, use of grammatical morphemes, use of *yes* and *no*, and use of self-initiated question-asking (Goldstein, 2002). Massed trials are an important aspect of this approach. The primary use of PRT has been for the establishment of very specific language skills; however, PRT has also been used to increase the frequency and spontaneity of utterances.

In PRT, specific variables are manipulated in the natural language teaching condition such that (a) stimulus items are functional and varied, (b) natural reinforcers are employed, (c) any communicative attempts are reinforced, and (d) trials are conducted within a natural interchange. Because PRT was designed to be used in the natural environment, it is ideally suited for parent training and home use.

Applied Verbal Behavior

Applied verbal behavior (AVB) is a specialized form of ABA for the development of communication and language skills based on Skinnerian operant learning principles, or discrete trial training. AVB views language functionally with each verbal response defined by its antecedent and consequences. Consequently, AVB language instruction targets the acquisition of functional and distinct verbal *operants* (e.g., mands) rather than *topographies* (i.e., words). The *mand* is distinguished from other verbal operants in that it evokes a response that relates to a specific consequence and is the only verbal operant that directly benefits the speaker. The clinician arranges a child's environment to create the optimal condition under which the child will mand for preferred items, missing items, and/or information.

A final common feature of the AVB approach is pairing antecedents of strong verbal operants with stimuli that weakly control other verbal operants (i.e., stimulus transfer procedures) to teach new verbal operants. For example, a picture that evokes a *tact* (or label), such as *cat*, will be used to teach the intraverbal "Can you name an animal?" and subsequently faded to transfer control to the verbal antecedent. AVB or related forms of discrete-trial training have been successfully used to teach children with ASD to produce spoken words, to use questions, to use four-term sentences (*verbs* + *colors* + *shape/size* + *labels*) and to answer *what, how,* and *why* questions using single or multiple sentences. AVB has been less successful at teaching children with ASD to initiate communication and to generalize the communication behaviors to other contexts, unless the instruction is embedded within the child's daily activities.

Traditional Speech-Language Therapy

High-functioning children with ASD, or children who have at least sentence-level speech, are candidates for more traditional forms of speech-language therapy. "Traditional" means a process in which the child participates in formal and standardized testing, and then the intervention is individually designed based on the child's performance (profile of strengths and weaknesses) and needs. Typically, this intervention will address both comprehension and expression of spoken language. For school-age children, written forms of communication (reading comprehension and writing) may also be incorporated into the intervention process because difficulties in these areas are now understood to be related to a broader problem with language development.

Pragmatics, or the social use of language, is typically a major area of focus of language intervention for high-functioning children with ASD. Even if the child has fluent discourse, he or she must learn to use language skills to successfully participate in academic and social settings. Standard approaches include situational role-playing and practicing skills in real-world environments. Frequently, visual cues such as picture symbols and written reminders are used to help the children learn and remember appropriate behaviors. Social stories (Gray, 2002) may also be incorporated into therapy activities. Another approach that has been successfully used to teach appropriate pragmatic behaviors to children with ASD is video modeling, in which peers are shown performing the social script being taught to the child (Brunner & Seung, 2009).

It is important to note that even highly verbal children and adults with ASD may have subtle impairments in language production and comprehension that interfere with their adaptive functioning. These deficits may go undetected by the standardized instruments that are typically used by SLPs. Sampling of language during conversation or interactions in the real world, and interviews with the child and his or her communication partners, are more likely to identify areas of difficulty for individuals with ASD at this level of function. Assessment of skills during narrative discourse—which requires the integration of language, knowledge, and an understanding of what the communication partner knows and does not know—is particularly important. Language intervention would then focus on the aspects of discourse comprehension (e.g., contextually based word meanings, inferencing) and expression (e.g., sequential presentation, organization, needs of the listener) that are problems for the child or adult with ASD.

Key Fact Box

- 20% of individuals with autism are nonspeaking (defined as fewer than five words per day).
- 50% of individuals with autism develop some usable spoken language.
- 30% of individuals with autism develop fluent spoken language.
- SLPs are the primary service providers of communication and language intervention for children with autism.
- Early intervention should begin as soon as a problem is detected, even if the child is not yet speaking and even before the child receives a definitive diagnosis.
- Language interventions should be selected based on an individual child's needs, not based on the child's diagnosis of ASD.

Summary

Deficits in social communication are almost universally characteristic of individuals with ASD. Social communication includes nonverbal aspects of language (e.g., eye gaze, facial expression) as well as the use of spoken language to interact with others (pragmatics). Weaknesses in language comprehension are also common in this population. Addressing social-communication deficits should begin early in the child's life, shortly following the initial ASD diagnosis. The role of the speech and language therapist can change over time, based upon an individual child's needs. These can include individual and group therapy as well as classroom consultation. A wide range of language-based interventions and programs are available, including a number that have been shown to meet best-practice criteria.

Further Reading

1. Fombonne, E. (2005). Epidemiological studies of pervasive developmental disorders. In: F. R. Volkmar, R. Paul, A. Klin, & D. Cohen (Eds.), *Handbook of autism and pervasive and developmental disorders* (pp. 42–69). Hoboken, NJ: John Wiley & Sons.

2. Lord, C., Risi, S., DiLavore, P., Shulman, C., Thurm, A., & Pickles, A. (2006). Autism from 2 to 9 years of age. *Archives of General Psychiatry, 63,* 694–701.

3. American Speech-Language-Hearing Association (2006a). Guidelines for speech-language pathologists in diagnosis, assessment, and treatment of Autism Spectrum Disorder across the life span [Guidelines]. Available from www.asha.org/policy.

4. Romski, M., Sevcik, R., Cheslock, M., & Barton, A. (2006). The system for augmenting language. In R. McCauley & M. Fey (Eds.), *Treatment of language disorders in children,* (pp. 123–148). Baltimore, MD: Paul H. Brookes.

5. Goldstein, H. (2002). Communication intervention for children with autism: A review of treatment efficacy. *Journal of Autism and Developmental Disorders, 32,* 373–396.

6. Frost, L., & Bondy, A. (2002). *Picture exchange communication system.* Newark, DE: Pyramid Educational Products.

7. Prizant, B., Wetherby, A., Rubin, E., Laurent, A., & Rydell, P. (2006). *The SCERTS model: A comprehensive educational approach for children with Autism Spectrum Disorder.* Baltimore, MD: Paul H. Brookes Publishing.

8. Koegel, L., Koegel, R., Harrower, J., & Carter, C. (1999). Pivotal Response Intervention I: Overview of approach. *Journal of the Association for Persons with Severe Handicaps, 24,* 174–185.

9. Gray, C. (2002). *The new social story book.* Arlington, TX: Future Horizons.

10. Brunner, D., & Seung, H. (2009). Evaluation of the efficacy of communication-based treatments for Autism Spectrum Disorder: A literature review. *Communication Disorders Quarterly, 31,* 15–42.

Questions

1. Which of the following is an example of a problem with verbal communication frequently observed in children with ASD?
   a. echolalia
   b. perseveration
   c. repetitive, stereotyped movements
   d. poor eye contact
   e. a & b

2. Which of the following statements is NOT TRUE about speech-language pathologists (SLPs)?
   a. SLPs have specialized training in the assessment and diagnosis of communication and language disorders
   b. SLPs can implement behavioral intervention programs
   c. SLPs are trained to work with individuals on communication development from birth through adulthood
   d. SLPs can only work with individuals with autism after spoken language develops
   e. SLPs provide training to the significant communication partners of the individual with ASD

3. Which of the following is an example of an augmentative and alternative communication system?
   a. Sign language
   b. Electronic speech output device
   c. Picture Exchange Communication System (PECS)

d. a and c

e. All of the above

4. The following therapeutic program focuses on the development of social communication skills while helping the child develop and maintain a well-regulated emotional state, as well as supporting the child's communication partners by providing specific tools to enhance learning.

a. SCERTS

b. PECS

c. Pivotal response training

d. Applied behavioral analysis

e. Applied verbal behavior

5. Which of the following statements is TRUE in regards to assessment and treatment of communication and language skills for individuals with autism?

a. The most appropriate treatment approach should be based on the child's age and verbal abilities only.

b. Communication and language intervention should be addressed separately from other intervention programs like applied behavioral analysis.

c. Some individuals with high-functioning autism will have impairments in language production and comprehension that may not be detected by standardized testing.

d. Non-verbal children with ASD should all be taught sign language.

e. Treatment approaches that use typically developing peers as communication models have not been effective.

Answers

1. e. a & b Both echolalia and perseverative utterances are typically observed in the spoken language of children with ASD.

2. d. Speech-language pathologists work with individuals with the development of communication. Therefore, it is particularly important for individuals without spoken language as a means of communication to be seen by the SLP.

3. e. All of the above. Any means of communication other than speech is considered an augmentative communication system.

4. a. Emotional regulation is a central feature of the SCERTS therapeutic program.

5. c. Some individuals with high-functioning autism will have impairments in language production and comprehension that may not be detected by standardized testing.

Feeding, Sleep, and Toileting Interventions

Kristine Kielar, Cynthia R. Johnson, and
Benjamin L. Handen

Feeding Disorders *196*
Sleep Disturbances *201*
Toileting Issues *206*
Further Reading *212*
Questions *212*
Answers *213*

This chapter will cover three commonly associated problems experienced by children with Autism Spectrum Disorder (ASD): feeding disorders, sleep disturbances, and toileting issues

Each section will describe the problem area, methods of assessment, and treatment options. These problems are usually reported to the primary care doctor or pediatrician, preschool teacher, speech and language pathologist, occupational therapist, or child and adolescent psychiatrist, if serving young children. These professionals may provide recommendations to help problem-solve with the parents. The physician may also refer the child to medical specialists to rule out medically treatable causes. Often, if the problems persist and intensify, then it is the psychologist, behavioral specialist, or therapist, with experience in applied behavioral analysis and functional behavioral assessment, who can develop and implement a behavior plan with the parents and the other professionals. It is important for the child and adolescent psychiatrist and other physicians who work with children with ASD to understand the severity of the problems and the best practice approaches.

Feeding Disorders

Feeding Disorders

Description of the problem and prevalence

Children with ASD commonly present with food-related difficulties. A recent study by Schreck, Williams, and Smith (2004) found that children with ASD, in comparison with neuro-typical children, have more general feeding problems. These include refusing foods, needing to have food presented in a particular way or with specific utensils, accepting only low texture foods, and eating only a narrow range of foods. This section will address feeding issues in four areas:

- Food selectivity/texture problems
- Difficulty sitting for meals
- Eating too quickly or too slowly
- Eating too much

There has been a considerable amount of research in regard to these areas, mostly within the behavioral literature. However, speech and language therapists and occupational therapists (OT) also have expertise in this area and often collaborate with behavioral psychologists in the treatment of feeding disorders. In addition, a nutritionist also can be helpful in planning dietary changes, and gastroenterology (GI) may be needed to rule out medical contributions to feeding problems.

Assessing feeding problems

Food Selectivity and/or Texture Problems: Many children with ASD are extremely picky eaters, limiting their preferences to only one or two foods. In addition, such children also can be extremely picky about a particular brand or way of preparing their food (e.g., only eating chicken nuggets or macaroni and cheese). Sometimes there is an additional problem of texture preferences, where a child will only eat a certain texture of food (e.g., stage-three baby foods). A possible consequence of being a picky eater or having food texture problems is that overall food and caloric intake may be limited, or that certain nutrients are not at recommended levels. In addition, some children may engage in behaviors such as vomiting, gagging, or throwing a tantrum when unfamiliar foods are introduced by parents or school staff. Finally, such limitations may make it difficult for the child to join the family at restaurants or eat at the homes of friends and relatives (further limiting community experiences).

It may be helpful to obtain enough general information about a food selectivity problem to:

(1) determine if the problem presents significant health risks,
(2) determine if additional referrals are needed, and
(3) determine if the problem warrants establishing a treatment plan.

There are also a number of possible medical factors that could be impacting a child's feeding problems that may need to be assessed:

- Is the child underweight and young enough to possibly be diagnosed as "failure-to-thrive"?
- Should the child be seen for a GI consultation to rule out possible gastro-esophageal reflux disorder (GERD) or other structural problem?
- Should the child be seen by a speech or OT to assess chewing and swallowing skills?

- Is the child "tube-dependent" at this time (i.e., receiving a significant portion of the daily nutritional intake via g-tube or nj-tube) and requires a more specialized feeding team evaluation?

Difficulty Sitting for Meals: Difficulty remaining seated at a table for meals can be a problem for many children with ASD. For some, problems with overactivity and inattention may make it difficult to sit anywhere (at school, at meals, at church) for any length of time. Other children with ASD may have developed habits such as only eating while watching videos, or they may simply "graze" throughout the day (taking food from the refrigerator at will). Attempts to change this pattern may result in an escalation of inappropriate behavior, and families may have found it easier to maintain the current situation. There are several areas to explore:

- Does the family have regular, structured meals where there are clear cues that the child needs to remain seated?
- Is overactivity a significant concern in multiple environments that might require specific treatment?
- Is the child hungry? Is it possible that a medication regimen needs to be adjusted (e.g., if a child is on a stimulant) or that the family needs to limit access to food at other times to better insure that the child will be hungry during scheduled meals?
- What prior attempts has the family made to address the problem?

Eating Too Quickly: Eating too rapidly is also a common problem for children with ASD. This may make it difficult to keep the child at the dinner table, as once the child has finished eating s/he has no reason to remain. Proper assessment should follow some of the same steps as discussed above, under "Difficulty Sitting" In addition, the clinician will want a very specific description of how the meal works (e.g., is the child served first, how much is s/he given, does the child self-feed?). Finally, it may be useful to know if the child swallows each bite as it is taken, or if the child stores multiple bites in his/her mouth and then swallows later.

Eating Too Much: While restricted eating patterns are a common feature among children with ASD, some children also have problems with too high a caloric intake. This tends to occur quite frequently when children are prescribed psychotropic medications, such as atypical antipsychotics. Other children may exhibit restrictive eating patterns that tend toward high-calorie foods. In addition, many children with ASD may lead somewhat sedentary lives and have only limited opportunities for physical activity. Consequently, their weight may become an issue over time. Attempts to control food intake can be challenging for a family.

As discussed in the earlier problem areas, it will be important to obtain a clear description of the problem (not simply that "he's always eating") as well as what has already been attempted to address the concern. Areas to inquire about include:

- Is the child on a medication regimen that could affect satiety?
- When does the child eat (at mealtimes or throughout the day)?
- Does the child have free access to food?
- What types of foods are available to the child (and are there any restricted food preferences)?
- What types of physical activities does the child enjoy or engage in?

Treating feeding problems

Food Selectivity and Texture Problems: If the problem is related to difficulty with chewing or swallowing, OT and speech are typically the specialists who are best equipped to deal with this concern. If the problem is felt to be more behavioral (e.g., a child will eat chicken, but refuses any other foods), then a behavior analyst is best trained to address such concerns. The behavioral literature is replete with papers in which food selectivity and texture problems are treated. For example, in one of the earlier papers describing behavioral interventions, Handen, Russo, and Mandell (1987) described the use of behavioral procedures to gradually wean eight children (many of whom had developmental disabilities or ASD) from feeding tube dependence. Many of the principles outlined in that paper continue to be used today for treating food selectivity.

- Use preferred foods to reinforce acceptance of less preferred foods. For example, if a child loves to eat macaroni and cheese, a bite of this food can be given if the child takes a small bite of spaghetti.
- Select new foods that are in same food group and that have similar characteristics to preferred foods. If a child will only eat chicken nuggets, consider a different brand of chicken nuggets or other type of nugget. This is often referred to as a "lateral move."
- Go slowly. This is referred to as "shaping" in the behavioral literature, where only small, gradual changes in demands are made. Some children can handle a "bite for a bite" contingency in which a bite of less preferred food is required to earn access to highly preferred food. Other children need a smaller step, such as only being asked to lick the less preferred food (or even allow it to be present on the same table). Introducing new foods requires a fair amount of skill and experience. Consequently, it may require the assistance of school staff or clinicians who have considerable experience working in this area.
- Some children may require the use of non-food reinforcers, such as watching 30 seconds of a favorite video.
- Behaviors such as tantrums or crying are best ignored (rather than giving in and ending the meal).

Note: Treating limited food preferences is an extremely challenging task. It often requires more than providing general suggestions during a single consultation. Problems with "packing" food (keeping food in the mouth, but not swallowing), a child's refusing to open his or her mouth to accept less desired foods, or vomiting and regurgitation will probably require consultation and assistance from an experienced clinician. Resources can sometimes be found through the child's school, specialty clinics, or outpatient OT, or speech and language programs.

Difficulty Sitting for Meals: There are a number of fairly simple suggestions that can be provided to a family prior to suggesting more intensive consultation with another behavioral health professional.

- Establish a mealtime routine (see below).
- Reconsider the timing of medication (or the timing of meals) if a child is prescribed medication that might affect their appetite.
- Consider treating overactivity in general if it appears to be a problem in multiple environments (keeping in mind that the side effects of some medications include decreased appetite).

- Have the family limit access to food during the day (this may require locking cabinets in the kitchen or even changing some of the purchasing habits of the family, such as buying unhealthy snack foods).
- Consider some preventive strategies, such as seating the child in such a way that it is more difficult for them to get up. Also, slow down the meal by providing smaller portions and then providing "seconds" after the child has finished what was given. Finally, some children may require other activities at the table to keep them interested and busy (e.g., drawing, books). Many families have learned to use such strategies as a means of keeping a child at a table at restaurants.
- Consider setting contingencies and using reinforcement. Higher-functioning children may be able to "make a deal" that requires that they sit at the table for the entire meal in order to have dessert. Lower-functioning children may need more frequent use of reinforcement, such as access to favorite toys for sitting for a specified period of time (e.g., three minutes, as signaled by a timer). Other children may simply start by having meals that last a few minutes and then slowly and gradually increasing meal length.
- Always remind families to start small. By this, we mean that the behavioral requirement should initially be close to the child's current abilities or behavior. For example, if a family decides to teach a child to remain seated at meals, they may want to start with a requirement of sitting for only five minutes. Then the requirement can be gradually increased as the child succeeds.

Eating Too Quickly: Simple treatment options include structural changes in how the meal is served as well as the teaching of appropriate eating skills.
- A structural strategy is to slow down the meal by providing smaller portions and then providing "seconds" after the child has finished what was given. One extreme would be to provide single bites at a time to the child.
- A teaching strategy would be to reinforce taking one bite at a time and swallowing before taking a second. This could be done in combination with a structural strategy of providing only a single bite at a time. Other children may need to be taught to put their utensil down after taking a bite, or even counting between bites.

Eating Too Much: Many of the prior treatment suggestions also apply for overeating. These include:
- Establishing a mealtime routine (see below).
- Limiting access to food except during meals (which may include locking up food). This may also require discussion with school staff.
- Purchasing more healthy foods (which may require consultation with a nutritionist).
- Reconsidering the current medication regimen if that is felt to be contributing to the problem.
- Increasing the activity level by enrolling the child in karate or swimming, purchasing a trampoline for the home, taking walks, etc.

Combination Problems: Oftentimes a child presents with a combination of feeding problems (e.g., the child eats too much but also refuses to sit during meals). Our advice is to attempt to address only one problem at a time, as mealtime programming can be extremely taxing for families. However, the good news is that it is often possible to address two problem areas with the same program. For example, limiting access to food except during mealtimes can address many of the feeding problems that have been discussed. Similarly, the child who is taught to eat more slowly will probably remain at the dinner table for a longer period of time.

Establish a Mealtime Routine: Establishing a consistent mealtime routine is one of the best ways to begin to address many of the feeding problems addressed in this section. Below are some tips for how to guide parents.

- *Schedule snacks and meals at about the same time every day:* This will help establish a new pattern for the child with ASD, limit food intake to these times, and increase the chances that the child will be hungry at mealtime.
- *Eating or drinking should only occur at a table:* Parents should only allow eating or drinking when the child is seated at the appropriate table. If the child gets up, food should not be available elsewhere. Access to food may need to be controlled as well (e.g., locking up cabinets).
- *Limit number and size of snacks:* This will also increase the child's desire for food during scheduled meals.
- *Limit the amount of time for snacks and meals:* Snacks can be fairly short (e.g., 10 minutes) so that the child cannot fill up on snack foods. The child should also not be allowed to remain seated for a meal any longer than the rest of the family. Sometimes the use of a timer can be helpful.
- *Meals should be positive:* Meals should not be a time for parents to fight with their children. Of course, eating problems can lead to many anxieties for parents (with concerns that a child may be eating too much or too little). However, if the mealtime demands are changed using small steps, both parent and child will experience some successes. Also, parents should be encouraged to use lots of praise for appropriate behavior ("Great! You remembered to put your fork down") and to make mealtimes fun.
- *Limit distractions:* Remind parents to limit distractions so that the child can concentrate on eating or on developing new eating skills. This may require that the TV be turned off and other toys and objects be removed.

Sleep Disturbances

Description of the problem and prevalence

It has long been a widely held belief that children with ASD commonly experience poorly regulated sleep patterns and habits. In fact, it has been suggested that sleep dysfunction in ASD may be an indicator of neural dysfunction, along with seizure disorders and cognitive disability. This body of literature has reported that a large percentage of children with ASD experience sleep disturbances of some type (Liu et al., 2006). The sleep problems identified in this research have primarily been **dysomnias**—including bedtime resistance and struggles, delayed sleep onset, difficulty maintaining sleep with night awakenings, early morning waking, and decreased total sleep time.

Children with ASD have also been reported to have **parasomnias**—sleep-related breathing disorders, sleep-related movement disorders, and circadian rhythm sleep disorder. However, this is a very under-studied area. While earlier study samples included children with ASD with co-occurring developmental delays or intellectual disabilities, recent reports of children with ASD and typical cognitive development reported sleep disturbances at a rate commensurate with that of lower-functioning individuals with ASD.

Vulnerability for sleep disturbances in children with ASD

Over a decade ago, Johnson (1996) suggested that children with ASD may be vulnerable to sleep problems due to their core deficits and associated features. Core social and communication deficits and often co-occurring cognitive deficits potentially interfered with a child's early learning to engage in self-soothing and self-comforting. This leaves the child with ASD less able to promote sleep onset independently. For these same reasons, the child with ASD may have a poorer ability to understand what is asked of them and lack understanding of social and environmental cues, which may negatively affect the development of the sleep/wake cycle, due to lack of appropriate stimulus-control in learning. Increased sensitivity to environmental changes around bedtime (e.g., the change to Daylight Savings Time) and changes in bedtime routine may result in sleep disruption. Ritualistic behaviors and a need for sameness may interfere with sleep as well.

Medically, children with ASD are also at increased risk for seizure activity, and nocturnal seizures may interfere with sleep. Along with these vulnerabilities, there is emerging support in the literature that children with ASD may have altered sleep architecture (Richdale & Schreck, 2009). Finally, children with ASD often have comorbid psychiatric diagnoses associated with sleep problems such as anxiety, depression, and ADHD.

Sleep problems are usually discussed with the primary care doctor or pediatrician, neurologist, or child and adolescent psychiatrist. After initial recommendations are made, and if the problem persists and intensifies, then referral to a sleep clinic can be made. In specialized programs or university settings, there may be a neurologist or pulmonologist, and a psychologist or other healthcare professional who can help rule out organic etiology and set up a sleep assessment and intervention plan. The following sections will describe examples of approaches to assessment and treatment, which

Table 9.1 – Common Sleep Problems Reported in ASD

1. Bedtime Resistance and Challenging Behaviors
2. Delayed Sleep Onset
3. Sleep Association Problems
4. Night Awakenings
5. Early Morning Awakenings

can be used by a variety of professionals in working with parents and their children with ASD.

Assessing bedtime and sleep problems

Sleep problems are assessed using many different methods.

- There are several *sleep questionnaires* that have been used in individuals with ASD. These questionnaires attempt to determine the types of sleep problems observed, as well as gauge their severity. Two sleep questionnaires used with children with ASD include the Children's Sleep Habit Questionnaire (Owen et al., 2000) and the Modified Simond & Parraga Sleep Questionnaire (Wiggs & Stores, 1998).
- *Sleep diary data* are the most common type of sleep assessment information collected. These data include information on when an individual goes to bed, when they fall asleep, and when they wake at night, along with when they wake in the morning.
- For children with behavioral issues, information about the *antecedents and consequences* of problem behaviors at bedtime and throughout the night might also be collected.
- Detailed information about the current *bedtime routine*, if there is one, is also important for making recommendations to improve bedtime problems. Collectively, this information can inform what recommendations to make as well as what sleep problems are most interfering and should be targeted first. The shortcomings of theses measures are that they are subjective and not always accurate if a third party is recording. Parents may not be aware when their child wakes at night. They may only be aware when the child is disruptive and wakes the caregivers.
- *Actigraphy* is an objective measure of sleep that can add to what parents report. This measure of body movements is a widely accepted measure of *sleep* versus *wake*.
- *Polysomnography* (PSG), however, remains the gold standard assessment in the assessment of sleep problems. While this level of testing is not always warranted, PSG has detected abnormalities in sleep structure in children with ASD (see Richdale & Schreck, 2009).

Behavioral treatments of sleep problems with ASD

Sleep problems among children with ASD have been treated with many of the same behavioral interventions that have proven to be successful among typically developing children. However, there remains a striking paucity of empirical studies specifically targeting sleep disturbances in children in this population. There are a few reports involving children with intellectual disabilities, some of whom had comorbid diagnoses of ASD, suggesting the effectiveness of behavioral procedures. Procedures have included the use of bedtime routines, faded bedtime procedures, extinction and reinforcement procedures, stimulus fading, and scheduled waking. These procedures, along with general sleep hygiene guidelines, can address the common sleep problems reported in children with ASD.

General Sleep Hygiene Guidelines
- Consistent sleep times (bedtime and morning waking and daytime naps for young children) should be adhered to in order to promote better sleep.
- Children should also be exposed to morning sunlight to promote the sleep-wake cycle.
- Regular exercise and eating meals at a regular time are also part of a healthy sleep hygiene regimen.
- Bright light exposure along with "screen" light (TV, DVDs, computers, videogames) should be avoided close to bedtime.
- The bedroom should be conducive to sleep (e.g., comfortable temperature, limited light, quiet).

Addressing bedtime resistance and sleep onset problems

It is often the case, by *establishing a consistent bedtime routine* or making some changes to a routine, that problems around bedtime and falling asleep may be improved.
- A bedtime routine should include a regular bedtime.
- It is also recommended that activities that are calming or soothing be included.
- Activities such as physical exercise or play should be avoided at least 30 minutes before bedtime.
- Watching TV or playing games on the computer should also be avoided with a general recommendation of 45 minutes prior to bedtime.
- For children on medication which may interfere with sleep, rearranging the dosing schedule should be considered.
- The use of a visual schedule of the bedtime routine may be considered. Visual schedules, commonly used with children with ASD, are intended to provide visual reminders of upcoming events and expectations of the day. A pictorial, visual schedule of the specific steps in the bedtime routine could be a component.

A child might still have difficulty falling asleep despite the implementation of a consistent bedtime routine. It is typically recommended that a child fall asleep within 20 minutes of being placed in their bed. If a child can eventually fall asleep by themselves, a *faded bedtime procedure* is a common strategy to decrease sleep latency. With this procedure, a later bedtime is initially set. For example,

Step 1—Collect sleep diary data.

Step 2—If the child's bedtime is 8:30 p.m., but he never falls asleep until 9:30 p.m., then his bedtime would be set at 9:30 p.m.

Step 3—Once the child is consistently falling asleep before 10:00 p.m., then move his bedtime up by a small increment (e.g., 10 to 15 minutes).

Step 4—This "fading" of the bedtime would be systematically moved up until the target bedtime is achieved.

This procedure obviously should consider a child's developmental age as well as parental goals with respect to bedtime.

Addressing nighttime awakenings and difficulty maintaining sleep

The most common approach to getting a child to go back to sleep after awakening is to simply ignore her or him. This *simple extinction procedure* is a common recommendation pediatricians make to young mothers when their babies are crying at night. However, this seemingly simple approach is often very difficult to do as parents may find it very uncomfortable to just "ignore" their child. Furthermore, a crying child may wake not only the parents but also others in the house. An approach to avoid some of the problems with placing a child's night waking on extinction is a modified strategy referred to as "graduated extinction" in the literature. In *graduated extinction*, the parent is instructed to take the following steps.

Step 1—Check on the child at a specific time interval (e.g., every five minutes). Hence, when the parent enters the bedroom is not contingent on the child's behavior but on a set schedule.

Step 2—The parent should be instructed to briefly go in to check on the child, reassure the child that everything is okay, and give a quick back rub or other physical contact the child likes.

Step 3—This time interval is slowly and gradually increased.

This approach not only avoids the pitfalls of a pure extinction approach (i.e., extinction burst of worsening behaviors), but it does not result in a child's becoming increasingly distressed and thus engaging in behaviors incompatible with sleep. Furthermore, parents are more likely to find gradual extinction acceptable.

Addressing sleep association problems

Many children with ASD have *sleep association problems*. For example, they may require that a parent lie with them until they fall asleep or they may fall asleep in places other than their bed (such as in the family room with the TV on or in their parents' bed). All of these examples would be considered sleep association problems as the child is only able to fall and remain asleep independently in places other than his/her bed.

In these situations, *"stimulus fading" strategies* should be considered. For example, if a child can only fall asleep with a parent in his bed or with the TV on, there are three suggested strategies:

Strategy I
"Fade" by having the parent sleep on a mattress next to the bed of the child. Once this is completed, further "fade" by having the parent remain in a chair in the room until the child falls asleep.

Strategy II
Another way to fade is for the parent to slowly remove herself or himself from the bed by introducing a replacement, such as a full-size pillow or body pillow.

Strategy III
Systematically "fade out" the TV while "fading in" more appropriate sleep association, such as listening of soothing music.

Table 9.2 – Example of an Initial Behavior Plan for a Young Child with ASD

Description of Child: Ethan is a 3½-year-old child with ASD. He lives at home with his parents and younger sister. He attends an inclusive preschool and receives intensive behavioral intervention in the home as well. He receives speech therapy both in preschool and at a private clinic. While he has limited verbal skills, he is able to use pictures to communicate, and he is able to understand what is asked of him. Ethan's parents resorted to taking him downstairs if he did not fall asleep in his room by 7:00 p.m. so he would not wake his brother. Ethan would typically fall asleep around 9:00 p.m., and his parents would then carry him into his room around 11:00 p.m.

Initial Behavioral Bedtime/Sleep Plan: As Ethan never fell asleep before 9:00 p.m., a faded bedtime procedure was used by which his bedtime was set later. His bedtime routine was started at 8:30 p.m., and he was to have no access to the television or computer after 7:45 p.m. At 8:30 he was transitioned from downstairs to upstairs. A visual picture of this transition was used. If Ethan complied with making the transition upstairs, he was allowed to complete a puzzle, a very favorite activity. Using Ethan's bedtime routine visual schedule, he was prompted through the steps: 1) bathe, 2) brush teeth, and 3) read books, including one on expectations around bedtime. Once upstairs, parents were asked to avoid any transitions downstairs. Ethan was allowed to sleep in the beanbag or rocking chair, BUT only in his room. As he had been allowed to sleep downstairs on a beanbag chair, the first goal was to develop a sleep association with his room and then to systematically fade to the bed. A reinforcement system was added whereby Ethan earned access to a favorite puzzle in the morning if he remained in his room after transitioning upstairs.

Toileting Issues

Description of the problem and prevalence

Most parents look forward to the day when their child is toilet trained. No more diapers! The parent of a child with ASD is no different. According to recent survey studies, more than half of parents of children with ASD report toileting and urination problems (LeBlanc et al., 2005). The *average age for toileting a neuro-typical child is 2.5 years old*. Neuro-typical children prepare themselves for toileting through natural observation; however, children with ASD may not be able to do this. For children with ASD, difficulties in comprehending language and logic may hinder the ability to understand what is expected of them; they may not understand why they need to void in the toilet and not in a diaper. An attachment to routines and resistance to change may make the transition from diapers to the toilet even more difficult. These children may not like the bathroom environment with its bright lights and echoes or the change in temperature when they remove their clothing.

Children with ASD may be further impeded by their idiosyncrasies. They may not know how to read bodily cues and are therefore not aware of the urge to use the toilet. In addition, they may not mind the sensation of being soiled. All of these factors must be taken into account when toilet training the child with ASD. It is also important to determine if a child is to be **schedule trained** (i.e., will successfully void on the toilet when taken by an adult) or to be **trained for independence** (both initiating and indicating to others the need to void). Oftentimes, families will report that a child is toilet trained, when, in fact, only schedule training has taken place. This information will assist in developing an appropriate intervention.

Assessing toileting problems

The initial step to any toileting procedure is assessment of readiness, data collection, and the establishment of a realistic goal (taking into account that independent toileting may be many steps down the road). The following questions should be addressed to determine if a child possesses the prerequisite skills necessary for toilet training to be *schedule trained*:

- Is the child able to remain dry for 60 to 90 minutes at a time?
- Can the child stay seated for three to five minutes at a time? If not, it will be important to determine if this is a problem with compliance or a fear response, as the treatments would differ.
- Are there any concerns with constipation or diarrhea? Does the child take any medication for constipation or diarrhea? This may need to be appropriately treated before toilet training can be attempted.

Medical referral may need to be made to the child's primary care doctor or pediatrician and/or gastroenterologist (GI) in order to evaluate and treat severe or chronic constipation or diarrhea or both. It is important to assess whether any medications or diet are contributing to the constipation or diarrhea.

Addressing the above three areas should indicate that a child is ready to be schedule trained. The next set of questions can assist in determining if a child is ready for *independent toileting* (which includes initiation and alerting to others the need to void).

- Does the child display any warning signs to signal an adult that s/he must void? These can include increased fidgetiness, touching their diaper, crossing of the legs, etc.
- Does the child indicate when s/he is wet or soiled? This can involve behaviors similar to warning signs above or that the child appears uncomfortable.
- Does the child engage in excessive tantrums or self-stimulatory behavior? These types of behaviors could impede the training process and prevent learning.
- Does the child possess any independent self-help skills, such as pulling her or his pants up and down and hand-washing and drying? Please note that lack of these skills should not hinder independent training, but will require that an adult assist the child.

> **Treatment of Toileting Problems**
> In the ASD field, two widely used methods for toilet training are **schedule training** and **independent toilet training** (either intensive or extended). Both methods are acceptable and should be selected based upon the (readiness) skills the child possesses at the time of training.

Please keep in mind that not all children respond to the same teaching techniques; a method that is helpful for one child may not be useful for another. However, this section will cover some of the basic toileting training procedures.

Schedule Training: Schedule training is the easiest way to begin toileting and could serve as the first step to independence. However, being "schedule trained" is not the same as independent toilet use (which includes initiation as well as indicating the need to void). Schedule training requires that an adult be responsible for the child's toileting and results in the child's depending on others to tell them when to toilet. The overall goal of schedule training is to teach the child to void when s/he is placed on the toilet and to withhold urine and wait until taken to the toilet at all other times.

Independent Training: Independent training can be achieved in one of two ways—intensive training or extended training. Intensive independent training is just that, *intensive* with the end result being independent initiation and voiding in the bathroom. Extended training is far less intensive and can take longer; however, the result is still independent initiation and voiding on the toilet.

Schedule Training
- Create a prompting schedule; use a timer
- Take child to the toilet to void every 60 to 90 minutes
- Child should sit for three to four minutes to attempt voiding
- Complete "dry pants" checks. A "dry pants" check involves the adult periodically checking the child to see if s/he is wet or dry. If dry, child is reinforced for having "dry pants." If wet, child is taken to the bathroom and prompted through the established toileting routine.
- Be consistent across environments

Intensive Independent Training (Recommend seeking professional for
   guidance)
   • All sessions take place in the bathroom
   • Intensive sitting schedule
   • Child is frequently given liquids to promote urination
   • High reinforcement for successful urination
   • Be consistent across environments
Extended Independent Training
   • Training occurs in the natural environment with trips to the bathroom
     as needed
   • Less-intensive sitting schedule
   • Liquids are not offered more frequently than normal
   Table 9.3 (below) describes the pros and cons about each method.
   Regardless of which technique is selected for toilet training the child with
ASD, it can be helpful to establish a positive bathroom routine. This will
help the child become familiar with the bathroom and what this particular
room is used for. A positive bathroom routine includes prompting the child
through a series of consecutive toileting steps. A picture schedule is useful
to visually represent a chain of steps:
Step 1—Enter bathroom
Step 2—Pull down pants
Step 3—Sit on toilet
Step 4—Wipe
Step 5—Stand up and pull pants up
Step 6—Flush toilet
Step 7—Wash hands
   Data Collection: As with any behavior intervention, data collection
is prudent. A simple tracking chart should be used to determine the
effectiveness of any intervention. In addition, the chart can also be used
to collect baseline data to determine toilet training readiness. Table 9.4
(below) is an example of elimination record data collection.
   Associated Problems: As with any behavioral intervention for a child
with ASD, associated problems can be present. Two common problems
associated with toilet training include *refusal to sit* and *diaper rituals*.
1. *Refusal to Sit*: This includes noncompliance surrounding the toilet. When
   or if this occurs, refusal to sit must be addressed prior to any training
   technique. Shaping is the most effective way to address this behavior.
   Shaping includes establishing a short-term goal and then building on that
   goal. Each short-term goal is reinforced and mastered before moving on.
   • Child is required to sit on the toilet for three to five seconds,
     reinforcement is given, and child is removed from the toilet. Once
     the child is able to sit for three to five seconds, increase the required
     sitting time by three to five seconds.
   • Continue to increase the time intervals in this manner until the child
     is able to sit on the toilet compliantly for three to four minutes.
2. *Diaper Rituals*: This typically occurs when a child is urine trained, but
   not bowel trained. Children with diaper rituals are often able to urinate
   in the toilet, but require a diaper/pull-up for bowel movements. Again,
   shaping is the most effective way to address diaper rituals.
   • Allow the child to defecate in the diaper as long as s/he is physically
     in the bathroom. Please note that at this stage, the child does not

Table 9.3 –Toilet Training

Schedule Training		Intensive Independent Toilet Training (Must seek professional for guidance)		Intensive Extended Toilet Training	
PROS	CONS	PROS	CONS	PROS	CONS
Child is not required to possess all readiness skills.	Will most likely result in prompt dependence for toilet use.	Does not cause prompt dependence.	Child must possess all readiness skills prior to implementation.	Less time-consuming for the adult.	Can take months to reach independence.
Easier method and an alternative to intensive toilet training.	Must separately train for independence later on	Promotes independent toilet use from the start.	Intensive training for 4 to 7 days; 7 to 8 hours each day.	Does not require professional guidance.	Must be very aware of child's toileting cues. If not, frequent accidents can occur.
Teaches control over bladder and bowel function in preparation for independence.					

Table 9.4 – Elimination Record

Child's Name: _____   Date Begun: _____

Time	Day 1 Pants	Day 1 Toilet	Day 2 Pants	Day 2 Toilet	Day 3 Pants	Day 3 Toilet	Day 4 Pants	Day 4 Toilet	Day 5 Pants	Day 5 Toilet	Day 6 Pants	Day 6 Toilet	Day 7 Pants	Day 7 Toilet
7:00	D	NV	U/BM	U										
8:00	U	NV	D	NV										
9:00	D	NV	D	U										
10:00	D	U	U	NV										
11:00			D	NV										

Pants column = Record every hour; **D** for dry pants–**U** for urinated in pants–**BM** for bowel movement in pants–and **U/BM** for urinated and bowel movement in pants.
Toilet column = Record each bathroom visit; **U** for urinated on toilet–**BM** for bowel movement on toilet–**NV** for did not void on the toilet.

have to sit on the toilet. Once the child is able to do this consistently, move on to the next step.

- Allow the child to defecate in the diaper as long as s/he is sitting on the toilet. It may be necessary to leave the lid down at first until the child becomes accustomed to having a bowel movement while seated. Once the child is able to do this consistently, move onto the next step.
- Begin cutting a small hole in the bottom of the diaper/pull-up prior to placing it on the child for a bowel movement. Gradually make the hole bigger and bigger until the diaper/pull-up is no longer needed for bowel movements.

As with any behavioral intervention, consistency, patience, and practice are key elements. This is especially true of toilet training. These methods, when properly implemented, can lead to any child's achieving success in toilet training.

Key Fact Box

I. Children with ASD commonly present with food-related difficulties:

1 Food selectivity/texture problems
2 Difficulty sitting for meals
3 Eating too quickly or too slowly
4 Eating too much

II. A large percentage of children with ASD experience sleep disturbances:

a) *Dysomnias*
   Bedtime resistance and struggles, delayed sleep onset, difficulty maintaining sleep with night awakenings, early morning waking, and decreased total sleep time.
   Children with ASD have also been reported to have:
b) *Parasomnias*
   Sleep-related breathing disorders, sleep-related movement disorders, and circadian rhythm sleep disorder.

III. More than half of parents of children with ASD report toileting problems:

It is also important to determine if a child is to be
- *schedule trained* (i.e., will successfully void on the toilet when taken by an adult), or
- *trained for independence* (both initiating and indicating to others the need to void).

Further Reading

1. Handen, B. L., Mandell, F., & Russo, D. C. (1986). Feeding induction in children who refuse to eat. *American Journal of Diseases of Children, 140,* 52–54.
2. Johnson, C. R. (1996). Sleep problems in children with mental retardation and autism. *Child & Adolescent Psychiatric Clinics of North America, 5,* 673–683.
3. LeBlanc, L. A., Carr, J. E., Crossett, S. E., Bennett, C. M., & Detweiler, D. D. (2005). Intensive outpatient behavioral treatment of primary urinary incontinence of children with autism. *Focus on Autism and Other Developmental Disabilities, 20,* 98–105.
4. Liu, X., Hubbard, J. A., Fabes, R. A., & Adam, J. B. (2006). Sleep disturbances and correlates of children with Autism Spectrum Disorder. *Child Psychiatry Human Development, 37,* 179–191.
5. Owens, J. A., Spirito, A., & McGuinn M. (2000). Sleep habits and sleep disturbance in elementary school-aged children. *Journal of Developmental and Behavioral Pediatrics, 21,* 27–36.
6. Richdale, A. L., & Schreck, K. A. (2009). Sleep problems in Autism Spectrum Disorder: Prevalence, nature, and possible biopsychosocial etiologies. *Sleep Medicine Reviews, 13,* 403–411.
7. Schreck, K. A., Williams, K., & Smith, A. (2004). A comparison of eating behaviors between children with autism and without autism. *Journal of Autism and Developmental Disorders, 34,* 433–438.
8. Wiggs, L., & Stores, G. (1998). Behavioural treatment for sleep problems in children with severe learning disabilities and challenging daytime behaviour: Effect on sleep patterns of mother and child. *Journal of Sleep Research, 7,* 119–126.

Questions

1. Which is NOT a common feeding problem associated with ASD?
   a. Food selectivity
   b. Texture problems
   c. Refusal to eat meals at table
   d. Limited feeding skills
   e. All of the above

2. What is an accepted treatment for food selectivity?
   a. Present the child with as many food options as possible
   b. Use preferred foods to reinforce taking small bites of less preferred foods
   c. Limit access to favored foods, hoping the child will become hungry
   d. There is not really a good treatment at this time

3. What are some prerequisites for a child being ready to be toilet trained?
   a. Ability to sit on the toilet for 3–5 minutes
   b. Ability to remain dry for 60–90 minutes
   c. Ability to sit on the toilet for 10–15 minutes
   d. Ability to remain dry for 30–45 minutes
   e. a and b

4. Which is NOT an option for toileting training a child with ASD?
   a. Schedule training
   b. Intensive independent training
   c. Intensive schedule training
   d. Extended independent training

5. What is NOT a common sleep problem in children with ASD?
   a. Bedtime resistance
   b. Excessive nighttime and daytime sleep
   c. Night awakening
   d. Sleep association problems

6. Which intervention is NOT recommended to address sleep problems in ASD?
   a. Use of a visual schedule
   b. Structured bedtime routine
   c. Graduated extinction
   d. Timeout

Answers

1. d. Limited feeding skills
2. b. Use preferred foods to reinforce taking small bites of less preferred foods
3. a and b
   • Ability to sit on the toilet for 3–5 minutes
   • Ability to remain dry for 60–90 minutes
4. c. Intensive schedule training
5. b. Excessive nighttime and daytime sleep
6. d. Timeout

Educational Issues: School-Age

Michelle Lubetsky, Virginia Martin, and Benjamin L. Handen

Educational Law 218
The IEP Process 222
School Placement 226
Summary 228
Further Reading 228
Questions 228
Answers 229

In working with children and adolescents with ASD, it is important to understand the educational system. This chapter will provide an overview of educational law, the individual education plan (IEP) and school placement issues. The initial section will discuss The Individuals with Disabilities Education Act (IDEA), previously Public Law 94-142, and its implications and effects on the provision of educational services for children with ASD and other developmental disorders. The subsequent section will review the IEP process and the types of questions that parents and professionals should be asking in order to provide appropriate services to the child with ASD. Finally, information regarding possible school placements, as well as examples of supplementary aids and services within general and special education, are discussed.

- IDEA: child must have one or more disabilities identified in IDEA and demonstrate a need for special education (e.g., autism spectrum disorder, intellectual disability, learning disability).
- IEP: if specified, related services can be provided such as speech and language therapy, occupational therapy, counseling, and behavioral supports.
- 504 plan: a document that delineates specific accommodations that will be implemented by the school, based upon written evidence of need that does not meet IDEA requirements.

Educational Law

What the law says

The Individuals with Disabilities Education Act explains the educational rights of students with disabilities and describes eligibility requirements for children to receive special education supports and services. IDEA is the reauthorization of Public Law 94-142, which was first adopted in 1975. Amendments in 2004 were designed to align special education law more closely to No Child Left Behind, federal educational legislation that seeks to improve academic outcomes for all students.

Students who are eligible for special education supports and services

A two-pronged requirement applies to determine if a child can receive special education services:

1. The child must have one (or more) of the specific disabilities identified in IDEA.
2. The child must, as a result of that disability, demonstrate a need for specially designed instruction.

The protections that are available for students under IDEA

The following components of IDEA represent significant protections for students with disabilities:

- *Free and Appropriate Public Education—FAPE*: It is every child's right, including those with disabilities, to receive a free and appropriate public education. In some cases, the term "appropriate" can lead to different interpretations.
- *Least Restrictive Environment—LRE*: Children are to be educated in a setting with children without disabilities, to the maximum extent possible. The provision requires that the IEP team address individual educational placement decisions.
- *Individual Education Plan—IEP*: This legal document is designed to represent individualized instructional programming for the student. It should be reviewed annually and modified as needed to promote progress towards goals.

Students with ASD can be included in regular education

Least Restrictive Environment requires that the general education classroom be considered when placement decisions are made. All students must have access to the general education curriculum, to the extent appropriate. The team should determine if the addition of supplementary aids and services could allow the students to meet their goals within the general education setting. If the student requires supports and services that cannot be delivered in the general education classroom, then other options, such as receiving instruction outside of the regular classroom, may be considered.

Support services are available in schools for students with ASD

"Supplementary Aids and Services means aids, services, and other supports that are provided in regular education classes, other education-related settings, and in extracurricular and non-academic settings, to enable children with disabilities to be educated with nondisabled children to the maximum extent appropriate…" (IDEA 300.114–300.116). Aids and services include specially designed instruction, such as accommodations and modifications to instruction. They can also include the manner in which content is presented, how a child's progress is measured, direct supports to the child, and support and training for staff who work with the child. Often, children with ASD benefit from additional itinerant services such as speech and language therapy, occupational therapy, and counseling. Types of services are individually determined from evaluation data.

The student with ASD may require behavioral support

If an IEP team determines that general classroom management techniques are insufficient to ameliorate challenging behavior and a *student's behavior is interfering with his/her learning or the learning of others*, then the IEP team should consider implementing a functional behavioral assessment to guide the development of a *positive behavior support plan* (see Chapter 5 on functional behavioral assessment). A positive behavior support plan should include methods that utilize positive behavioral techniques to shape a child's behavior. Using information derived from the functional behavioral assessment, the least intrusive interventions should be selected for inclusion in the plan. The positive behavior support plan should be included in the IEP, and everyone involved should be familiar with the implementation strategies in order to promote successful outcomes (300.324[2][I]).

If the student does not meet the two-pronged criteria for special education

The Rehabilitation Act of 1973 protects the rights of qualified individuals by prohibiting discrimination based on their disability. Section 504 of the Rehabilitation Act states that organizations that receive federal funds are required to make their programs accessible by providing reasonable accommodations to individuals with disabilities. Students with disabilities who do not qualify for the protections of IDEA may benefit from the development of a 504 plan with the school's 504 coordinator, committee, or team.

Definition of a 504 plan

The 504 plan is a document that delineates *specific accommodations* that will be implemented by the school. All staff should be made aware of the accommodations, and the plan should be reviewed annually. After implementing an initial 504 plan, a meeting should be scheduled within six weeks to review progress. Issuing a 504 plan does not provide the same level of protections as found in an IEP, but it can inform teachers of specific areas of need and direct them to implement accommodations that promote equal access to the curriculum.

A parent or school personnel can request a 504 plan, which is based upon the legal protection of Section 504 of the Rehabilitation Act. Accommodations may be necessary for students with ASD, psychiatric symptoms, medical illness, or other disabling conditions, and a written recommendation may be provided by the child and adolescent psychiatrist, other physicians, psychologists, or other service providers including school personnel.

Recommended interventions for children with ASD

The National Standards Project was developed to examine research in interventions for children with ASD (www.nationalautismcenter.org):

- Its primary goal is to provide critical information about which treatments have been shown to be effective for individuals with ASD.
- The project examined and quantified the level of research supporting interventions that target the core characteristics of ASD in children, adolescents, and young adults (below 22 years of age) on the autism spectrum.
- The National Standards Report offers a single, authoritative source of guidance for parents, caregivers, educators and service providers as they make informed treatment decisions.
- It is important to note that research studies supporting established treatments include multiple variables such as age, location, and intensity, among others, which may have an impact on outcomes.
- The National Standards Project committee recommends that service begin as soon as a child is suspected of having ASD.
- They further state that services should be provided at least *25 hours a week, 12 months a year*.
- The intervention should be systematically planned, engaging, and developmentally appropriate, and should focus on spontaneous functional communication and social instruction.

Findings

- *Established*—Treatments that produce beneficial outcomes and are known to be effective for individuals on the autism spectrum. The majority of these interventions are rooted in applied behavior analysis, behavioral psychology, and positive behavior supports.
- *Emerging*—Treatments that have some evidence of effectiveness, but there is not enough evidence to warrant complete confidence in these treatments. Examples of treatments with emerging research include: language training, including augmentative and alternative communication and social communication; motor/imitation interaction; structured teaching; and multi-component approaches.
- *Unestablished*—Treatments for which no sound evidence could be identified. Findings include: facilitated communication, auditory integration, diet, and sensory integrative approaches.

The IEP Process

An Individual Education Plan is a written document that delineates the educational program that is designed to meet a child's individual educational needs. Every child who receives special education services must have an IEP.

Referral process for an IEP

A child who already has an identified disability, such as ASD, might transition from early intervention services (typically ages neonate to three) into school-age services through *Child Find* as they near three years of age. Child Find is a component of the IDEA that requires states to identify, locate, and evaluate all children with disabilities, aged birth to 21, who are in need of early intervention or special education services. If a child is transitioning from early intervention services, an evaluation will occur and an IEP may be developed around age three as the child prepares to enter preschool. If a child has not yet been identified as having a disability, Child Find can make a referral for an evaluation. Parents, teachers, and other school personnel can also make a referral for an evaluation at any time. It is best for parents to put their request in writing when submitting their referral for evaluation to the school or school district. The child and adolescent psychiatrist, other physicians, psychologists and related service professionals can advise the parent to request an evaluation to begin this process.

The evaluation for an IEP

Parental consent is always required before an evaluation can be done. The school or school district has 60 days after the parent[s] gives consent to complete the evaluation (check individual state guidelines; if the state requirements are more stringent, they prevail). The evaluation is typically completed by a certified school psychologist and typically takes place in the child's school. This evaluation must be individualized for the child and be comprehensive. The goals of the evaluation are to determine if the child has a disability that requires special education services, identifying the child's educational needs, and identifying which special education services are appropriate for the child.

Information is obtained from standardized assessments (generally cognitive, adaptive and achievement testing); functional behavior analysis (analyzing patterns of a child's behavior, including antecedents and consequences); baseline data collected throughout the evaluation using behavioral data (to describe the frequency, duration, or intensity of behavior); and parent and teacher reports. Prior evaluations and diagnoses (e.g., a psychological evaluation report indicating a diagnosis of ASD) may also be integrated into the evaluation.

How disability is determined

The school psychologist will submit the *Evaluation Report* (ER) which includes background information about the child, a summary of the evaluation results, determination of disability, and recommendations for services. The child's parents have the right to challenge the results. Within 30 calendar days after a child is determined to be eligible for special education services, the IEP team must meet and write an IEP for the child.

The IEP meeting

The school staff will coordinate participants of the IEP team, including parents, teachers, and other school personnel, to set a date and time for the IEP meeting. Parents are given ample notice of the meeting and are allowed to invite other individuals to the meeting who might have knowledge of or special expertise about the child. The IEP team gathers to discuss the results of the evaluation and to address the child's needs, services, and placement. Parents (and the student, if appropriate) are able to be actively involved in this discussion. Parents must be able to understand the diagnosis and the child's educational needs. They should have an opportunity to collaborate with school personnel and be able to resolve differences with others on the IEP team. Parents must provide consent before services can begin. If parents do not agree with the IEP team's decisions, they can try to resolve the problem within the team, participate in mediation, file a complaint, or request a due process hearing. The child and adolescent psychiatrist, other physicians, psychologists, and related service professionals can provide input to the parent for the IEP meeting.

Attendees at the IEP meeting

Parents are permitted to bring others with them to the IEP meeting. Many parents utilize the services of an educational advocate. An Educational Advocate is a person who will provide parents with assistance in advocating for their child for educational services, supports, and special education programs. Advocates also often have general knowledge about special education law. They can attend the IEP meeting with parents and act on the child's behalf or help negotiate for services. Parents can also bring friends or relatives to the IEP meeting.

The IEP document

The IEP includes information about the child and the results and recommendation of the evaluation. It also includes detailed goals for the child's education and creates an individualized plan for educational services. It must specifically state the services that will be provided. The IEP must include:
- Baseline data about the child's academic achievement and functional performance
- Annual goals (what the child can reasonably accomplish in one year)
- The services to be provided to the child (including supplemental aides, supports, accommodations)
- How much of the day, if any, the child will be educated separately from non-disabled students
- When services or modifications will begin, how they will be provided, where they will be provided, and how long they will last
- How the school will measure progress toward annual goals
- Discussion of the child's transition plan if they are age 14 or older (see section on transition planning for more information)

Table 10.1 (below) delineates some of the questions that parents should ask as part of the IEP process.

The IEP review

The IEP is reviewed annually; however, the family should be informed of the child's progress through periodic progress reports throughout the year.

Table 10.1 – An IEP Checklist

Present Level of Performance

a. Is there sufficient information on what the child is doing now?
- are strengths identified?
- are needs specified?
- are parental concerns considered?.
b. How does the child's disability affect their progress in the general curriculum?
c. Does the IEP establish a baseline of information about the child?
- are special factors identified (e.g., hearing, vision, behavior, communication)?
- does the disability affect their progress in the academic curriculum?
- are both academic and non-academic needs described?
- are results of the most recent evaluation(s) included?

Annual Goal

a. What can the child accomplish within the legal time frame (typically one year)?
- are goals aligned with academic standards/general curriculum?
- if appropriate, are functional goals addressed?
- are the goals measurable?
- are they meaningful?
b. Is the goal stated in the following terms?
c. The child—will do what—to what degree—measured how?
d. Does the goal apply to a variety of situations and activities?

Short-Term Objectives/Benchmarks

a. What will the child need to do to achieve each annual goal?
- is the objective/benchmark aligned with a goal statement?
- does it represent a precursor step or building-block skill?
- is the objective/benchmark measurable?

The IEP team will meet again to review the IEP at least once per year, or more often if the parents or the school personnel ask for a review. Parents should be active members of the team and offer information and suggestions. They have the right to agree or disagree with the IEP, including decisions regarding the provision of specific services or placement recommendations. The parent can ask to reopen the IEP process if they have concerns and would like to discuss possible changes.

Reevaluation

A reevaluation should occur at least every three years. However, the child must be reevaluated more often if the condition warrants or if the parent or teacher requests an updated evaluation.

Transition Planning (see Chapter 11 on transition-age and adult interventions)

When a *child turns 14*, a statement of transition must be included in the IEP to describe how the school will prepare the child to move from school into adult life. This transition plan is updated annually along with the IEP. The IEP team will consider post-secondary education, vocational training, employment or supported employment, adult services, independent living, and community participation. Since special education services can continue until age 21, a long-range plan is developed to promote progress toward transition goals that consider strengths, needs and interests.

School Placement

The IEP team determines the student's school placement based on the evaluation report and the specific needs of the child. They must always consider the Least Restrictive Environment factor first.

Least Restrictive Environment

The Least Restrictive Environment is a standard based on the IDEA that states that every effort should be made so that a child may be educated, to the maximum extent possible, with non-disabled students in a typical classroom setting. The use of special classes, separate schooling, or the removal of children with disabilities from the regular education classroom should occur only if the nature and severity of the disability is such that education in a regular education classroom with supplementary aides or services is not appropriate. The Least Restrictive Environment is determined individually by the IEP team and parents. This determination should not be made solely on diagnosis (i.e., if a child has a diagnosis of ASD, s/he should not automatically be placed in an Autism Support Classroom), the location of staff, availability of funds, or convenience. Generally, placement in the regular education classroom is considered first. The IEP team should discuss the types of *supports* (e.g., a classroom aide) that would be required for the child to remain in the regular classroom setting before alternatives are considered (see table 10.2 below). If a new school placement is proposed, close proximity to the child's home is an important consideration. A child's placement cannot be changed without parental agreement (or if the school district chooses to initiate a due process hearing to make its case for the need for a placement change).

School placement determination

The child's educational placement will first be determined at the initial IEP meeting by the IEP team. After the initial IEP is in place, placement determinations will be made annually (during the annual IEP meeting). The determination is based on the child's IEP and specific needs and progress.

Types of school placements

The following is a sample of educational placement options.
- Regular education/typical classroom
- Special education classroom (i.e., learning support, life skills support, autistic support) within a typical school
- Special education school (a center-based program run by the public school or affiliate)
- Home instruction/cyber school
- Approved private school program

Options as students reach middle to late adolescence

The transition plan is updated annually along with the IEP. The IEP team will consider post-secondary education (e.g., community college, local college), vocational training (e.g., sheltered workshop), employment or supported employment (e.g., job coach, accepting employer), adult services, independent living, and community participation. Since the adolescent has the right to continue in the educational system *until age 21*, the IEP team should develop a long-range, individualized transition plan, and learn skills

---

Table 10.2 – Examples of Supports and Services for Children with Disabilities

---

Autism Spectrum Disorder in the Regular Education Classroom

- Speech therapy, occupational therapy, physical therapy
- Social skills groups/support
- Accommodations/modifications to curriculum
- Adjustments in the manner in which material is presented (i.e., enlarged text, text to speech, with visual cues)
- Adjustments in the manner in which progress is measured
- Accommodations to the environment (i.e., seating, room setup, wheelchair accessibility, sensory room)
- Support and/or training for teaching staff
- Specialized equipment (i.e., augmentative communication device, sensory materials)
- Pacing of instruction (i.e., frequent breaks, extra time for homework, home set of materials/books)
- Testing adaptations
- Instructional content should be meaningful and should consider interests and long-term goals, especially for students who are transition age

---

to prepare them for adulthood. The content should be meaningful and should consider interests and passions and long-term goals, especially for students who are later transition age, 18 to 21.

Often adolescents with ASD and intellectual disability stay in school until age 21, and learn skills appropriate for their developmental level that will prepare them for their transition. Adolescents with ASD who want to graduate at age 18 end their federally funded education, and must seek services from local agencies based on eligibility standards. Note: Check with state regulations about the age limit for such assistance in each state.

Summary

This chapter reviewed the basics of educational law, the Individual Education Plan (IEP), and school placement issues. It is important to understand the provision of educational services for children with ASD and other developmental disorders, the IEP process, and the types of issues that parents and professionals should be considering in order to provide appropriate services to the child with ASD.

Further Reading

1. Buron, K. D., & Wolfberg, P. (2008). *Learners on the autism spectrum*. Shawnee Mission, KS: Autism Asperger Publishing Company.
2. National Autism Center (2009). National Standards report: Addressing the need for evidence-based practice guidelines for Autism Spectrum Disorder. Retrieved October 2010 from http://www.nationalautismcenter.org/pdf/NAC%20Report.pdf.
3. National Research Council (2001). *Educating children with autism*. Washington, DC: National Academy Press.
4. Office of Special Education Programs (OSEP)—U.S. Department of Education. Retrieved October 2010 from http://www2.ed.gov/about/offices/list/osers/osep/index.html.

Questions

1. What protections are available to students with disabilities under IDEA (Individuals with Disabilities Education Act)?
   a. A free and appropriate public education, least remedial education, and an individual education plan
   b. A free and appropriate public education, least restrictive environment, and an individual education plan
   c. A free and accurate public education, least restrictive environment, and an individual education plan
   d. A free and accurate public education, least remedial education, and an independent education plan

2. What is meant by "the two-pronged criteria" for special education?
   a. Students must have autism and intellectual disability to qualify for educational support services
   b. Students must have autism and emotional support needs to qualify for educational support services
   c. Students must have a disability that is recognized by IDEA, and also demonstrate a need for specially designed instruction
   d. Students must have a diagnosis and demonstrate severe behavior challenges to qualify for educational support services

3. Which of the following are *true* about a 504 plan?
   a. The 504 plan is a document that delineates specific accommodations that will be implemented by the school
   b. All staff should be made aware of the accommodations, and the plan should be reviewed annually

c. Issuing a 504 plan does not provide the same level of protections as found in an IEP, but it can inform teachers of specific areas of need and direct them to implement accommodations
d. All of the above

4. Which of the following are *true* about Least Restrictive Environment?
   a. The Least Restrictive Environment is determined individually by the IEP team and parents.
   b. This determination should not be made solely on diagnosis, the location of staff, availability of funds, or convenience
   c. Placement in the regular education classroom is considered first, and the IEP team should discuss the types of supports required
   d. A child's placement cannot be changed without parental agreement
   e. All of the above

5. Which of the following is *NOT* true about IEP (Individual Education Plan)?
   a. The IEP includes detailed goals for the child's education and creates an individualized plan for educational services
   b. It must specifically state the services that will be provided
   c. The IEP includes baseline data about the child's academic achievement and functional performance
   d. The school does not need to measure progress toward annual goals
   e. The IEP includes discussion of the child's transition plan if they are age 14 or older

Answers

1. b. A free and appropriate public education, least restrictive environment, and an individual education plan
2. c. Students must have a disability that is recognized by IDEA, and also demonstrate a need for specially designed instruction
3. d. All of the above
4. e. All of the above
5. d. The school does not need to measure progress toward annual goals

Transition-Age and Adult Interventions

John J. McGonigle, Allen Meade Gregory, and Martin J. Lubetsky

Transition-Age Skills Assessment and Training *234*

College Preparation and Support/Post-Secondary Education *236*

Job-Finding and -Coaching *238*

Social Competency Training and Activities *243*

Independence Skills Training *243*

Housing Options *244*

Diagnostic Clarification, Identification and Treatment of
   Comorbid Disorders *246*

Summary *248*

Further Reading *249*

Questions *250*

Answers *251*

The previous chapter focused on educational issues for the school-age child up through adolescence. This chapter will briefly discuss transition-age issues for adolescents through adults. Transition goals are developed in order to obtain services and funding for transition-age youth. Young adults have a wide range of options when planning for transition, including day activity programs or vocational training settings, jobs, junior college, college, and community living. Future planning starts with a fundamental premise of making choices: choices in education, employment, housing, health decisions, and social relationships.

The topics discussed in this chapter include:

Transition-age skills assessment and training
College preparation and support/post-secondary education
Job-finding and -coaching
Social competency training and activities
Independence skills training
Housing options
Diagnostic clarification, identification, and treatment of comorbid
disorders.

With the increased rate of children identified with ASD over the past 10 years, the number of adults with ASD is now growing. Systems have been focused on improving early identification of ASD and developing educational programs to meet the needs of this population. Educational funding provides services for individuals with ASD up to age 21. However, the transition from school services to adulthood can be difficult for the young adult and family.

Transition planning refers to the process that uncovers, develops, and documents the skills, challenges, goals, and tasks that will be important for a person with ASD to move from childhood supports to adult services. Planning for transition requires knowledge of systems and teamwork. There are several questions that the student, parents, and transition team need to answer in order to develop an effective transition plan: Where will this individual be at the end of this process? What skills will this student need to develop? What setting will be the best for this student to apply these skills? How will these skills be generalized? These are questions that the transition team should begin to address as the child with ASD approaches early adolescence.

It is important for the psychiatrist, primary care doctor, neurologist, psychologist, other health care and related services providers to understand the transition issues and planning for adulthood. Most often, adults with ASD need to transition all of their health care and behavioral health care to adult practitioners.

Transition-Age Skills Assessment and Training

Transition planning begins in school with the child, family, and education team. The Individuals with Disabilities Education Act (IDEA 04) was signed into law in 2004 and became effective in 2005. The Act states that when a student turns 16 years of age, transition planning must be in effect in the student's Individual Education Plan (IEP). The process often begins with early discussion and planning by age 14 (IDEA, 2004; Wehman, 2006). IDEA 04 also requires the inclusion of a "statement of the student's transition goals and services" be included in the IEP packet. Transition Services continues in the educational system, for identified special needs students, until the age of 21.

The planning process introduces the student and parent to services, activities, instruction, and support designed to provide the skills necessary to succeed post–high school. A good transition plan will include both long- and short-term goals, identify the necessary supports, and be very specific to the interests, abilities, and desires of the student. The planning focuses on individualized transition goals. "Effective transition planning provides the opportunity for adolescents to learn about themselves and plan for their future" (Hendricks & Wehman, 2009).

Transition plans guide what the adolescent needs to learn and what supports are required. Transition planning often needs to occur across a range of anticipated changes in an adolescent's life. These may include the transition from elementary to middle school, middle school to high school, high school to college, high school to alternative day services, high school to adulthood, pediatrician services to adult doctor (family doctor) services, and child to adult psychiatric services. Seltzer and colleagues (2004) report that the earlier the evidence-based interventions, treatments, and supports are implemented, the better the outcomes for people with ASD.

Supports and services to be considered in transition planning:

- *Instruction*: Consider the academic or employment requirements for a chosen course of study or work activity; explore employment skills training, career technical education, social skills, driver's education, and college entrance preparation.
- *Related services*: Consider the need for occupational, physical, or speech therapy; medical services; therapy or counseling; special transportation or mobility training; explore disability support services in college or university or other professional supports; help with coordinating support services ("case management").
- *Community experiences*: Identify options for community work, recreation/leisure activities, tours of post-secondary education settings, residential and community tours, volunteering and training in accessing community settings, and joining a team, club, or organization.
- *Employment*: Identify options for career planning, job shadowing, guidance counseling, interest inventories, job placement, internship options, on-the-job training, on-campus jobs, or supported employment.
- *Adult living skills*: Explore vocational rehabilitation services or working with a life coach; apply to Local Management Entity (supports coordination) for services; research Social Security benefits and work

incentives; help the individual register to vote, file taxes, explore residential options, obtain marriage counseling, become involved in spirituality and the religious community, obtain training in renting a home and personal home management, increase community access, and obtain heath care benefits (including health insurance).
- *Activities of Daily Living (ADL) skills*: Provide self-care training, health and wellness training, independent living training, and money management.
- *Functional/situational vocational evaluation*: Conduct situational work assessments, obtain work samples, enroll in work adjustment programs, conduct aptitude tests and help arrange a series of job tryouts.

Characteristics of a good transition plan (OAR, 2006)—IDEA specifies that transition planning is a coordinated set of activities for a student with a disability that is:
- *Outcome-oriented*—involves a process with clear goals and measurable outcomes
- *Student-centered*—is based on specific skills that the student needs and reflects the young adult's interests and preferences
- *Broad-based*—includes instruction and related services, community experiences, development of employment and post-school living objectives, and acquisition of daily living skills and vocational evaluation
- *Working document*—outlines current and future goals, along with the specific strategies for achieving these goals and addressing changes over time. Identifies individuals, providers, and locations where specific services will be provided.

Transition planning often begins earlier than age 16, by engaging the student in activities that become part of an employability assessment. Such an assessment should address the following questions:
- Can the individual take and receive orders?
- Can the individual follow time concepts and naturally occurring rhythms during the day? (e.g., knows when to return from break and lunch and the bathroom.)
- Does the individual have a basic understanding of manners required for a successful interview (e.g., hand-shakes, eye contact, saying "Yes Sir," "No Sir," "Yes Ma'am," "No Ma'am")?
- Can the individual be responsible with the care of his or her belongings (e.g., a uniform may be required for employment)?
- Does the individual have a basic ability to answer simple questions about likes and dislikes?
- Can the individual be responsible in the restroom and with personal hygiene (e.g., hand washing; for males, using a urinal; for females, personal care)?

Who represents the *players and stakeholders* in transition planning?

Representatives include the student, teachers, parents, doctors and health care providers, therapists and behavior supports, and anyone else of value to the student and family.

College Preparation and Support/Post-Secondary Education

The transition to a college program can be difficult and requires different preparation and planning than for employment. Areas to address include:

- Choosing the right school, finding the best match
- Identifying the type of program—vocational school, community college, technical institute, small state school, large university
- Arranging for school support services—guidance counselor, disability office, accommodations
- Providing instruction in organization
- Providing instruction in time management
- Providing instruction in independent living skills for dormitory or apartment
- Developing self-advocacy skills

There are many programs and models designed to address the college preparation needs of individuals with ASD. For example, Achieving in Higher Education with Autism/Developmental Disabilities (AHEADD) model provides a comprehensive and effective private support structure for students with ASD who want to attend college (www.aheadd.org/model). The four core elements include:

- Professional staff involved on-site
- Development of campus and community support network (e.g., develop and implement accommodations)
- Utilization of campus resources (e.g., college disability and health services)
- Peer mentoring

It is helpful to begin exploring early, and to look into summer preparation programs, summer courses, vocational schools, technical or trade schools, or junior colleges. It is important to find the right match between the student with ASD and the school program (e.g., close to home, number of students, size of classes, school supports, accommodations, social atmosphere, clubs, etc.).

Job-Finding and -Coaching

Meaningful employment is one goal for individuals with ASD who choose to work. It is important to remember the psychological value of being employed. Learning specific work-related skills should include not only job-related tasks, but also developing interpersonal skills and personal strategies that will foster a positive work experience (Hendricks & Wehman, 2009). Employment for a person with ASD is a principal means to connect with co-workers and become involved with their community. In turn, being employed directly impacts the individual's self-esteem, self worth, and identity, and helps them establish friendships, which are all critical components of one's quality of life and satisfaction (Jahoda, 1981). Being employed is an essential determinant of happiness. Labor and industry and social psychology measures of unemployment have found that people who are unemployed have significantly lower well-being scores than people who are employed. Fryer and Payne (1986), Argyle (2001), and Lucas et al. (2004) found strong statistical evidence of a connection between employment and happiness and unemployment and depression. Having a job that is fulfilling and valued can be a preventative measure for depression.

The **Office of Vocational Rehabilitation** (OVR) is a nationwide federal program to help people find employment. OVR can provide vocational assessment, job-finding, and job-coaching. Job matching is the match between the individual's characteristics and the job's requirements.

Types of employment range from least to most supportive:

- Competitive employment—full-time or part-time job with responsibilities, competitive with other individuals, fully integrated, without long-term support.
- Supported employment—ongoing training and personalized support is provided in competitive employment setting.
- Secured or segregated employment—work in self-contained area not integrated with other workers without disabilities, with behavioral support in place.

Strategies for successful employment

The employment outcomes for individuals with high-functioning autism and Asperger's disorder are reported to be generally much lower than would have been expected on the basis of their intellectual functioning (Howlin, 2004). It is important to develop strategies that will allow the individual with ASD to succeed, such as:

- Fine-tuning where their interests lie is helpful to finding employment
- Teaching rudimentary interviewing skills, with manners present, goes a long way
- Assisting the individual to develop a basic résumé with references
- Keeping physicals current, with documentation, is important; include TB tests when nearing the age of 21, or sooner, if employment opportunities occur
- Keeping I-9 documentation at the ready
- Visiting day programs, and if this is the career pathway, asking to be placed on the waiting list
- Providing instruction on how to interview
- Providing instruction regarding rules for success on the job
- Working with employers to address needed workplace accommodations

Supported employment models

TEACCH (Treatment and Education of Autistic and related Communication Handicapped Children and Adults) Supported Employment Program (Keel, Mesibov, Woods, 1997)—offers three models of supported employment: individual placement model, dispersed enclave model with more support, mobile crew model with more support and less independence.

Project SEARCH (Cincinnati Children's Hospital)—combines employer's need for high-turnover, entry-level positions, with a supported employment provider specialized in working with individuals who have developmental disabilities (see websites http://www.cincinnatichildrens.org/svc/alpha/p/search/, http://projectsearch.info/apps/).

Suitable careers for people with ASD

A successful job is often one that will utilize the interests, talents, and strengths of the individual with ASD. Temple Grandin has made suggestions on career choices in ASD (Grandin, 2010). She describes "types of minds"—saying that there are three basic types of specialized minds in ASD (types of thinkers):

1). *Visual thinkers*—People who think in photorealistic pictures like Google for images. Visual thinkers are good at the following occupations:
   - Art and Graphic Design
   - Industrial Design
   - Architecture
   - Auto Mechanics
   - Drafting
   - Photography
   - Animal Trainer

2). *Pattern thinkers*—These are the individuals who are often very good at math and music. Reading may be their area of weakness. Pattern thinking is a more abstract form of visual thinking. They think in patterns instead of pictures. Some good occupations for pattern thinkers are:
   - Scientific Researcher
   - Statistics—Data Mining
   - Engineering
   - Music
   - Mathematics
   - Computer Programming
   - Chemistry

3). *Word fact thinkers*—These are the individuals who know all the facts about their favorite things such as movie stars or baseball players. History is often a favorite subject. They are NOT visual thinkers, and they are often poor in art. The following careers would be good choices:
   - Journalist
   - Blogger
   - Librarian
   - Record-Keeping Jobs
   - Special Education Teacher
   - Bookkeeping
   - Speech Therapist

Examples of good and bad job choices (Grandin, 2010):

Good jobs for Non-Visual Thinkers—These are individuals who are good at math, music, or facts. Some good occupations for these individuals include:

- Accounting—Develop skills in a specialized field, such as income taxes
- Library Science—Reference librarian. Help people find information in the library or on the Internet
- Computer Programming—Less visual types can be done as freelance work
- Engineering—Electrical, electronic, and chemical engineering
- Journalist—Very accurate facts, can be done as freelance
- Copy Editor—Corrects manuscripts. Many people freelance for larger publishers
- Taxi Driver—Knows where every street is
- Inventory Control—Keeps track of merchandise stocked in a store
- Tuning Pianos and Other Musical Instruments—Can be done as freelance work
- Laboratory Technician—Running laboratory equipment
- Bank Teller—Very accurate money counting, much less demand on short-term working memory than a busy cashier who mostly makes change quickly
- Clerk and Filing Jobs—Knows where every file is
- Telemarketing—Gets to repeat the same thing over and over, selling on the telephone

Jobs for Nonverbal People with Autism or People with Poor Verbal Skills:

- Reshelving Library Books—Can memorize the entire numbering system and shelf locations
- Factory Assembly Work—Especially if the environment is quiet
- Copy Shop—Running photocopies. Printing jobs should be lined up by somebody else
- Janitor Jobs—Cleaning floors, toilets, windows, and offices
- Restocking Shelves—Can be done in many types of stores
- Recycling Plant—Sorting jobs
- Warehouse—Loading trucks, stacking boxes
- Lawn and Garden Work—Mowing lawns and landscaping work
- Data Entry—Primarily for individuals with strong fine-motor skills
- Fast Food Restaurant—Cleaning and cooking jobs with little demand on short-term memory
- Plant Care—Watering plants in a large office building.

Bad jobs for People with High-Functioning Autism or Asperger's Syndrome (jobs that require high demands on short-term working memory):

- Cashier—Making change quickly puts too much demand on short-term working memory
- Short-Order Cook—Having to keep track of many orders and cook many different things at the same time
- Waitress—Especially difficult if they have to keep track of many different tables
- Casino Dealer—Too many things to keep track of
- Taxi Dispatcher—Too many things to keep track of
- Taking Oral Dictation—Difficult due to auditory processing problems
- Airline Ticket Agent—Having to deal with angry people when flights are canceled

- Futures Market Trader—Totally impossible
- Air Traffic Controller—Information overload and stress
- Receptionist and Telephone Operator—Would have problems when the switchboard gets busy.

Tips for preparing for transition across all age groups

It is important to provide clear and accurate information regarding both the skills and support needs of the individual with ASD. Such information should include presentation and degree of the core features of ASD, such as communication deficits, deficits in social skills and social reciprocity, restricted patterns of behavior, as well as passions and interests. Making a few accommodations to the environment can decrease the person's distraction and increase their compliance and productivity.

Need for sameness, and difficulty with transitions

- Match the person to the transition environment. Some individuals enjoy large, wide-open settings, while others prefer small settings
- People with ASD require predictability, consistency, and structure
- Clearly define expectations, schedules, and activities
- Develop a visual agenda/schedule
- Provide clear, concise directives to insure that individual understands expectations in advance

Table 11.1 – "I Do That for Everybody:" Supervising Employees with Autism (adapted from Hanger & Cooney, 2005)

Area	Strategy/Support
Job modification/ adaptation Accommodations	Provide structure and organization Provide consistency and predictability Limit down time between jobs and limit social demands
Supervision	Give specific, detailed directions regarding job responsibilities Meet periodically to review performance Establish trust Provide opportunities for self assessment/feedback Allow additional time for changes in jobs and new/ novel work activities
Co-worker relationship and social interactions	With the approval of the employee, inform co-workers about the worker's periodic need for assistance in social areas Team employees with co-worker[s] as mentors to assist with job-related questions/concerns Include the employee as part of a team
Support services	Provide assistance and support when difficulties arise Access the assistance of Employee Assistance Program (EAP) when necessary

Atypical responses to sensory experiences

For the –individual with ASD, there are particular issues to pay attention to and accommodate:

- Sensory issues (i.e., overstimulation, distraction):
  - Sensitivity to smells
  - Sensitivity to sounds
  - Sensitivity to light, particularly fluorescent lights
  - Sensitivity to temperature
  - Sensitivity to touch (i.e., may experience difficulty when being touched)
- Body positioning issues (i.e., standing too close to people, maybe too far away, or just having general difficulty with body placement)
- Transitioning between activities or tasks (i.e., rigid or flexible, is time needed between activities to adjust?)
- Small group vs. large group settings.

Job-matching and preparing employers

A key ingredient in successful employment is the willingness of the employer to accommodate the employee, and proper preparation of the supervisor and work setting. The employer's knowledge of individuals with ASD and the specific future employee is important to a successful match. The supervisor's ability to make personal accommodations or job modifications, if needed, and to respond to questions will allow the person with ASD to fit in the job. Appropriate mentoring and support, as well as building co-worker cooperation and relationships, will assist in successful job placement and retention.

Social Competency Training and Activities

Transition plans, such as school to college and school to work, require skill building in social competency in order to increase positive social interactions and prevent and limit negative interactions. The lack of social competency and difficulty in using social skills is a significant barrier that can interfere with a successful transition for an individual with ASD at any stage in the lifespan. Teaching and practicing these skills is an essential component of a successful transition. Throughout adulthood, developing a social network and accessing community resources will help the adult with ASD to succeed. If religious faith is important to the individual, then another goal should include building social linkage to a faith-based organization and peer group. Peer-to-peer support programs help the individual work with and learn from a peer. (Social competency and social skills interventions are discussed in Chapter 13.)

Independence Skills Training

Transition planning and services in adulthood can offer independence skills training, beyond basic activities of daily living and self hygiene skills. This is a brief list of skills to learn and practice, and domains in which to get organized and develop schedules.

- Identify individualized goals
- Develop ways to get organized
- Prepare a schedule
- Practice daily living skills
- Practice telephone skills
- Learn skills for cleaning and maintaining an apartment or home
- Learn laundry and clothing skills
- Learn nutrition and cooking skills
- Develop budgeting skills and money management
- Learn banking skills
- Learn mobility skills and use of public transportation
- Develop an exercise plan (utilize a personal trainer)
- Identify key health care providers, names, phone numbers, emergency number
- Develop appointment-keeping and time-management plan

Part of independence skill building should include social networking, social activity groups, and if desired, faith-based groups.

Housing Options

Residential and community living

Many individuals with ASD live at home with their families; however, an increasing number of young adults are being placed in a wide variety of living options with varying degrees of restrictiveness. Developing a housing plan involves the individual with ASD, family, supports coordinator, and services coordinator, depending upon funding from intellectual disability services or mental health services, or a case manager from Social Security office. Finding housing outside of the family is a difficult step both emotionally and financially.

Types of living arrangements
- Independent living—own apartment and support staff who provide independence and daily living-skills training on a time-limited basis
- Supported living—support staff provide individualized services in own apartment or home
- Supervised apartment living—staff provide direction and supervision and emergency response on-site within an apartment building
- Adult foster care or "life-sharing"—live with a family who is recruited by an agency who oversees and certifies the family
- Living in parent's home with supports
- Supervised group home living—agency-run home with several individuals and trained staff in the home
- Personal care home
- Nursing home

Supports coordination ("case management")

The Supports Coordinator (SC) plays a critical role in the transition from child to adult services and funding. Each state may have different terminology or organizational structure. The SC usually works out of the Office of Intellectual Disability (OID), which is a division of the Department of Public Welfare (DPW). If the individual with ASD does not have intellectual disability (ID), then supports and funding do not come out of this office. Some states are creating separate funding or waivers for individuals with ASD who do not have ID.

A waiver is a specific funding mechanism that depends upon the individual's meeting certain criteria of need and on the availability of funding in that state. State and federal budgets and guidelines for waivers may vary with each change in government leadership. Consolidated Waiver and Person/Family Directed Support (PFDS) Waiver services are available to people with ID aged three and older. However, services funded by the waivers are not available to people while they are living or staying in public or private intermediate care facilities, nursing homes, residential treatment facilities, or hospitals. There is an annual cap in the PFDS, but there is no similar cap associated with the Consolidated Waiver. Residential services are only available through the Consolidated Waiver.

Major responsibilities of the SC to foster transition include:
- Assessment of the individual and family needs
- Development of an Individual Support Plan (ISP), which is an individualized and comprehensive transition plan (with the involvement of the individual with ASD)

- Assisting the individual with self-advocacy and self-determination
- Linking the individual and family to services across systems
- Planning for advocacy and legal issues
- Monitoring and tracking outcome measures and transition plan goals.
- Ensuring health and safety by developing an individualized safety or crisis plan

Diagnostic Clarification, Identification and Treatment of Comorbid Disorders

Most individuals with ASD are diagnosed in early childhood or by school-age. Some young adults are evaluated for symptoms of high-functioning autism or Asperger's disorder that have not been identified earlier. The psychiatrist, primary care doctor, psychologist, and other health care and service providers need to be aware of the presentation of an adult with ASD and the range of comorbid medical and psychiatric symptoms displayed.

Diagnostic clarification of adult presenting with symptoms of ASD (see Chapter 2 on ASD diagnostic assessment). Information that is often needed for a psychiatric evaluation includes:

- Developmental history (parents, medical/psychiatric records, school reports)
- Vocational/work history
- Post-secondary education history (technical school, junior college, college)
- Current problem list
- Updated rating scales (e.g., SCQ, SRS, GARS 2, ASQ)
- ADOS, if needed

Some common characteristics seen in persons with ASD that may lead to difficulty coping include:

- Challenges in interpreting nonverbal language
- Rigid adherence to rules
- Poor eye-gaze or avoidance of eye contact
- Few facial expressions and trouble understanding the facial expressions of others
- Poor judge of personal space—may stand too close to other students
- Trouble controlling their emotions and anxieties
- Difficulty understanding another person's perspective or how their own behavior affects others
- Very literal understanding of speech; difficulty in picking up on nuances
- Unusually intense or restricted interests in things (maps, dates, coins, numbers/statistics, train schedules)
- Unusual repetitive behavior, verbal as well as nonverbal (hand flapping, rocking)
- Unusual sensitivity to sensations—may be more *or* less than typical students
- Difficulty with transitions, need for sameness
- Possible aggressive, disruptive, or self-injurious behavior; unaware of possible dangers

Situations that often increase anxiety for persons with Asperger's disorder and lead to difficulty coping include:

- When conversation involves multiple speakers
- Rapid shifting of topics
- Latency of response
- Difficulty in seeking clarification

- Lack of confidence
- Overabundance of irrelevant information

Identification and treatment of comorbid disorders (see Chapter 12 for behavioral and psychotherapeutic interventions)—The following are examples of difficulties encountered by individuals with ASD (Lovell & Reiss, 1993):
- Intellectual distortion—they are often unable to label and report on their own experience (from feelings to words)
- Psychosocial masking—as a result of improvised social skills, mis-assumption of psychiatric symptoms (anxiety/paranoia)
- Cognitive disintegration—a stress-induced disruption of information processing that presents as psychotic features (self talk, or imaginary friend, thinking out loud).

Co-occurring disorders in adults with ASD (Ghaziuddin, 2002)—Associated psychiatric and medical conditions (see Chapter 3 for medical and comorbid psychiatric disorders):
- Anxiety disorders—social anxiety, generalized anxiety, panic
- Obsessive-compulsive disorder (which is an anxiety disorder)
- Attention deficit hyperactivity disorder (usually without hyperactivity)
- Depression
- Bipolar disorder
- Tic disorders
- Psychotic disorder or schizophrenia
- Seizure disorder
- Sleep disorder
- Allergies
- Gastrointestinal disorders
- Movement disorders

Since there are limited services for adults with ASD, especially psychiatric and mental health providers, it is important to teach key people in the individual's life about signs and symptoms to watch for and significant changes in their usual functioning level. This group might include the family, support team, case manager, employer, job coach, college counselor, and student disability office.

Summary

Transition planning includes the individual with ASD, parents, and teachers, and requires knowledge of systems and teamwork. Some young adults with ASD are able to transition to a day activity program or vocational training setting, employment, technical school, junior college, college, and community living. It is important to focus on the individual's strengths, interests, and passions, and to be aware of their areas of weakness. There are many challenges for the individual with ASD in learning and using skills in order to succeed in employment, school, social, and community living settings. Often characteristics of ASD make coping and anxiety-management difficult. It can be helpful for the adult with ASD to seek out services such as skill building in social competency, and behavioral health services. The psychiatrist, primary care doctor, psychologist, and other health care and service providers need to be aware of the presentation of an adult with ASD and the range of comorbid medical and psychiatric symptoms displayed.

Key Fact Box

- Individuals with Disabilities Education Act states that transition planning begins by age 14, and when a student turns 16, transition planning must be in effect in the student's Individual Education Plan.
- The student with special needs such as ASD may continue in the educational system for transition services until the age of 21 (unless an individual state's regulation has a different age limit).
- Transition planning and transition services include a set of activities related to preparing a student to enter adult life, including employment, further education, and community living.
- Transition planning extends through all of life's passages and can include skills training in activities of daily living, healthcare, money management, leisure, social activities, dating, and marriage and child decisions, along with social and civic responsibilities.

Further Reading

1. Attwood, T. (2007). *The complete guide to Asperger's syndrome.* London: Jessica Kingsley Publishers.
2. Bashe, P., & Kirby, B. (2001). *The OASIS guide to Asperger's syndrome.* New York: Crown.
3. Grandin, T. Choosing the Right Job for People with Autism or Asperger's Syndrome. Autism Research Institute. Retrieved November 10, 2010, from http://www.autism.org/temple/jobs.html.
4. Grandin, T., & Duffy, K. (2004). *Developing talents, careers for individuals with Asperger syndrome and high-functioning autism.* Shawnee Mission, KS: Autism Asperger Publishing Co.
5. Hagner, D., & Cooney, B. F. (2005) "I do that for everybody": Supervising employees with autism. *Focus on Autism and Other Developmental Disabilities, 20*(2), 91–97.
6. Hendricks, D. R., & Wehman, P. (2009). Transition from school to adulthood for youth with Autism Spectrum Disorder. *Focus on Autism and Other Developmental Disabilities, 24*(2) 77–88.
7. Howlin, P. (2000). Outcome in adult life for more able individuals with autism or Asperger syndrome. *Autism, 4*(1), 63–83.
8. Howlin, P., Goode, S., Hutton, J., & Rutter, M. (2004). Adult outcome for children with autism. *Journal of Child Psychology and Psychiatry, 45*, 212–229.
9. Hurlbutt, K., & Chalmers, L. (2004). Employment and adults with Asperger's syndrome. *Focus on Autism and other Developmental Disabilities, 19*(4), 215–222.
10. Jahoda, M. (1981), Work, employment and unemployment: Values, theories, and approaches in social research. *American Psychologist, 36*, 184–1991.
11. Müller, E., Schuler, A., Burton, B., & Yates, G. (2003). Meeting the vocational support needs of individuals with Asperger syndrome and other autism spectrum disabilities. *Journal of Vocational Rehabilitation, 18*, 163–175.
12. Nesbitt, S. (2000). Why and why not? Factors influencing employment for individuals with Asperger syndrome. *Autism, 4*(4), 357–369.
13. Organization for Autism Research (OAR) & Danya International (2006). *Life journey through autism: A guide for transition to adulthood.* Arlington, VA: Organization for Autism Research, Inc.
14. Organization for Autism Research (OAR), Danya International, & Southwest Autism Research & Resource Center (SARRC) (2005). *Life journey through autism: An educator's guide to Asperger syndrome.* Arlington, VA: Organization for Autism Research, Inc.
15. Project SEARCH, Cincinnati Children's Hospital. See websites, http://www.cincinnatichildrens.org/svc/alpha/p/search/, http://projectsearch.info/apps/.
16. Seltzer, M.M., Shattuck, P., Abbeduto, L., & Greenberg, J.S.. (2004). Trajectory of development in adolescents and adults with autism. *Mental Retardation and Developmental Disabilities Research Reviews, 10*, 234–247.
17. Wagner, M., Marder, C., Blackorby, J., Cameto, R., Newman, C., Levine, P., & Davies-Mercier, E. (2003). The achievement of youth with disabilities during secondary school: A report from the National Longitudinal Transition Study—2. Prepared for the Office of Special Education Programs, U.S. Department of Education. Menlo Park, CA: SRI International. Retrieved February 12, 2003, from http://www.nlts2.org/reports/reports_collapsed.html.
18. Wagner, M., Cadwallader, T., Marder, C., Cameto, R., Cardoso, D., Garzo, N., Levine, P., & Newman, L. (2003). Life outside the classroom for youth with disabilities: A report from the National Longitudinal Transition Study—2. Prepared for the Office of Special Education Programs, U.S. Department of Education. Menlo Park, CA: SRI International. Retrieved February 12, 2004, from http://www.nlts2.org/reports/reports_collapsed.html.
19. Wehman, P. (2006). *Life beyond the classroom: Transition strategies for young people with disabilities.* Baltimore, MD: Brookes Publishing.

Questions

1. Which of the following is *true* about IDEA?
   a. IDEA stands for Individuals with Disabilities Education Act.
   b. The Act states that when a student turns 16, transition planning must be in effect in the student's Individual Education Plan (IEP).
   c. IDEA requires the inclusion of a "statement of the student's transition goals and services" in the IEP packet.
   d. Students with identified special needs such as ASD may continue in the educational system for transition services until the age of 21.
   e. All of the above.

2. Which of the following is *not* true of transition planning?
   a. The planning process is completed by the teacher without the student or parent's input.
   b The transition plan focuses on what skills are necessary to succeed post–high school.
   c. A good transition plan will include both long- and short-term goals.
   d. The transition plan should be specific to the interests, abilities, and desires of the student.
   e. Office of Vocational Rehabilitation (OVR) can provide vocational assessment, job-finding, and job-coaching, if not provided by the school.

3. Which of the following is *true* about employment for individuals with ASD?
   a. Job matching is the match between the individual's characteristics and the job's requirements.
   b. Competitive employment is a full-time or part-time job with responsibilities competitive with other individuals, without long-term support.
   c. In supported employment, ongoing training and support are provided in similar opportunities as competitive employment.
   d. Secured or segregated employment involves work in self-contained areas not integrated with other workers without disabilities.
   e. All of the above.

4. Which is *not* a common characteristic in persons with ASD that may lead to difficulty coping in a job?
   a. Rigid adherence to rules in spite of what the supervisor says
   b. Poor judge of personal space (stands too close to others), which may lead to accusations of sexual harassment
   c. Difficulty understanding another person's perspective (how their own behavior affects others), which may lead to conflict with supervisor
   d. Very literal understanding of speech (difficulty in picking up on nuances), which may lead to being teased by co-workers
   e. Ease with transitions and flexibility

5. Which might be a "bad job choice for people with high-functioning autism or Asperger's disorder" (per Temple Grandin)?
   a. Cashier—making change quickly puts too much demand on short-term working memory
   b. Short-order cook—have to keep track of many orders and cook many different things at the same time
   c. Waitress—especially difficult if they have to keep track of many different tables
   d. Airline ticket agent—dealing with angry people when flights are canceled
   e. All of the above

Answers

1. e. All of the above
2. a. Not true—the transition planning process is completed by the teacher, student and parents.
3. e. All of the above
4. e. Not true—people with ASD often have difficulty with transitions and need to work on flexibility in changing situations in order to cope on the job or in post secondary education.
5. e. All of the above

Addressing Behavioral and Emotional Challenges in School-Age Children and Adolescents with ASD

Carla A. Mazefsky and Benjamin L. Handen

Identify Function of Behavior to Determine Appropriate
    Intervention 258
Changing Motivating Operations and Antecedents 260
Teaching Alternative Behaviors 262
Changing Reinforcers and Consequences 264
Summary 266
Further Reading 267
Questions 268
Answers 269

This chapter will summarize how to address behavioral and emotional challenges in school-age children and adolescents with autism spectrum disorder. Chapter 5 focused on functional behavioral assessment as a means of providing the structure for implementing a behavioral treatment plan based on applied behavior analysis principles. Chapter 7 highlighted early childhood interventions within an educational and behavioral framework. Chapter 9 described interventions for specialized concerns, such as feeding, sleep, and toileting issues, in young children. Comorbid psychiatric disorders in individuals with ASD are defined in Chapter 3, and Chapter 11 focused on adults. Interventions that relate to social skills training and social competency are found in Chapter 13.

Treatment for children and adolescents with ASD necessarily goes beyond a sole focus on social interaction, communication, and repetitive behaviors. Many children with ASD have problematic emotional and behavioral reactions that require immediate attention during the course of other interventions. There are many different types of behavioral and emotional problems that could occur in ASD, such as self-injury, self-stimulatory behaviors, anxiety, aggression, noncompliance, and over-activity. Service providers for children with ASD need to be able to address these behavioral challenges quickly and efficiently in order to avoid further escalation of difficulties.

As discussed in Chapter 6's introduction to treatments, there have been two recent scientific treatment practice reviews with the goal of identifying evidence-based practices in ASD. Both the National Autism Center's (NAC) National Standards Project and the Maine Department of Health and Human Services (DHHS) with the Maine Department of Education have made their treatment recommendations available to the public. The two reports focused their efforts on examining well-controlled studies involving children with ASD and used fairly similar categories in which to rate the scientific research.

Categories used by the Maine DHHS report (2009)
- Level 1: Established Evidence
- Level 2: Promising Evidence
- Level 3: Preliminary Evidence
- Level 4: Studied and No Evidence of Effect
- Level 5: Insufficiently Studied
- Level 6: Evidence of Harm

National Autism Center's National Standards Project Scientific Merit Rating Scale Categories and Criteria (2009)

Category	Criteria
Established	• Merit ratings of 3 to 5 • Research supports the use of the treatment
Emerging	• Merit rating of 2 • Further research is necessary to support use of the treatment

Unestablished	• Merit rating of 0 to 1 • Further research is necessary to support the use of the treatment • Studies conducted provide treatment effects that show ineffectiveness or harm
Ineffective/ Harmful	• Merit ratings of 3 • Lack of positive treatment effects, or harmful effects found

Table 12.1 below lists the interventions that were determined to meet the definition requirements as "established treatments" or "established evidence" by the two reports.

Certainly, there were some commonalities as well as differences between the two reports. For example, the picture exchange communication system (PECS) was found to be well established by National Autism Center but actually was rated as "insufficiently studied" by the Maine group. This proved to be the exact opposite for story-based intervention packages.

However, the most important point is that both reviews found treatments based on the principles of *applied behavior analysis* to be most efficacious. These included discrete trial training, pivotal response treatment, and naturalistic teaching practices (described in Chapter 7, Early Childhood Interventions). The use of ABA procedures has been shown to be efficacious in dealing with a wide range of targeted behavioral concerns across the age spectrum in the fields of ASD and intellectual disability (mental retardation). Table 12.2 below contains a partial list of procedures and interventions that fall under the ABA umbrella.

Since the 1960s, behavioral journals have published hundreds of studies documenting the efficacy of ABA principles to address a wide range of concerns that typically affect children, adolescents, and adults with ASD. The following lists some of the areas that have been addressed by ABA.

Targeted behaviors to *eliminate*:
• Rumination/vomiting
• Sleep problems
• Feeding difficulties
• Self-injury
• Noncompliance
• Aggression/tantrums
• Repetitive/stereotypic behaviors
• Inappropriate speech (e.g., swearing, repetitive question asking)

Targeted behaviors to *strengthen*:
• Toilet training
• Communication skills
• Self-help skills
• Academic skills
• Social skills

The Key Fact Box below summarizes the primary components of effective interventions for behavioral and emotional problems in ASD, which are described in more detail in the following sections.

Table 12.1 – Established Treatments and Established Evidence

National Autism Center's National Standards Project Report:

http://www.nationalautismcenter.org/pdf/NAC%20Standards%20Report.pdf

Established Treatments

Antecedent Package
Behavioral Package
Comprehensive Behavioral Treatment for Young Children
Joint Attention Intervention
Modeling
Naturalistic Teaching Strategies
Peer Training Package
Pivotal Response Treatment
Schedules
Self-Management
Story-Based Intervention Package

Maine Department of Health and Human Services with the Maine Department of Education Report:

http://www.maine.gov/dhhs/ocfs/cbhs/ebpac/asd-report2009.pdf

Established Evidence

Applied Behavior Analysis for challenging behaviors
Applied Behavior Analysis for communication
Applied Behavior Analysis for social skills
Early Intensive Behavioral Intervention (UCLA/Lovaas model)
haloperidol (Haldol) - found effective for aggression
methylphenidate (Ritalin) - found effective for hyperactivity
Picture Exchange Communication System (PECS)
risperidone (Risperdal) - found effective for irritability, social withdrawal, hyperactivity and stereotypy

Table 12.2 – Examples of Behavioral Interventions

Token Economies	Response Cost
Extinction	Positive Reinforcement
Negative Reinforcement	Time Out
Differential Reinforcement	Shaping
Graduated Guidance	Fading
Video Modeling	Contracting
Functional Communication Training	Picture Exchange Communication
Discrete Trial Training	Delayed Prompting
Pivotal Response Training	Naturalistic Teaching Strategies

Key Fact Box: Primary Components of Effective Interventions

Assessment	Determine the function of the behavior and identify antecedents and motivating operations.
Changing motivating operations and antecedent management	Modify the environment to prevent behavior problems; change the trigger.
Teaching alternative strategies and behaviors	Identify deficits and teach child appropriate replacement behaviors/coping skills for a situation.
Consequences	Modifying consequences and reinforcement programs.

Identify Function of Behavior to Determine Appropriate Intervention

One of the hallmarks of ABA is proper assessment of the problem area, which is covered in Chapter 5 on functional behavioral assessment. Prior to implementing a program designed to decrease or eliminate a maladaptive behavior, a thorough analysis of the situation is required in order to determine the "function" of the behavior. Identifying the function should lead to a more appropriate intervention. Most behaviors serve either a social function (e.g., to get attention, to obtain an item, to avoid a demand) or a sensory function.

One concept that can be helpful to keep in mind when determining the function of the behavior is the distinction between "tantrums" and "meltdowns," summarized in Table 12.3 below. Temper tantrums are a purposeful behavior aimed at manipulating a situation to get what one wants. A behavioral or emotional "meltdown" in ASD can look like a tantrum, but is often quite different in nature. Specifically, meltdowns are generally thought of as extreme stress responses. Although children and adolescents with ASD can and do have temper tantrums, meltdowns are generally even more frequent and troublesome to providers. A meltdown, whether in the form of extreme anxiety or aggression, etc., would require a different type of intervention than a temper tantrum, given that it has a different function, often based on a setting event.

In addition to examining a behavior's function, the assessment should look at possible antecedents as well as setting events (called motivating operations). These are situations that can also impact a child's behavior—some of which situations may occur well before the behavior problem itself. For example, an adolescent who attends an autism classroom may display sporadic acts of aggressive behavior that the staff is unable to connect to anything that was going on in the classroom itself. It is possible that a motivating operation may be in effect that may make it more likely that the adolescent will be more irritable than usual (and not as responsive to classroom reinforcers). Below are some possible motivating operations that can either strengthen or weaken reinforcer effectiveness.

Biological: Hunger, sleep problems, menses
Medical: Pain, medication side effect
Social: Recent argument with family, having been teased

In addition to motivating operations, one also needs to examine other possible, more immediate antecedents to the behavior. Antecedents are typically something that occurs at the time of the behavior. Ongoing data-keeping that records information about the behavior can often assist in identifying possible antecedents. Table 12.4 below is a sample data sheet documenting incidents of aggression in class for an adolescent female, Susan C., with ASD.

Table 12.3 – Conceptual Difference between a Meltdown and Temper Tantrum

	Meltdown	Temper Tantrum
Level of internal regulation supporting the behavior	**LOW:** Uncontrolled, catastrophic reaction	**HIGH:** Goal-directed and purposeful
Function of the behavior	"Extreme emotional/ behavioral response to stress or overstimulation" (Lipsky & Richards, 2009, pp. 20)	Trying to get something pleasant or get out of doing something unpleasant

Table 12.4 – Data sheet documenting aggressive episodes for an adolescent female Susan C.

Date & Time	Activity/Situation	Staff	Behavior	Consequence
1/4/10 11:45 am	S asked to complete math sheet	SJ	Tore math sheet and flipped table	Sent to principal's office
1/5/10 2:45 pm	S told to stop playing on the computer and start to finish the math assignment	LS	Flipped chair	Staff spent 10 minutes talking with S about her behavior.
1/7/10 3:15 pm	S told to put game away and finish the math assignment from the morning	LS	Threw game and attempted to hit another student	Staff spent 10 minutes talking to S to calm her down.
1/12/10 11:15 am	S told to get out math book	SJ	Screamed and hit student sitting nearby	Sent to principal's office

Changing Motivating Operations and Antecedents

The purpose of conducting a functional analysis and collecting antecedent data is to provide hypotheses that can lead to the development of preventative strategies. As Table 12.3 above highlights, meltdowns are often a "reaction" or "response" that implicates some type of trigger in the environment. Therefore, often the first corrective step is to change the environment. This can involve either changing an actual aspect of the environment (e.g., finding a quieter space for learning if the child is becoming overwhelmed by too much chaotic noise) or teaching the people who interact with the child new skills. In fact, most interventions often focus on changing something about the behavior of the people working with the child as a means of changing the child's behavior.

For example, Bobby was a 12-year-old boy with high-functioning ASD. He did well in school all day long, but was very aggressive and defiant when he came home. After doing a functional assessment to identify antecedents and motivating operators, it was discovered that Bobby had to ride the bus nearly an hour and a half each way to and from school. Bobby had many noise sensitivities, and the bus was not only a socially strenuous environment, but very loud. Therefore, it seemed that one possible explanation was that he was becoming over-stimulated on the bus ride home and then was unable to effectively cope with demands placed on him by family members, such as homework or further interaction. A prevention strategy for Bobby thus involved having his parents drive him to and from school instead of taking the bus, which was much faster, quieter, and less stimulating. With this change, Bobby's behavioral problems after school at home quickly remitted.

Often the trigger or antecedent is somewhat less clear. For example, the above data for Susan C. suggest that one of the antecedents to problem behavior for this adolescent is being given task demands or being told to stop engaging in an enjoyable activity (in order to do something less desirable). There do not appear to be any particular patterns about time (the problem occurs both in the morning and the afternoon or evening) or day of the week (it seems to occur at different days). However, there may also be some clues to antecedents based upon what is not on the data sheet. For example, her problem behavior seems to only occur with staff members "SJ" and "LS." If other staff also interact with her, is it possible that they do so in a different way that avoids problems (perhaps there are ways to approach this adolescent that increase the likelihood that she will or will not respond by being disruptive)?

From an *antecedent* standpoint, data in the above case suggests that math may be difficult for Susan and that modifying the math demands may prevent some of the problems. It is also possible that the way this adolescent is instructed to stop or start an activity could impact her response. From the standpoint of motivating operations, there are also some interesting things to consider.

Notice that the behavior problem seems to occur in the late morning or mid-afternoon. If the adolescent were taking a short-acting stimulant, it is possible that it might be losing its effect by late morning. Conversely, if a longer-acting stimulant (e.g., Adderall XR) were being prescribed, that might explain problems in the mid-afternoon. Other possibilities are that the she is getting hungry and irritable by late morning or mid-afternoon (and needs a small snack at around 10:00 a.m. and/or 2:00 p.m.).

Teaching Alternative Behaviors

The data collected can also be used to develop a skills-building strategy for the adolescent that can be used to replace the maladaptive behavior. This may seem obvious for children and adolescents whose distress manifests as anxiety, in which case teaching anxiety-management strategies can be helpful. However, the concept of teaching a new skill can also be applied to many other manifestations of behavior problems that are less traditionally thought of as the focus of a "therapy," such as learning to wait or accept no, and how to appropriately get one's attention needs met.

General Concepts for Teaching Alternative Behaviors

The selection of an alternative behavior to teach should meet the following criteria:

- The alternative behavior should be more efficient. That is, it should quickly result in what the individual is communicating that they need (e.g., getting help).
- The alternative behavior should work consistently for the individual, especially in the beginning, in all situations and with all adults working with the individual.
- The alternative behavior should be less effortful than the challenging behavior.

When teaching alternative behaviors, it is important to *distinguish skill-acquisition deficits from performance deficits* (Bellini et al., 2007). In a skill-acquisition deficit, the child does not have the skill or behavior. Thus the goal is to teach a new skill or further develop recently acquired skills. In a performance deficit, the skill is present but is not being demonstrated or performed. This may be due to the child's being unaware of when to apply a skill or it may be due to their lack of motivation to perform the skill. The goal is to enhance performance of these existing skills.

There are many methods for teaching alternative behaviors and skills to address behavioral and emotional problems. Two main types of teaching strategies are incidental teaching and structured learning (Baker, 2008). *Incidental teaching* is experiential in nature and occurs as the event or behavior unfolds, typically in the natural environment. This could include prompting a child or pointing out cues in the child's environment, etc. *Structured learning* is probably what most providers are more familiar with, in that it involves didactic instruction of skill steps. Structured learning can occur one-on-one, in small groups, or with an entire class of children. With ASD, structured learning that uses a concrete, stepwise method is typically most effective. Many specific structured learning tools may be applicable, depending on the particular skill being taught, such as role-playing, modeling, psychoeducation, utilizing games, etc.

Functional Communication Training

One structured teaching approach that is often used is called *functional communication training* (Durand, 1999). Functional communication posits that an individual's maladaptive behavior serves a communicative function. Therefore, if a more efficient and appropriate means of communicating is taught, the maladaptive behavior should lessen. In the case of Susan C., the student appeared to be engaging in disruptive behavior to communicate her desire to avoid a challenging task. She could be taught a more appropriate way to manage the situation. For example, if the math were too difficult, she could be taught to request help.

Cognitive-Behavioral Therapy

Another example of a more structured teaching approach is the use of cognitive-behavioral therapy (CBT) strategies with individuals with ASD. CBT has been used in ASD for depression and mood concerns, generally as a framework to address skill deficits such as social skill weaknesses, and most commonly for anxiety-related problems. Atwood (2004) has suggested that CBT for children, adolescents, and adults with ASD should include affective education, cognitive restructuring, and teaching them how to use an "emotional toolbox" (strategies for handling negative emotions).

Research supporting the use of CBT in ASD is limited, but growing. Studies that have been published typically include younger children and usually involve modifying CBT programs for anxiety to have more structure, use more visual aids, and have increased parental involvement (e.g., Sofronoff et al., 2005). Recently, White and colleagues (2009) published preliminary findings for a CBT treatment targeting high-functioning adolescents with ASD and anxiety. At this stage, it remains difficult to make strong conclusions regarding the efficacy of CBT in people with ASD, but it does seem to be a promising approach and is a form of structured teaching that can be potentially quite useful for teaching alternative behaviors for anxiety-based maladaptive behaviors in particular.

Changing Reinforcers and Consequences

Reinforcers

Finally, the program should include the specific reinforcement of appropriate behavior (in Susan C.'s case, completing math and other assignments). This could involve a specific contract for completing work, a token economy (e.g., awarding points, stars), as well as staff attention for working. Higher-functioning adolescents can often participate in a contingency contract or token system.

Such programs involve the writing of a specific contract that outlines:
a) the specific work/task to be completed or rules to be followed,
b) the time period covered, and
c) the specific reinforcer that will be earned if the contract is met.

Table 12.5 below is an example of a contract written for an adolescent with ASD. It is important that the contract be signed by all parties and a copy be given to the student.

Many individuals are also placed on a token economy, which involves the awarding of points, stars, checks, signatures, etc., based on following specified rules or behavior. One frequently used point system involves the awarding of points at the end of each class period for following a set of specified rules. The point card below in Table 12.6 is for an adolescent with ASD who must follow three rules in each class period. Her teacher awards either 0 points (did not follow the rule), 1 point (partial following of rule) or 2 points (followed the rule) at the end of each class period. At the end of the day, the adolescent is able to exchange points for time on the computer (each point is good for 30 seconds of computer time).

Table 12.5 – Contract for Susan C.

Goal: To do better in math.

Responsibility: I will complete all daily math assignments with 70% accuracy and follow the classroom rules during math class (remain in my seat, work quietly, raise my hand to ask questions or for help).

Time Period: All assignments must be completed during the math class (from 11:15 a.m. to 12:00 noon).

Reinforcer: I will receive one check for each day that the above responsibilities are met. If I have at least four checks by the end of the week, I can go to the computer lab for the last school period.

Bonus: If I have a perfect week (all five checks), I can select a friend to join me in the computer lab.

_____	_____
Student Signature	Date
_____	_____
Teacher Signature	Date

Table 12.6 – Susan's Daily Point Card

Rule/ Period	Period 1	Period 2	Period 3	Period 4	Period 5	Period 6	Total
Complete work	2	2	1	2	0	2	9
Raise hand before talking	2	2	2	1	1	2	10
Keep hands to self	2	1	2	2	2	1	10
							Grand Total: 29

Consequences

"Consequences" include everything that follows a behavior. This could include attention, punishment, or nothing. In the example from the earlier data sheet for Susan C., it appears that the student was experiencing a number of consequences that could be inadvertently maintaining the behavior. In all cases, the consequence seems to involve escaping from the task demand. In addition, the student is provided with individual attention by either classroom staff or the school principal. So the final part of the program for this student would be to attempt to eliminate these potential sources of reinforcement. One option is to instruct staff not to "counsel" the student after an incident. Instead, staff can have a standard daily meeting time with the student at the end of the day when they can discuss both appropriate and problem behavior. This session is not contingent upon the student's behavior that particular day. Second, the student probably should not be sent to the principal. Third, it will be important to maintain the task demand so that the student does not learn that disruptive behavior will end the demand (even if it takes the student some time to calm down, the work must be completed).

In addition to eliminating consequences that may be reinforcing the behavior, there are several other consequences that can be put into place, such as:

- *Time-out*: This can involve removing the student to a quiet area of the classroom or even out of the room for a designated period of time contingent upon the occurrence of a specific maladaptive behavior. It is important that time-out not be used for escape-motivated behavior. It is best used for behavior whose function appears to be attention-motivated (since time-out should be a place where no attention is given).
- *Extinction/ignoring*: This involves having staff and other students ignore the behavior until the student is once again behaving appropriately. Again, this consequence should only be used for maladaptive behaviors that are attention-motivated.

- *Response cost*: This involves the loss of access to a reinforcing activity. The most frequent response cost intervention used by parents is grounding (loss of TV, car privileges, etc.). In the classroom, this can involve loss of recess time, computer time, etc. If the student is using a token economy, this might also involve the loss of a point when the maladaptive behavior occurs.

Summary

Children and adolescents with ASD present with a variety of emotional and behavioral challenges that often need to be addressed during the course of treatment. While ABA may be more traditionally thought of as a treatment for very young and low-functioning children, using an ABA framework can be quite beneficial in the development of interventions for problematic behavioral and emotional reactions in school-aged children and adolescents. This framework can be flexibly applied to a host of presenting concerns, including aggression, self-injury, hyperactivity, noncompliance, anxiety, and so forth.

As summarized in the *Key Fact Box*, the primary steps involved include:

- Assessment of the problem to identify underlying functions and motivating operators,
- Changing antecedents or triggers in the environment as a means of preventing the problematic behavior in the first place (ranging from changing aspects of the environment, to demands placed on the child, to ways that others interact with the child),
- Teaching the child or adolescent replacement behaviors to more appropriately meet their needs, either through structured teaching such as cognitive-behavioral interventions or teaching and prompting discrete skills in the natural environment; and
- Developing a reinforcement program and set of consequences to manage and support the use of the more appropriate replacement behaviors.

This approach recognizes that every person with ASD is unique and maladaptive problems may take many forms, thus an individualized strategy is required. The strategies described have been evidence-based and can be applied to develop an individualized intervention to promote behavioral and emotional stability across a variety of presenting concerns stems from the strongest evidence base.

Further Reading

1. Atwood, T. (2004). Cognitive behaviour therapy for children and adults with Asperger Syndrome. *Behaviour Change, 21*(3): 147–161.
2. Baker, J. E. (2008). *No more meltdowns.* Arlington, TX: Future Horizons.
3. Bellini, S., Peters, J., Berner, L., & Hopf, A. (2007). A meta-analysis of school-based social skills interventions for children with Autism Spectrum Disorder. *Remedial and Special Education, 28*(3): 153–162.
4. Durand, V. M. (1999). Functional communication training using assistive devices: Recruiting natural communities of reinforcement. *Journal of Applied Behavior Analysis, 32,* 247–267.
5. Lipsky, D., & Richards, W. (2009). *Managing meltdowns: Using the S.C.A.R.E.D. calming technique with children and adults with autism.* Dexter, MI: Thomason-Shore.
6. Sofronoff, K., Attwood, T., & Hinton, S. (2005). A randomized controlled trial of a CBT intervention for anxiety in children with Asperger syndrome. *Journal of Child Psychology and Psychiatry, 46,* 1152–1160.
7. White, S.W., Ollendick, T., Scahill, L., Oswald, D., & Albano, A.M., (2009). Preliminary efficacy of a Cognitive-Behavioral Treatment program for anxious youth with Autism Spectrum Disorder. *Journal of Autism and Developmental Disorders, 39,* 1652–1662.
8. Wolfe, M. M., Risley, T. R., & Mees H. (1964). Applications of operant conditioning procedures to the behavior problems of an autistic child. *Behavior Research and Therapy, 1,* 305–312.

Questions

1. Which of the following statements is true of functional behavioral assessment?
   a. Prior to implementing a program designed to decrease or eliminate a maladaptive behavior, a thorough analysis of the situation is required.
   b. The primary goal of such an analysis is to determine the "function" of the behavior.
   c. Identifying the function should lead to a more appropriate intervention.
   d. Most behaviors serve either a social function (e.g., attention, to obtain an item, to avoid a demand) or a sensory function.
   e. All of the above

2. The selection of an alternative behavior to teach should meet which of the following criteria?
   a. The alternative behavior should be more efficient (i.e., it should quickly result in delivering what the individual is communicating they want).
   b. The alternative behavior should work consistently for the individual, in all situations and with all adults working with the individual.
   c. The alternative behavior should be less effortful than the challenging behavior.
   d. None of the above
   e. All of the above

3. The specific reinforcement of appropriate behavior might include:
   a. A specific contract for completing work
   b. A token economy (e.g., awarding points, stars)
   c. Staff attention for working
   d. Time-out
   e. a, b, and c

4. An applied behavior analysis's primary steps include:
   a. Assessment of the problem to identify underlying functions and motivating operators
   b. Changing antecedents or triggers in the environment as a means of preventing the problematic behavior
   c. Teaching the child or adolescent replacement behaviors to more appropriately meet their needs
   d. Developing a reinforcement program and set of consequences to manage and support the use of the more appropriate replacement behaviors
   e. All of the above

5. The use of cognitive-behavioral therapy strategies includes:
   a. Used in ASD for depression/mood concerns
   b. To address skill deficits such as social skill weaknesses and for anxiety-related problems
   c. To provide affect education

d. Teaching of an "emotional toolbox" (strategies for handling negative emotions)
e. All of the above

Answers

1. e. All of the above
2. e. All of the above
3. e. a, b and c
4. e. All of the above
5. e. All of the above

Social Challenges and Social Skills Interventions

Michelle Lubetsky, Melissa Smiley Jacobson, and Benjamin L. Handen

Individuals with ASD Have Problems with Social Skill
   Development 274
Social Development Theories 276
Social Motivation 278
Building Social Competence 280
Social Intervention Strategies 282
How to Determine the Appropriate Social Skills Program 290
Summary 292
Further Reading 293
Questions 294
Answers 294

This chapter will provide many clinical recommendations on how to do social skills training and improve social competency in individuals with autism spectrum disorder. Previous chapters have described behavioral, educational, language, and therapeutic approaches from early childhood to adulthood. The primary impairment in ASD is the social and communication areas. Key concepts in ASD such as "theory of mind" and "executive function" deficits will be defined. Examples of social intervention strategies will be shown. Social skills instruction can be provided by a range of trained service providers for children, adolescents, and adults with ASD.

Individuals with ASD Have Problems with Social Skill Development

One of the hallmarks of ASD, as stated in the DSM- IV-TR, is the atypical development of social relatedness. However, it is important to understand the etiology of social skill deficits in order to provide compassionate and competent treatment. Many people with ASD have a combination of strengths and weaknesses that, together, cause a unique range of social skill difficulties.

Importance of teaching social skills

In addition to acquiring social skills with the goal of meeting typical social expectations, gaining social competence has an added benefit for overall physical and emotional health. When individuals are socially connected and have a system of social support, they develop a greater ability to cope with stress. Also, socially competent individuals develop an enhanced sense of communality, which has a positive effect on emotional health (Cohen, 2004).

Social Development Theories

There are currently three well-accepted theories of social development in ASD. Each will be briefly described below.

Theory of Mind deficit

Definition: Difficulty with both awareness and understanding of another individual's perspective. This was later referred to as "mind blindness." Research has shown that most typical children learn this skill by age four, while children with ASD learn this much later, between the ages of nine and 14 years.

The social implications of Theory of Mind deficits (Cumine et al., 1998)

- Difficulty predicting the behavior of others, leading to the avoidance of anxiety-producing situations
- Difficulty reading the intentions of others and understanding motives behind their behavior
- Difficulty explaining their own behavior
- Difficulty understanding emotions, their own and those of others, leading to the appearance of lack of empathy
- Difficulty understanding how their behavior affects how others think or feel, leading to an apparent/perceived lack of conscience or motivation to please others
- Difficulty taking into account what other people know or can be expected to know, leading to the appearance of disorganized cognitive processing
- Inability to read and react to the listener's level of interest in what is being said
- Inability to anticipate what others might think of one's actions
- Inability to deceive or understand deception
- Poor sharing of attention
- Lack of understanding of social interactions that enable the initiation and maintenance of social relationships
- Difficulty in understanding "pretending" and difficulty differentiating fact from fiction

> **Clinical example:** A teenager had a passion for politics and has a particular fascination with the Kennedy family. As a result, this young Midwestern teen began speaking with a Boston accent both at home and in school. This illustrated his Theory of Mind impairment, as he had not thought about how his peers would react to this behavior.

Central Coherence deficit

Definition: Difficulty drawing multiple sources of social and environmental information together, causing problems with understanding the larger contextual picture.

The social implications of Central Coherence deficits (Cumine, et al., 1998)

- Idiosyncratic focus of attention
- Imposition of the individual's own perspective onto others' experiences
- A preference for the known

- Inattentiveness to new tasks
- Difficulty choosing and prioritizing
- Difficulty organizing themselves, materials, and experiences
- Difficulty seeing social connections, thus causing problems with generalizing skills and knowledge
- Lack of compliance with directives that they do not understand

Clinical example: A boy with ASD with an average or above average IQ reads a story and has the ability to report the content to his teacher in detail. However, if the teacher asked him to explain the symbolism of a character's behavior and how it relates to a personal experience, he would be stumped. Therefore, when asked to use the information in new and novel ways, he would be confused and might refuse to comply, as he may have little or no understanding of the story's overall concept.

Executive Functioning deficits

Definition: Difficulty with the following executive functioning skills:
- Planning
- Self monitoring
- The ability to inhibit various social responses
- The ability to express behavioral flexibility
- Processing and expressing information in an organized and fluid manner

The social implications of Executive Functioning deficits (Ozonoff, 1995)

Causes difficulties with the following:
- Perceiving others' emotions
- Imitation of social behaviors
- Pretend play, which is essential to early learning
- Planning, organizing, and prioritizing
- Starting and stopping activities, behaviors, and thoughts

Clinical example: An adolescent is in advanced placement classes in high school. He is fastidious regarding completing all homework assignments on time and correctly. However, he continues to get poor grades. His Executive Functioning deficits are demonstrated by his inability to keep track of when his assignments are due, in addition to where he has placed his work once it has been completed.

Social Motivation

Just as there is a spectrum of autism, there is also a range of social motivation. Some individuals are extremely interested in engaging with their peers,
but struggle to appropriately initiate or maintain social connectedness.
Others with ASD have very little social motivation. These individuals often
report extreme anxiety when engaging with people for a variety of reasons.
For example, it may be difficult to predict how the people around them will
behave and, therefore, individuals on the spectrum may chose to avoid all
anticipated anxiety-provoking social environments.

Caution

Many people assume that a lack of social initiation and reciprocal communication indicates that individuals with ASD lack the desire to engage
in social interaction. On the contrary, many individuals with ASD lack
the skills to be successful socially, yet they desire to be a part of social
relationships (Bellini, 2006).

Building Social Competence

Building Social Competence

Bellini (2006) identifies three specific components of social interactions that need to occur in a balanced manner in order for individuals to have a successful social experience.

Three Components of Social Interactions
- Knowing what to do and how to do it based on understanding another person's perspective
- The ability to regulate responses to one's own emotional state, which may hinder successful social performance
- The execution of the social performance

Individuals with ASD are challenged to coordinate these components. In schools, these components can be integrated into goals within the child's individualized educational plan (IEP).

Reasons for including social skills instruction in an IEP
- A diagnosis of ASD includes a "qualitative impairment in social functioning" (DSM IV-TR), indicating that children with ASD will experience challenges in meeting typical social benchmarks.
- Social competence is a fundamental skill that is necessary for navigating changing environments.
- The breadth of academic skills that an individual may possess will never be recognized if basic social skills are not evident. Practitioners must recognize that academic and social skills are not mutually exclusive; they are mutually dependent.

Methods to teach social skills

Although much research exists to support specific approaches for teaching academics, fewer data are available in the area of social skills instruction. However, it is clear that intervention methodologies must be designed to address the unique difficulties of individuals with ASD. Complicating matters further, characteristics of learners with ASD render traditional social skills curricula ineffective. Lack of insight and concrete thinking are two issues that challenge practitioners to find appropriate materials to teach social competence. The need for direction in teaching social competence has led to the investigation of social skills programs within school settings. A recent meta-analysis of 55 single-subject research studies revealed that "social skills programs for children with autism are largely ineffective" (Bellini, 2007). It is important to note that this research established strict inclusion criteria, eliminating many studies that remain relevant for practice, if not for research.

Bellini points to the need for additional research and indicates that "there is no single intervention strategy that will teach the child with ASD to be successful socially!" (Bellini, 2007). He explains that several strategies, based on behavioral, cognitive, and social-learning theory, and can be effective within a broader individualized plan that includes assessment, implementation, monitoring, and evaluation.

Some of the strategies that warrant consideration include:
- Social narratives
- Social problem solving
- Emotional regulation techniques
- Visual strategies
- Video modeling/video self-modeling (Bellini, 2006; Gray, 2000; Attwood, 2007).
- ABA strategies (which can also be effective when teaching discrete skills such as initiation of conversation, staying on topic, responding to greetings, and others)

Why traditional therapeutic techniques fail

Traditional therapeutic techniques, such as individual psychotherapy, group therapy, and character education, often fail because they are not focused on the unique deficit areas that are common in individuals with ASD. These approaches require the following skills, which represent challenges for individuals with ASD:
- Insight into feelings
- Ability to understand their role and others'
- Ability to communicate experiences, thoughts
- Ability to see connections, generalize
- Understanding of abstract concepts
- Awareness of social context, motivating factors

Social Intervention Strategies

Despite the fact that individuals with a diagnosis of ASD have many common core characteristics, the manner in which these qualities are expressed is unique to the person. This often leaves clinicians confounded about how they should proceed, as one strategy may be successful with one client but may cause significant behavioral problems with another. Therefore, a wide variety of social skill strategies and interventions have been developed to assist clinicians with this task. Some of the more frequently used social intervention strategies are described below.

Social narrative interventions

Definition: A variety of strategies that focus on teaching new social skills and encourage individuals to regulate their behavior through the use of reasonably short sentences or phrases known as *social stories* and *comic strip conversations*. These narratives can then be utilized as a starting place to practice developing social skills via social scripting and role plays.

Examples of social narrative strategies
Social Story (1991, copyright Carol Gray)
A social story explicitly describes the process of a social situation. It not only highlights the actual steps one needs to learn to perform in the social situation effectively, but also focuses on why the skill is needed and how the behavior will directly affect the people and environment around them. When writing a social story, a clinician must utilize a format that includes the following three types of sentences.

Descriptive sentences: These are described as the "backbone" of the social story, and include the answers to the who, what, where, and why of the social situation.
Examples:
1. My name is _____.
2. Often, my mother takes me to the doctor.

Perspective sentences: These express thoughts, feelings, mood or motivation. These statements focus on helping the individual learn how their behavior affects others.
Examples:
1. My mother takes me to the doctor because she cares about me and wants me to be healthy. (motivation)
2. When I go to the doctor, I often feel scared that he will have to do something to me that hurts. (feeling)

Directive sentences: These illustrate the desired positive response that should be demonstrated within the context of the indentified social situation.
Examples:
1. When I am scared, I can ask for a squeeze or my favorite toy,
2. When I hear I am going to the doctor, I can decide what I need to take with me to help me stay calm.

Comic Strip Conversations (1994, copyright Carol Gray)

This technique is used to visually illustrate all aspects of conflict (actions, feelings, thoughts, and intentions) in order to help individuals with ASD identify misunderstandings and misinterpretations that might have occurred during social interactions (see Figure 13.1 below for example).

The main components of comic strip conversations:

- **Word bubbles:** used to illustrate what was actually said
- **Thought bubbles**: used to help the child express his/her perception of what others were thinking
- **Colors:** used to represent feelings (example: red is used for anger)

Social Scripting and Role Play

Social scripting involves creating a specific language-based guide for an iden- tified situation that is to be learned. These scripts are then practiced or role-played. Role play involves the clinician and child assuming the role of those in the scripted situation, thus allowing the child to rehearse the new language.

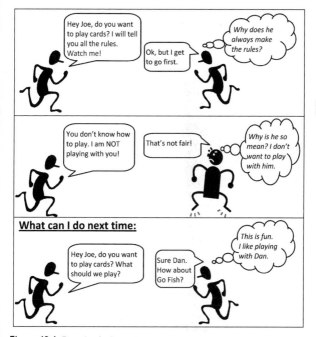

Figure 13.1 Example of a Comic Strip Conversation
Use visuals and words to identify misunderstandings and misinterpretations that might occur during social interactions, and to create strategies to resolve the conflict.

Example of a social script:
When I am opening presents at my birthday party, I will say "thank you", when someone hands me a gift. Then, as I am opening the present, even if it is something I already have or do not particularly want, I will say: "This is great," "I really wanted one of these," or "You know me so well, I really like _____ (the type of toy I just received)."

Social problem solving—social cognition interventions

Teaching a finite set of social skills is not sufficient to develop social competence. Similarly, acquiring a repertoire of skills is not sufficient to navigate complex social situations. The ability to *analyze* social scenarios and select from an array of possible social responses leads to socially competent behavior. Social cognition strategies help to teach children to "think socially" by using a variety of tools to build core skills. Social thinking helps learners become social problem-solvers and teaches them to match the right social response to the situation (Winner, 2005).

ILAUGH Model of social cognition (Winner, 2005)

Definition: Developed to explain the coordination of a wide variety of skills and concepts needed to successfully process information and react appropriately in social situations.

I = Initiation of communication—the ability to begin the social connection with others. More specifically, the skills needed to enter a group or ask for assistance, if needed.

L = Listening with your eyes and brain—how to utilize and coordinate information received both verbally and visually when in a social situation.

A = Abstract and inferential language/communication—learning to understand and utilize the concept that there are two "codes of language": literal/concrete and figurative/illustrative.

U = Understanding of perspective—the ability to understand that other people think differently than oneself.

G = Gestalt processing/getting the big picture—learning that a social situation is not just made up of specific facts but of larger social concepts.

H = Humor and human relatedness–learning to understand and use humor to enhance or correct social situations. Learning how to connect with others is the core to creating meaningful relationships.

Steps of perspective taking (Winner, 2005)
Perspective taking is the ability to consider your own and other people's thoughts and emotions.
Step 1: When two people share a space, they have a little thought about each other.
Step 2: Once they have had a thought about each other, they can evaluate the motivation of the person sharing their space.
Step 3: The people now assess what the other person in their space might be thinking about them.
Step 4: As a result of this information, the people now modulate and monitor their own behaviors in an attempt to maintain how they would like to be perceived.

Social autopsy (La Voie, 1994)

Definition: A visual examination of a social error used to help the individual with ASD determine the cause and the extent of the damage caused by the problematic social interaction. The goal is to help the individual prevent the same or similar social problem from occurring in the future. This is accomplished as the therapist and client write a flowchart of each step that led to the social problem. Then the therapist guides the client to evaluate where he/she could have made different choices at each step that may have changed the outcome of the social situation. The beauty of this technique is that it also illustrates that the clients have many opportunities in the future to change a negative situation (see Figure 13.2 below for example).

Situation Options Consequences Choices Strategy Simulation, or SOCCSS (Roosa, 1995)

Definition: This is a specific formula used to put interpersonal relationships in sequential form in order to help illustrate that everyone has choices and each choice has a consequence. This should be utilized when an individual needs to problem-solve a social situation. The individual is asked to express all of their ideas regarding how to resolve the problem without being guided by the clinician. The therapist then helps the individual evaluate, step by step, the consequences of the solution ideas. The goal is that individual will learn how to identify a solution that leads to a positive outcome (see Figure 13.3 below for example).

Emotional regulation techniques—self-rating scales/thermometers

Definition: As anxiety is often a significant obstacle to successful social interactions, learning how to identify, communicate, and manage anxiety is paramount to the ability to utilize social skill strategies. A "thermometer" chart is one way to develop a personalized self-rating scale, as it provides a concrete description of emotions. One way to create the thermometer is to develop a numerical rating system that incorporates special interests. Using the individual's interests allows the formation of a common language. The scale should rate both positive and negative feelings so it can be utilized in a variety of settings (Buron & Curtis, 2003) See Figures 13.4 and 13.5 below for examples.

Visual supports (Hodgdon, 2001)

Definition: These are strategies that represent information through pictures, images, symbols, or written words to promote communication and understanding. While spoken language is fleeting, visual information is static and remains available to the learner for reference. Interacting with information visually can work in several ways, to help individuals to:

- focus their attention on what is being communicated
- comprehend what is happening, what is not happening, and what is changing
- organize their thoughts and events
- be more engaged

Examples may include daily schedules, mini-schedules, written directions, work systems, choice boards, and communication symbols. See Figure 13.6 for example.

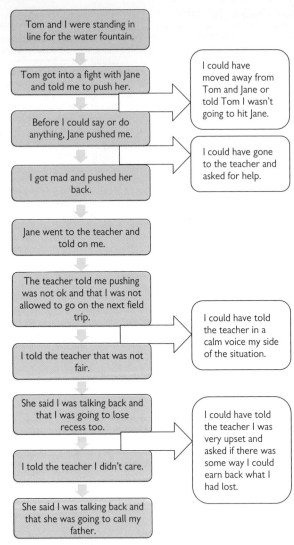

Figure 13.2 Example of Social Autopsy

Problem situation: Jane is spreading a rumor about me that I like Larry

OPTION 1: I could call Jane a liar to her face	OPTION 2: I could never go to school again	OPTION 3: I could practice what I'm going to say before I go to school
• Jane could say something mean back to me	• My parents would get called by the school and other authorities to find out why I'm missing	• Then I would know what I am going to say before I see Jane
• The teacher could see us and Jane can tell the teacher that I started the problem	• The authorities will make my parents send me to school or they will get in trouble	• I would be more prepared to deal with Jane when she teases me again
• The teacher could give me detention for starting a conflict with Jane	• I would not be able to graduate from high school	• Then I can walk away and ignore any more teasing
• Jane will tell all the kids in the class what happened	• Then I would not be able to go to college	• Then I will continue going to school
• The kids will still tease me about liking Larry	• If I don't go to college I can't become an anthropologist	• I would graduate high school
		• I can get into a good college
		• I can become an anthropologist

Figure 13.3 Example of SOCCSS

Rating	Looks like	My scale	I can try
5	Wild	Thunderstorm	Go to quiet spot
4	Mad	Pouring rain	Deep breathing
3	Wiggly	Showers	Ask for a break
2	So-so	Sprinkles	Ask for help
1	Calm	Rainbow	Awesome

Figure 13.4 Example of a Self-Rating Scale
This sample was created by a second-grader. He compared his emotional states to feeling like a rainbow or a thunderstorm. He used the following table to practice labeling emotional states and to practice the techniques to return to calm. He also completed a visual reminder by drawing the components of his scale.

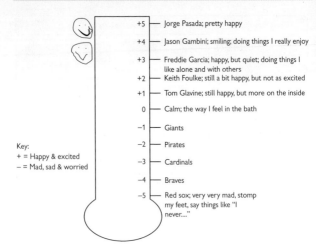

Key:
+ = Happy & excited
– = Mad, sad & worried

Figure 13.5 Example of a Self-Regulation Thermometer

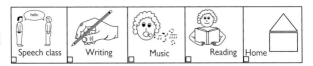

Figure 13.6 Example of a Visual Support

How to Determine the Appropriate Social Skills Program

It is important to note that there is no one right way to work with an individual with ASD who is struggling with social skills development. Therefore, it is helpful to have a basic system for deciding what course of treatment to engage in with the individual and family. Bellini (2006) outlined the following comprehensive five-step model for social skills programming to assist clinicians who are working to identify the strategies that will most effectively address each individual's needs.

Step 1: Social skills assessment

When beginning to evaluate social competence, it is vital to identify the individual's baseline strengths and weaknesses. As a result, a variety of tools should be utilized to assess the individual in the following areas:

- Current social skill aptitude
- Ability to modulate emotional and affective status
- Behavioral functioning level
- Self-concept and perceived competence

When completing the assessment process, it is vital to get information from the individual as well as her or his parents and teachers. The following is a sample list of behavioral and diagnostic scales that include the core areas discussed above.

- Social Responsiveness Scale (SRS)
- Social Communication Questionnaire (SCQ)
- Asperger Syndrome Diagnostic Scale
- Gilliam Asperger's Disorder Scale
- Nisonger Child Behavior Rating Form
- Behavioral Assessment Scale for Children (BASC)
- Adaptive Behavior Assessment System (ABAS-II)
- Multidimensional Self Concept Scale (MSCS)

Step 2: Distinguish between skill acquisition deficits and performance deficits

Skill Acquisition Deficit

Definition: When a person simply does not possess the social skill needed and, therefore, cannot successfully perform the skill.

> **Clinical example:** When an individual with ASD does not understand how to effectively initiate a conversation and, as a result, stands near a group of his peers silently while they discuss his favorite topic.

Performance Deficit

Definition: This occurs when an individual possesses the social skill but does not perform the skill effectively. These are the most challenging for a clinician to evaluate, as they significantly affect the intervention if the skill is present but is not being utilized, rather than never acquired at all.

> **Clinical example**: This person understands how to start a conversation but has difficulty maintaining the social interaction. Therefore, when he attempts to talk about his favorite topic with some peers in his class, he experiences some difficulty. First, he walks up and waits for a break in the conversation before he starts talking. However, he has missed the social cues that his classmates are not interested in what he wants to discuss. As a result, his peers tease him and walk away.

Step 3: Select intervention strategies

As stated earlier, there is no one intervention strategy that will teach successful social competence. However, it is possible to identify effective strategies to address each individual's specific needs.

> A good guide when selecting an intervention strategy is to answer the following questions:
> - What skills will be targeted?
> - Does the strategy match the type of skill deficit?
> - What is the individual's developmental level?
> - What is the strategy or logic for using the intervention?
> - What components of the social interaction skills does it address?

Step 4: Time to implement the intervention

After the clinician identifies the intervention strategy, it is time to determine the format of the intervention program. After learning about the individual, the clinician will evaluate and decide if the individual would benefit from individual or a group clinical experience. Some interventions are best implemented in a classroom or other social environment.

The following are other items to consider and plan for when putting a social skills program into action:
- Training the team
- Selecting peer models
- Selecting materials and resources
- Determining when and where it will occur
- Developing a schedule

Step 5: Evaluate and monitor progress

The final step to a comprehensive social skills development program is monitoring the individual's progress. It is vital that every social skills curriculum be reviewed regularly in order to make the changes needed to positively impact treatment outcome. This can be done through a variety of data collection methods, including:
- Observational data collection, such as frequency recording, duration, and time sampling
- Interviews with parents and teachers
- Use of pre- and post-rating scales

> **Key Fact Box: Helpful Hints for Professionals Providing Social Skills Instruction**
>
> The following points can greatly affect the outcome of social skills intervention.
> - The activities used to teach social skills should incorporate each individual's unique areas of interest. The clinician can then expand social skills development to build new social repertoires.
> - The environment in which teaching occurs should be a place where the individual can be calm. It is vital to reduce anxiety in order to optimize performance and reduce possible behavioral issues.
> - Social skills training should include a balance of directive and facilitative interaction techniques which promote clear instruction, opportunities for practice, and a respectful partnership.
> - It is important not to rely solely on verbal communication. Teaching individuals to pay attention to non-verbal cues will enhance their success in untangling social confusion.
> - As social skills development may be intuitive for clinicians, it is easy to make learning objectives too complex. Develop a plan with concise, simple goals and be cautious of the tendency to address too many new skills at once.
> - Ultimately, the best method for generalizing skills and promoting success is to develop treatment goals that are meaningful to the individual and that afford him or her greater opportunities.

Summary

Social skills deficits are rooted in social learning theory and are the hallmark of an individual with ASD. When these challenges are significant, they can lead to misunderstandings that often trigger anxiety, frustration, anger, or even inappropriate social behavior. A number of instruction and cognitive strategies are available to minimize these potential problems.

Social skills interventions must begin with assessment and should be interactive for individuals to comprehend the material. Addressing social skills deficits can be included in a student's IEP as well as via community-based activities. This is an area that cannot simply be taught for a few minutes a week. Instead, instruction in social skills should be included in as many settings and situations as possible. Just like learning any new skill, progress toward meaningful goals should be monitored and evaluated. As individuals with ASD gain social competence, they may become more socially connected and develop their own system of social support.

Further Reading

1. Attwood, T. (2007). *The complete guide to Asperger's syndrome.* London: Jessica Kingsley Publishers.

2. Baker, J. (2003). *Social skills training for children and adolescents with Asperger syndrome and social-communication problems.* Shawnee Mission, KS: Autism Asperger Publishing Company.

3. Bellini, S. (2006). *Building social relationships.* Shawnee Mission, KS: Autism Asperger Publishing Company.

4. Buron, K. D., & Curtis, M. (2003). *The incredible 5-point scale–Assisting students with Autism Spectrum Disorder in understanding social interactions and controlling their emotional responses.* Shawnee Mission, KS: Autism Asperger Publishing Company.

5. Cohen, S. (2004). Social relationships and health. *American Psychologist, 59,* 676–684.

6. Cumine, V., Leach, J., & Stevenson, G. (1998). *Asperger Syndrome: A practical guide for teachers.* London: David Falton Publishers.

7. Gray, C. (2000). *The new social story book.* Arlington, TX: Future Horizons.

8. Gray, C. (1998). Social stories and comic strip conversation with students with Asperger syndrome and high functioning autism. In E. Schopler, G. B. Mesibov, & L. J. Kunce (Eds.), *Asperger syndrome or high functioning autism* (167–198). New York: Plenum Press.

9. The Gray Center for Social Learning and Understanding: Retrieved October 2010, from http://www.thegraycenter.org/.

10. Hodgdon, L. A. (2001). *Visual strategies for improving communication: Practical supports for school and home.* Troy, MI: QuirkRoberts Publishing.

11. Lavoie, R. D. (1994). *Learning disabilities and social skills, with Richard Lavoie: Last one picked . . . First one picked on* [Video and Teacher's Guide]. Available from PBS Video, 1320 Braddock Place, Alexandria, VA 22314-1698.

12. Ozonoff, S., & Miller, J. N. (1995). Teaching theory of mind: a new approach to social skills training for individuals with autism. *Journal of Autism and Developmental Disorders, 25*(4): 415–33.

13. Roosa, J. B. (1995). *Men on the move: Competence and cooperation "conflict resolution and beyond."* Kansas City, MO: Author.

14. Winner, M.G. (2005). *Think social! A social thinking curriculum for school-age students.* San Jose CA: Think Social Publishing.

15. Michelle Garcia. Winner–Social Thinking: Retrieved October 2010, from www.socialthinking.com.

Questions

1. Which theory describes the individual with ASD as having difficulty with: reading the intentions of others, understanding emotions, and responding to a listener's level of interest?
   a. Central coherence deficit
   b. Executive function deficit
   c. Theory of Mind deficit
   d. Social competence deficit

2. Individuals with ASD lack the desire to engage in social interaction.
   a. True
   b. False

3. Which provides an example of a social narrative?
   a. Writing a story to describe how to perform in a social situation
   b. Writing in a personal journal to describe your feelings
   c. Writing a story illustrating a conflict to help identify misunderstandings in social situations
   d. a & c

4. What components are important in the development of a social skills program?
   a. Using data collection to evaluate and monitor progress.
   b. Conducting a social skills assessment prior to implementing interventions
   c. Determining if there is a performance or an acquisition deficit
   d. All of the above

5. What is the key component in effective social skill instruction?
   a. Social skills should be taught exclusively in a one-to-one clinical setting
   b. Consider the client's unique areas of interest as a means to engage them
   c. Social skills training should include planned social opportunities that are meaningful to the client
   d. b & c

Answers

1. c. Theory of Mind deficit
2. b. False
3. d. a & c
4. d. All of the above
5. d. b & c

Pharmacological Interventions

**Benjamin L. Handen, Tiberiu Bodea,
Rameshwari V. Tumuluru, and
Martin J. Lubetsky**

Medications for Symptoms of Attention Deficit
  Hyperactivity Disorder *298*
Antipsychotic Medications in ASD *306*
Antidepressant Medications in ASD *310*
Mood Stabilizers/Antiepileptic drugs (AEDs) in ASD *316*
Sleep Medications in ASD *317*
Polypharmacy in ASD *318*
Complementary Alternative Medicine (CAM)
  Treatments *318*
Summary *319*
Further Reading *320*
Questions *322*
Answers *323*

Previous chapters have focused on diagnosis, assessment, various interventions from early childhood to adult. This chapter will review a selection of the more common medications used in individuals with ASD:

Medications for symptoms of attention deficit hyperactivity disorder:
a. Stimulants
b. Atomoxetine (Strattera)
c. Alpha-2-adrenergic receptor agonists
Antipsychotic medications
Antidepressant medications
Mood stabilizers/antiepileptic drugs (AEDs)
Sleep medications
Polypharmacy
Complementary Alternative Medicine (CAM) Treatments

In working with children, adolescents, and adults with ASD, medications are often used for reduction of specific target symptoms. The symptoms may be specific target behaviors in ASD such as irritability, self-injurious behavior, and aggression. Only two medications, risperidone and aripiprazole, have received Food and Drug Administration approval to treat these target behaviors in ASD. When medications are used for indications other than what they received FDA approval for, such use is considered "off-label." Also, individuals with ASD may have symptoms of a comorbid DSM Axis I disorder, such as the inattention, distractibility, hyperactivity, and impulsivity of attention deficit hyperactivity disorder (ADHD), depression, anxiety, mania, or psychotic disorder. Then medication choices are based on these comorbid psychiatric disorders rather than specifically for ASD. People with ASD may be more sensitive to dosing and side effects.

It is not uncommon to use more than one medication to target ASD symptoms and/or comorbid disorders. Complementary and alternative medicine approaches have also been tried with some children with ASD, but the efficacy research is very limited. It is important to remember that the child or adult with ASD should also be receiving appropriate psychosocial treatment, including educational and behavioral health services (many of which are described elsewhere in this book). Also, as with the use of any pharmacological treatment, it is expected that the prescribing clinician has also examined and addressed other possible factors (e.g., medical issues, new school, sleep issues, changes in work or home, etc.) that can impact behavior and might explain the reported symptoms.

Medications for Symptoms of Attention Deficit Hyperactivity Disorder

Symptoms associated with attention deficit hyperactivity disorder, such as inattention, distractibility, hyperactivity, and impulsivity, are the most frequently reported concern among children with ASD. For example, in a recent survey involving a non-clinical sample of 487 children with ASD, 41% of parents and 29% of teachers reported that their children/students displayed moderate to severe hyperactivity (Lecavalier et al., 2006). In addition, recent data on medication prescribing rates also indicate that behaviors associated with ADHD are the most commonly treated target symptom among children with ASD. Results of a survey conducted by Witwer and Lecavalier (2005) found that 24% of a non-referred sample of 352 school-age children with ASD had been prescribed stimulant medication in the past year. Despite the fact that a significant number of children with ASD exhibit and are treated for ADHD symptoms, DSM-IV-TR (APA, 2000) currently excludes a co-occurring diagnosis of ADHD and ASD. However, it is possible that the upcoming revised DSM-5 may eliminate this restriction.

While the approach for addressing ADHD symptoms in the ASD population is similar to that of typically developing children, the data in support of pharmacological treatment in ASD is more limited and equivocal. However, there have been several controlled trials that provide some guidance in treating ADHD symptoms in this population.

In general, studies of pharmacological treatment have found the following for children with ASD:

- Response rates tend to be lower than among typically developing children,
- Symptom improvement is often less robust,
- Side effects are more frequently reported, and
- Significantly more children are unable to tolerate commonly prescribed medications.

Therefore, the prescribing clinician should take an approach in which:
- Starting doses are lower and the titration is slower than would typically occur
- The child with ASD should also be receiving appropriate psychosocial treatment, including educational and behavioral health services
- As with the use of any pharmacological treatment, it is expected that the prescribing clinician has also examined and addressed other possible factors (e.g., medical issues, new school, sleep issues, etc.) that can impact behavior and might explain the reported symptoms
- As with typically developing children, hyperactivity, impulsivity, and inattention would be expected to be long-standing and present in multiple settings and situations

Stimulant medications
Short-acting (~2 to 3 times/day):
- methylphenidate (Ritalin, Metadate)
- dexmethylphenidate (Focalin)
- dextroamphetamine (Dexedrine)
- mixed amphetamine salts (Adderall)
Long-acting (~1 time/day):
- methylphenidate (Concerta)
- Metadate CD
- Ritalin LA
- Focalin XR
- Adderall XR
- methylphenidate (Daytrana patch)
- lisdexamfetamine dimesylate (Vyvanse)
Non-stimulant medications
- atomoxetine (Strattera)
Alpha-2-adrenergic receptor agonist medications
- clonidine (Catapres)
- guanfacine (Tenex)
- guanfacine extended-release (Intuniv)
- clonidine hydrochloride extended-release (Kapvay)

The next section will summarize the research findings for treating ADHD symptoms in ASD.

a. Stimulants

Stimulants remain that first-line option for treating ADHD symptoms in ASD. While large-scale studies of typically developing children with ADHD, such as the Multimodal Treatment Study for Children with ADHD (MTA), have found response rates to stimulants of around 77% (Greenhill et al., 2007), stimulants appear to be considerably less efficacious in treating ASD. While the preceding box lists most of the currently available stimulants, research among children with ASD has tended to be limited to methylphenidate (MPH) (although there is no reason to assume similar response rates for other stimulants). Stimulants work by blocking the reuptake of norephinephrine and dopamine. Since 1995, there have been three double-blind, placebo-controlled trials of MPH in ASD, all indicating that MPH can be efficacious in this population (Handen et al., 2000; Quintana et al., 1995; Autism RUPP 2005). An open-label, retrospective study of 195 children with ASD who had been treated with stimulants found only a 24.6% response rate to the first drug choice and an even smaller rate of response when patients were prescribed an alternative stimulant (Stigler et al., 2004).

Children with Asperger's disorder tended to respond better than children diagnosed with PDD, NOS, or autistic disorder, and high rates of side effects were noted. Conversely, a second recent open-label study comparing 113 typically developing children with ADHD and 61 children with ASD and ADHD symptoms found response rates of 63% and 51%

respectively (based upon a retrospective Clinical Global Impressions Improvement scale—Santosh et al., 2006).

> The largest and most recent controlled trial was a crossover study of MPH involving 72 children, ages five to 14 years, with ASD (Autism RUPP, 2005). Twice-daily doses (8:00 a.m., noon) of low, medium, and high (approximated to 0.125, 0.25, and 0.5 mg/kg per dose) were used, along with a third dose (4:00 p.m.) that was approximately half of the earlier doses. The doses ranged from 7.5 mg/day to 50 mg/day in divided doses. Using a criteria of a "1" or "2" rating on the Clinical Global Impressions Improvement Scale *and* a >25% decrease on *both* parent and teacher Hyperactivity subscales (or a >30% decrease on *either* the parent or teacher-completed Hyperactivity subscale) of the Aberrant Behavior Checklist,
> - 49% of study participants were labeled as responders.
> - 18% of subjects were discontinued from the trial due to adverse events.
>
> Treatment response was unrelated to IQ and ASD diagnostic category. As with all children, there should be an exam and a review of personal and family history for relevant cardiac events prior to starting stimulant treatment.

b. Atomoxetine (Strattera)

Atomoxetine (ATX) was approved by the FDA in 2002 as an alternative to stimulants for the treatment of ADHD in individuals over six years of age. It is generally considered to be a second-line alternative for children who are stimulant nonresponders or who have had side effects that preclude the use of this class of medication. Prescribed once per day, this agent works via blocking the reuptake of norepinephrine (Pliszka, 2005). ATX efficacy among typically developing children is supported by a number of large, controlled, multicenter trials. It appears to be well tolerated with response rates similar to those of immediate-release MPH.

As far as we aware, research support for ATX in the treatment of ADHD

> - However, studies have shown that ATX efficacy does not match that of extended-release mixed amphetamine salts (Adderall XR) or osmotically released MPH (Concerta); (see review by Garnock-Jones & Keating, 2009).

symptoms in ASD is limited to one open-label report, two prospective open-label studies, and one, relatively small double-blind, crossover study (Jou et al., 2005; Troost et al., 2006; Posey et al., 2006; Arnold et al., 2006). Both open-label studies included children with ASD who were not taking concomitant medications (or discontinued medications prior to beginning the trial), and used a flexible dosing schedule. The first, conducted by Troost and colleagues (2006), included 12 children (ages six to 14 years) with ASD and borderline to normal intellectual functioning. Dependent measures included the Clinical Global Impressions (CGI) Severity Scale for ADHD symptoms, and the Hyperactivity subscale and ADHD Index of the Conners' Parent Rating Scale–Revised. While statistically significant decreases were noted on all three measures, gastrointestinal side effects led to five subjects' discontinuing the trial. Doses ranged from 17.5 to 80 mg per day.

The second prospective trial was conducted by Posey and colleagues (2006) and included 17 subjects (ages six to 17 years) with ASD. Two subjects discontinued the trial due to increased irritability and two due to their inability to swallow pills. Statistically significant decreases were noted on a Parent and Teacher–completed SNAP-IV Hyperactivity-Impulsivity subscale (www.adhd.net) and the Hyperactivity subscale of the Aberrant Behavior Checklist (Aman, 1985). The mean final dose across subjects was 1.2 mg per day. Neither study reported an overall response rate.

Finally, Arnold and colleagues (2006) conducted a double-blind, placebo-controlled, crossover study of ATX with a sample of 16 children with ASD (ages five to 15 years). Concomitant medications were not discontinued (except β-blockers and systemic drugs), as long as doses had been stable and there were no changes planned during the course of the trial. The two study conditions lasted six weeks each, involving a three-week titration period. Final doses ranged from 20 mg to 100 mg (mean highest dose = 44.2 ± 21.9 mg/day). Statistically significant gains were noted on a Parent ABC Hyperactivity subscale and a DSM-IV-based ADHD rating scale (ABC Hyperactivity: 24.69 to 19.31; DSM-IV Hyperactivity: 17.31 to 10.40). However, improvement on a DSM-IV-based Inattention rating scale failed to be statistically significant. Nine subjects were deemed ATX responders (based upon a >25% improvement on the ABC-H subscale and a score of "1" or "2" on the CGI-I), and four were placebo responders. Hence, there was an overall response rate of around 50% with a placebo response rate of 25%. A high rate of gastrointestinal problems and fatigue was reported among subjects. One child was removed at week four from the active medication arm of the trial following a severe adverse event. ATX has some similarities to antidepressants, and the child should be monitored for any increased risk of suicidal ideation (FDA Medication Guide, 2009).

c. Alpha-2-adrenergic receptor agonists

Prescribed alone and in combination with stimulants, alpha-2-adrenergic agonists (clonidine and guanfacine) have a long history of use in the treatment of ADHD. Their mechanism of action involves inhibition of the locus coeruleus, which appears to decrease norepinephrine function and reduce hyperactivity. Attention may also be improved via changes in both the serotonergic and dopaminergic systems (Poncin & Scahill, 2007; Werry & Aman, 1999). FDA-approved as anti-hypertensive medications:

- Clonidine and guanfacine use for the treatment of ADHD symptoms is off-label. (Similarly, clonidine has long been used as an off-label treatment for Tourette's syndrome.)
- Guanfacine XR (GXR: Intuniv) recently received FDA approval as a monotherapy for treatment of ADHD in children ages six to 17 years (however, short-acting guanfacine use for ADHD remains off-label).

While no studies have been published with GXR involving children with ASD, two large randomized trials have shown GXR to be efficacious for treatment of ADHD among typically developing children (Biederman et al., 2008; Salee et al., 2009). Short acting guanfacine has a longer duration of action and is less sedating than clonidine.

Over the past two decades, there have been a few small trials of clonidine (Catapres) and guanfacine (Tenex) for the treatment of ADHD symptoms in ASD. Among the earlier trials, a double-blind, placebo-controlled study by Jaselskis and colleagues (1992) involved a crossover trial of clonidine in a sample of eight children diagnosed with ASD (ages 2.8 to 8.1 years). Doses were given three times a day and were gradually titrated during the first two weeks of treatment. After being held steady for four weeks, the medication was tapered and the six-week crossover arm begun. Doses ranged from 0.15–0.20 mg/day. Statistically significant decreases on a teacher-completed ABC Hyperactivity subscale (placebo, 28.4 ± 10.8; clonidine 24.9 ± 11.1) and Connors Parent-Teacher Questionnaire (placebo = 12.9 ± 5.5; clonidine = 10.1 ± 4.9) were noted.

- The clinical significance of the changes remains questionable.
- Side effects, such as hypotension and drowsiness, led to doses' being decreased for three subjects.

A retrospective chart review of 80 children and adolescents with ASD (ages three to 18 years of age) found only 23.8% to be responders (Posey et al., 2004). However, target symptoms included not only ADHD symptoms, but insomnia and tics. Over 30% of patients complained of transient sedation, and approximately 15% of patients reported increased irritability, nocturnal enuresis, headache, or constipation. A prospective, open-label study of guanfacine was conducted by Scahill and colleagues (2006) involving 25 children (ages three to nine years) with ASD who had failed a prior MPH trial. Medication doses were gradually increased over a five-week period to a maximum of 3.0 mg/day (in two to three divided doses) and then remained stable for an additional three weeks.

- Parent ratings were the most improved (36% decrease on the SNAP-IV, 39% decrease on the ABC Hyperactivity subscale), with more modest decreases noted on the teacher SNAP-IV (18%) and ABC (27%).
- Increased irritability led to three subjects' discontinuing the trial, and a number of subjects had their guanfacine doses adjusted due to irritability, sedation, or sleep disturbance.

Finally, Handen and colleagues (2008) conducted a double blind, placebo-controlled crossover trial of guanfacine in 11 children (ages five to nine years) with intellectual disability (n = 4) and/or ASD (n = 7). Seven of the subjects were taking concomitant medications (held constant during the trial). Eight subjects were titrated to the maximum dose of 1 mg, three times per day. The remaining three subjects received doses ranging from 1.0 to 2.5 mg/day as a result of side effects. Four of the seven subjects with ASD were "medication responders," based upon a decrease of ≥50% on the parent and teacher ABC Hyperactivity subscale. Guanfacine side effects included fatigue, lethargy, diarrhea, social withdrawal, and constipation.

Atypical antipsychotics (see Section below)—For patients with ASD who fail to respond to the more traditional pharmacological treatment options for ADHD symptoms, atypical antipsychotics are the class of medications with the most empirical support for successfully treating selected behavioral symptoms in ASD. There is some evidence that both irritability and ADHD symptoms are similarly improved (the specific effects on symptoms of irritability are covered later in this chapter).

The first large-scale study of risperidone in ASD was published in 2002 in the *New England Journal of Medicine* (McCracken et al., 2002). In that paper, a mean decrease of 46.5% was noted on the ABC Hyperactivity subscale for subjects on risperidone (N = 49) in comparison to a 14.5% decrease for placebo (N = 52). Doses ranged from 0.5 to 3.5 mg/day. A subsequent multicenter Canadian trial of risperidone in ASD (N = 79) documented a mean decrease of 54.6% on the ABC Hyperactivity subscale for those prescribed risperidone versus 23.9% for those on placebo (Shea et al., 2004). Doses for the Canadian trial ranged from 0.01 to 0.06 mg/kg/day (mean 1.17 mg). Finally, a recently published multicenter trial of aripiprazole documented significant decreases on the Hyperactivity subscale of the ABC (using fixed doses of 5, 10, and 15 mg/day) in comparison to placebo (Marcus et al., 2009).

- Atypical antipsychotics should probably be reserved for children with comorbid irritability, aggression, and/or self-injurious behavior, and whose hyperactivity and impulsivity are severe and/or extremely dangerous.
- Two medications, risperidone (Risperdal) and aripiprazole (Abilify), are approved by the U.S. Food and Drug Administration for treatment of irritability in ASD.
- Both antipsychotics have been shown to be efficacious in treating irritability in large, multicenter trials, which have included measures of ADHD symptoms.

Summary—Medications for symptoms of attention deficit hyperactivity disorder

In summary, there is considerable support for the treatment of ADHD in the typically developing population. However, the extant literature is more limited in children with ASD. This limitation may be explained by various factors, including the exclusion of children with ASD from most large studies, the exclusion of ADHD as a comorbid disorder for children with ASD (per DSM-IV-TR guidelines), and earlier reports that the use of stimulants with this population was contraindicated. Despite this, there has been more interest in the treatment of overactivity and inattention in individuals with ASD. However, the rate and robustness of treatment response may be less than that seen among typically developing children. Side effects are also more likely to occur, and questions remain regarding possible cardiac side effects with the use of stimulants and ATX, as well as possible increased suicidal ideation with ATX (antidepressant warnings) for both the typical and ASD population.

- The first line of treatment should be with the use of stimulant medication, where at least three double-blind, placebo-controlled trials have been conducted.
- The support for alternative options, such as ATX, is limited to a handful of open-label studies and a single double-blind, placebo-controlled trial.
- The use of alpha-2 agonists also has some research support in ASD, with a group of small, double-blind trials having been conducted.
- Once the use of stimulants, ATX, and alpha-2 agonists are found to not be efficacious for an individual with ASD who has ADHD symptoms,

there is support for the use of risperidone or aripiprazole for irritability, aggression, or self-injurious behavior in ASD. Secondary effects on measures of hyperactivity were also robust. This option should be reserved for individuals who present with symptoms of irritability, aggression, self-injurious behavior, and severe hyperactivity and impulsivity that has not responded to other pharmacological treatment (see Section below).

Finally, there is limited support at this time for the use of antimanics, naltrexone, or amantadine for the treatment of ADHD. Some increasing interest in the use of cognitive enhancing agents, such as cholinesterase inhibitors, may lead to additional data on the effects of this class of drugs on activity and attention.

Key Fact Box Summary of Treatment Options for ADHD Symptoms in ASD
- *Stimulants*: First-line treatment option. Response rates of <49%, with 18% unable to tolerate medication.
- *Atomoxetine*: Second-line treatment option. Response rates of <50%; data are more limited.
- *Alpha-2-adrenergics*: Second- or third-line treatment option. Response rates of <50%; data are more limited.
- *Atypical antipsychotics*: Third-line treatment option. Response rates 60%, but reserved for children with irritability, aggression, self-injurious behavior, and severe dangerousness with ADHD symptoms (see Section II below).

Antipsychotic Medications in ASD

Antipsychotic medication has been used more frequently in treating patients with ASD, especially for aggression. There has been limited evidence on the use of medication treatment for the core features of ASD, which include impairments in social relatedness and language (i.e., changes in Aberrant Behavior Checklist subscales). However, various medications have been used to treat behavioral symptoms in ASD, including poor attention, hyperactivity, repetitive/stereotypic behavior, aggression, impulsivity and self-injurious behavior. The following discussion will focus on the use of atypical antipsychotic agents in ASD.

Selected antipsychotic medications have been approved for use in the treatment of psychoses as well as mania in adults and adolescents.

There are two types of antipsychotics: *typical* or *conventional*, such as haloperidol (Haldol), thioridazine (Mellaril), and chlorpromazine (Thorazine);

> More recently, two atypical antipsychotic agents have been FDA-approved for use in children and adolescents with ASD (risperidone and aripiprazole).

and *atypical* antipsychotics which include risperidone (Risperdal) and aripiprazole (Abilify).

Mechanism of Action: Conventional antipsychotic agents block dopamine receptors, which are thought to be their primary mechanism of action. Atypical antipsychotic agents block dopamine receptors but also block serotonin receptors, which may play a role in their therapeutic and side-effect profile.

Early studies by Campbell and colleagues in the 1970s and 1980s supported the use of haloperidol in children with autism (Campbell et al.,1978; Anderson et al.,1984; Cohen et al., 1980; Perry et al., 1989), which indicated that haloperidol was effective in decreasing activity level, irritability, and stereotypies in children with autism. However, sedation and extra-pyramidal symptoms (EPS) such as dyskinesia were serious side effects. The atypical antipsychotic agents presented a better side-effect profile, making them more attractive for use in children with ASD. Several studies have been conducted detailing the use of atypical antipsychotic agents in ASD.

> Typical antipsychotic medications
> - haloperidol (Haldol)
> - thioridazine (Mellaril)
> - chlorpromazine (Thorazine)
>
> Atypical antipsychotic medications
> - risperidone (Risperdal)
> - aripiprazole (Abilify)
> - Olanzapine (Zyprexa)
> - quetiapine (Seroquel)
> - ziprasidone (Geodon)
> - clozapine (Clozaril)

Risperidone (Risperdal)

Risperidone is an atypical antipsychotic that was approved for use in 1993. Risperidone has a high affinity for serotonin receptors, dopamine receptors, Alpha-1 receptors, and H-1 histamine receptors, and a slight affinity to the muscarinic receptors. The use of risperidone in treating children with ASD has been well studied. Targeted symptoms include irritability, aggression, hyperactivity, and self-injurious and ritualistic behaviors. A number of open-label and case reports detailing the use of risperidone were published. The first double-blind placebo-controlled study of risperidone in ASD was conducted by McDougle and colleagues in 1998. In this study of 31 adults, risperidone was shown to be more effective than placebo, with somnolence being the most common side effect.

The largest study conducted was the RUPP Autism Network study, a double-blind placebo-controlled multi-center study in children with ASD (McCracken et al., 2002). Irritability, aggression and self-injurious behavior were targeted in n=101 subjects. Children were randomly assigned to either placebo or active medication. A total of 69.4% of the children assigned to risperidone were noted to be "responders" with significant decrease in symptoms of irritability.

During the placebo-discontinuation phase of the RUPP study, most of the children who were gradually switched to placebo from the active drug relapsed, which further supported the efficacy of active medication risperidone in targeting these specific behavioral symptoms in ASD.

The main side effects noted following these studies were sedation and weight gain. The most common adverse events with risperidone that occurred in these studies included: somnolence, increase in appetite, fatigue, upper respiratory tract infection, increase in saliva, constipation, dry mouth, tremor, muscle stiffness, dizziness, involuntary movements, repetitive behavior, rapid heartbeat, confusion, and increase in weight; as well as possible hyperprolactinemia, which could result in gynecomastia or galactorrhea. In the RUPP study, the dose range was 0.5–3.5 mg per day with a mean of 1.8 mg per day. Dose titration should be individualized and cautious, with a focus on target symptoms and side effects.

> Risperidone received FDA approval on October 10, 2006 for the treatment of irritability associated with autistic disorder, including symptoms of aggression, deliberate self-injury, temper tantrums, and quickly changing moods in children and adolescents aged five to 16 years. This is the first time the FDA has approved any medication for use in children and adolescents with ASD.

Aripiprazole (Abilify)

Aripiprazole is a partial dopamine agonist and a serotonin antagonist. In a case series reported by Stigler and colleagues, five patients who received aripiprazole showed significant improvement in symptoms of aggression, self injury, and irritability. The main side effect noted in this study was transient sedation. Owen, Sikich, and colleagues (2009) reported the results of a double-blind placebo-controlled study using aripiprazole in n=98 children ages six to 17 years. In this study, the children assigned the active drug showed a significant decrease in irritability. The main side effect noted was sedation followed by extrapyramidal side effects. Marcus, Owen, and colleagues (2009) reported the results of a double-blind placebo-controlled study using aripiprazole in n=218 children ages six to 17 years. In this study, the children assigned the active drug showed a significant decrease in irritability. Dose titration should be individualized and cautious, with a focus on target symptoms and side effects. This study suggested a starting dose of 2 mg per day, then increasing to 5 mg per day, with subsequent increases to 10 or 15 mg per day if needed. Dose adjustment of up to 5 mg per day at a time should occur gradually at intervals of one week or greater.

> Aripiprazole received FDA approval on November 24, 2009, for the treatment of irritability associated with autistic disorder, including symptoms of aggression towards others, deliberate self-injurious behavior, temper tantrums, and quickly changing moods in children and adolescents aged 6 to 17 years. This was the second time the FDA has approved a medication for use in children and adolescents with ASD.

Olanzapine (Zyprexa), quetiapine, ziprasidone, and clozapine

Olanzapine has a high affinity for dopamine, serotonin, alpha-1, histaminic, and muscarinic receptors. Several open-label studies have been reported with the use of olanzapine. However, sedation, increased appetite, and weight gain appear to be significant side effects, despite its improvement in reducing symptoms such as aggression, hyperactivity, and irritability.

Open-label reports have been published describing the use of quetiapine (Seroquel) and ziprasidone (Geodon).

The only published reports on the use of clozapine (Clozaril) are case reports. The lack of published studies may be a reflection of its side-effect profile, which includes development of seizures at a high dose, as well as the development of agranulocytosis, requiring the need for regular venipuncture for lab testing, which may be difficult in individuals with ASD.

Potential side effects of antipsychotic medications

The extant literature supports the use of both typical and atypical antipsychotics. However, the same literature supports the use of atypicals over the typical or conventional, due to a better side-effect profile. They should be used with caution. All atypical antipsychotics can cause significant increases in appetite and weight gain. In addition, the use of risperidone (and olanzapine at higher doses) can lead to increase in prolactin, which can cause galactorrhea, amenorrhea, and gynecomastia. Fatigue, sedation, dizziness, drooling, and EPS can occur with all antipsychotics, including aripiprazole. Tardive dyskinesia can potentially occur with atypical antipsychotics, and monitoring for abnormal movements should be performed periodically. Long-term data are limited, but a recent meta-analysis study of risperidone showed that the annual rate of tardive dyskinesia is approximately 0.3% (Correll, 2007). Clozapine use may result in seizures as well as life-threatening agranulocytosis (which requires frequent blood draws). Neuroleptic malignant syndrome is a rare but potentially serious side effect that can occur with typical and atypical antipsychotics. Acute onset of fever, confusion, and rigidity, and signs of autonomic activation (sweating, tachycardia, etc.) require emergent evaluation to determine whether neuroleptic malignant syndrome is present.

Though effective, antipsychotic medication must be used with caution in children, adolescents, and adults with ASD. Due to the risk of increased appetite, weight gain, and metabolic changes that could impact glucose metabolism, it is *recommended* to monitor baseline and subsequent measures, including, but not limited to, the following: height, weight, BMI (body mass index—table found on the CDC website); and laboratory measures including a fasting serum glucose and a fasting lipid profile. Given the possibility of medication-induced weight gain, it is important to educate parents and patients about healthy eating, exercise, monitoring food intake, and behavior management plans.

Summary—Use of antipsychotic medications in ASD

Risperidone and aripiprazole received FDA approval for the treatment of irritability associated with autistic disorder, including symptoms of aggression, deliberate self-injury, temper tantrums, and quickly changing moods in children and adolescents. Though effective, antipsychotic medication must be used with caution in children, adolescents, and adults with ASD, due to the risk of increased appetite, weight gain, and metabolic changes that could impact glucose metabolism.

Antidepressant Medications in ASD

Antidepressants have been studied as a possible pharmacological intervention for depression and anxiety symptoms and obsessive-compulsive behaviors in individuals with ASD who are diagnosed with these DSM psychiatric disorders. There have been several studies evaluating the efficacy of antidepressants in treating repetitive, perseverative, and ritualistic (compulsive-like) behaviors in individuals with ASD. In addition, the child, adolescent, or adult should be monitored for any increased risk of suicidal ideation (FDA Medication Guide, 2009). The following section will focus on the use of antidepressants in individuals with ASD.

Selective serotonin reuptake inhibitors (SSRIs)

The use of SSRIs has been studied as a possible psychopharmacological intervention for mood and anxiety symptoms and compulsive-like behaviors among individuals with ASD. There have also been several studies evaluating the efficacy of SSRIs in treating repetitive behaviors in individuals with ASD. These repetitive, ritualistic behaviors can be understood as either intrinsic to the condition, or a secondary adaptation, or sometimes as a manifestation of a coexisting OCD. The Interactive Autism Network (IAN) reported in 2009 that, out of 5,174 children diagnosed with ASD, 12.2% of them are taking antidepressant medication. Among them, the following three SSRIs were the most commonly prescribed: fluoxetine (Prozac) 3.5%, sertraline (Zoloft) 3.0%, and escitalopram (Lexapro) 1.4%.

Antidepressant Medications

Selective Serotonin Reuptake Inhibitor (SSRIs)
- fluoxetine (Prozac)
- sertraline (Zoloft)
- escitalopram (Lexapro)
- citalopram (Celexa)
- fluvoxamine (Luvox)

Tricyclic antidepressant
- clomipramine (Anafranil)

Serotonin–Norepinephrine Reuptake Inhibitor (SNRI)
- venlafaxine (Effexor)

Noradrenergic and Specific Serotonergic Antidepressant (NaSSA)
- mirtazapine (Remeron)

Fluoxetine (Prozac)

Class: SSRI

Fluoxetine and its active metabolite norfluoxetine have a slow elimination from the body that distinguishes it from other antidepressants.

A double-blind, placebo-controlled study has been conducted for fluoxetine in children with ASD (Hollander et al., 2005). This study examined the efficacy of liquid fluoxetine in the treatment of repetitive behaviors in childhood and adolescent ASD. Forty-five patients with ASD were randomized in a double-blind placebo-controlled crossover study of low-dose liquid fluoxetine. Outcome measures included measures of repetitive behaviors and global improvement. Low-dose liquid fluoxetine was superior to placebo in the treatment of repetitive behaviors, and it was only slightly, and not significantly, superior to placebo on global improvement score. Liquid fluoxetine did not significantly differ from placebo on treatment-emergent side effects. This study was the first controlled trial of liquid fluoxetine in children and adolescents and also provides evidence for the use of lower doses in the younger population.

Several other studies of fluoxetine have demonstrated efficacy in treating ASD symptoms. Cook and colleagues (1992) reported that fluoxetine (at doses of 20–80 mg/day) was effective in 15 of 23 subjects (age range, seven to 28 years) with autism.

DeLong and colleagues (2002) reported a positive response rate of 69% (89 of 129 children), with treatment duration ranging from five to 76 months. They also reported a high variability of dosing, with some patients responding best to 4–8 mg/day and others needing 15–40 mg/day.

Case reports have documented decreases in symptoms such as outbursts (Mehlinger et al., 1990; Todd, 1991), rituals/OCD behaviors (Cook et al., 1990; Mehlinger et al., 1990; Todd, 1991), depressive symptoms (Ghaziuddin et al., 1991; Hamdan-Allen, 1991), and trichotillomania (Hamdan-Allen, 1991) following treatment with fluoxetine.

Fluvoxamine (Luvox)

> **Class: SSRI**
> Fluvoxamine has the shortest half-life of all SSRIs; its mean serum half-life is 15.6 hours.

McDougle and colleagues (1996) conducted a double-blind, placebo-controlled trial in 30 adults. Eight of 15 subjects given fluvoxamine evidenced significant improvement in ratings of social relatedness and language usage, along with decreased repetitive thoughts, aggression, and maladaptive behavior. There were no placebo responders. Side effects were mild.

In a double-blind, placebo-controlled study of fluvoxamine in 18 children with autism, Fukada and colleagues (2001) found significant gains on measures of eye contact and language use without side effects.

A case study of the use of fluvoxamine with a seven-year-old Caucasian girl with severe pervasive developmental disorder, Kauffmann and colleagues (2001) demonstrated that fluvoxamine was significantly effective in reducing stereotypical and repetitive behaviors, anxiety, and aggression, and in improving prelinguistic and social behaviors.

Yokoyama and colleagues (2002) found three of five children with autism to evidence partial or significant decreases in aggression and self-injury when treated with open-label fluvoxamine. Only one subject, who was also prescribed haloperidol, experienced side effects (drowsiness). Conversely, McDougle (1998) reported significant side effects (e.g., aggression, agitation, anxiety, insomnia, hyperactivity), and only one in 16 children with autism demonstrated a positive clinical response following treatment with fluvoxamine.

Citalopram (Celexa)

> **Class: SSRI**
> Citalopram is highly selective for serotonin reuptake.
> It has a 35-hour half-life in children and adolescents and minimally inhibits the major cytochrome P450 drug-metabolizing enzymes with low potential for drug–drug interactions.

A retrospective chart review of 15 children and adolescents with pervasive developmental disorders treated with citalopram revealed a moderate improvement in anxiety and mood. Dose ranges were 5 to 40 mg daily. No association was detected between dose and response. Duration of treatment was positively correlated with outcome (Namerow et al., 2003).

In a double-blind, placebo-controlled study of citalopram in 149 children with ASD, Autism RUPP and Hollander and colleagues (2009) found that there was no significant improvement on the Clinical Global Impressions Improvement subscale or the Children's Yale-Brown Obsessive Compulsive Scales modified for pervasive developmental disorders. The results of this trial did not support the use of citalopram for the treatment of repetitive behavior in children and adolescents with Autism Spectrum Disorder.

Escitalopram (Lexapro)

> **Class SSRI**
> Escitalopram is the S-stereoisomer (enantiomer) of citalopram.
> Escitalopram has a high selectivity of serotonin reuptake inhibition, as it has the highest affinity for the serotonin transporter.

An open-label trial of escitalopram in ASD conducted by Owley and colleagues (2005) demonstrated that escitalopram both improved the CGI severity of illness ratings as well as decreased the scores on the Aberrant Behavior Checklist–Community Version (ABC-CV)—Irritability Subscale. Twenty-five percent of the subjects responded at a dose less than 10 mg and did not tolerate the 10 mg dose, and an additional 36% responded at a dose greater than or equal to 10 mg.

A wide variability in dose was found that could not be accounted for by weight and only partially by age. This is consistent with previous prospective, open-labeled studies that found that slower and individualized titration of medication doses in the ASD population can lead to decreased side effects.

Sertraline (Zoloft)

> **Class: SSRI**
> The elimination half-life of sertraline ranges from 22 to 36 hours.
> Sertraline has minimal inhibitory effects on the major cytochrome P450 enzymes, and few drug–drug interactions of clinical significance have been documented.

The use of sertraline in treating repetitive thoughts, repetitive behaviors, and aggression, with improvement of social functioning, was studied by

McDougle and colleagues (1998) in an open-label trial of 42 adults with ASD. Doses ranged between 50 and 200 mg as tolerated, with the maximum dose reached in three weeks and maintained for nine weeks. 57% of the subjects were considered improved or much improved, especially in the aggressive and repetitive behaviors domains.

Another open-label study was conducted by Steingard and colleagues (1997), this time including children with ASD and targeting symptoms of transition-associated anxiety and agitation. They were started on doses of 25 to 50 mg daily. Symptoms had improved as 89% of the subjects displayed response to treatment. The study reports that higher doses resulted in significant worsening of symptoms and have concluded that small doses of sertraline may be effective with fewer chances of resulting in unwanted side effects.

A case report of sertraline in two males with Asperger's disorder documented significant decreases in compulsive and repetitive behaviors (Ozbayrak, 1997).

Other antidepressant medications

Clomipramine (Anafranil)

> **Class: TCA**
> Clomipramine is a potent serotonin reuptake inhibitor with additional norepinephrine reuptake inhibitor; antiadrenergic, antidopaminergic, antihistamine, and anticholinergic properties; and associated side effects.
> Its plasma half-life after a single oral dose is approximately 21 hours.

Treatment trials have been for symptoms of depression, anxiety, obsessions/compulsions, and repetitive/ritualistic behaviors. Gordon and colleagues (1993) conducted a double-blind comparison of clomipramine, desipramine, and placebo in the treatment of autistic disorder and concluded that clomipramine was superior to both placebo and desipramine on ratings of autistic symptoms (including stereotypies), anger, and compulsive, ritualized behaviors, with no differences between desipramine and placebo. Clomipramine was equal to desipramine and superior to placebo for amelioration of hyperactivity.

Among open-label studies, Brasic and colleagues (1994) demonstrated decreased tic-like movements and compulsions with the use of clomipramine in a group of five children with autism. No significant side effects were noted. Conversely, Sanchez and colleagues (1996) found no therapeutic gains and considerable side effects with the use of open-label clomipramine in a group of seven children with autism. Case reports of clomipramine in children with autism have found decreased compulsive behavior and the elimination of trichotillomania (McDougle et al., 1992) as well as improved play, communication, hair pulling, and appetite (Holttum et al., 1994). Conversely, Magen (1993) found switching from haloperidol to clomipramine resulted in the re-emergence of self-injury, screaming/crying, and sound sensitivity in a 12-year-old male with autism. There have been no large double-blind placebo controlled studies to show evidence-based use.

Venlafaxine (Effexor)

> Venlafaxine is a serotonin–norepinephrine reuptake inhibitor (SNRI). Its active metabolites Desvenlafaxine and Duloxetine are also SNRIs.
>
> It is reported that in high doses it weakly inhibits the reuptake of dopamine.

Carminati and colleagues (2006) published three case reports on the use of low-dose venlafaxine (18.75 mg daily) in adolescents and young adults with ASD. Venlafaxine was prescribed to improve self-injurious behavior and attention deficit/hyperactivity disorder (ADHD)-like symptoms in ASD.

Hollander and colleagues (2000) conducted a retrospective clinical study of venlafaxine in a group of children with autism. Six of ten were rated as responders, with improvement noted in repetitive behaviors, restricted interests, social deficits, communication, inattention, and hyperactivity. Side effects included activation, nausea, and polyuria.

Mirtazapine (Remeron)

> Mirtazapine is noradrenergic and specific serotonergic antidepressant (NaSSA). Mirtazapine is not a reuptake inhibitor. Its antidepressant activity may be related to a direct enhancement of noradrenergic neurotransmission by blockade of alpha-2 autoreceptors.
>
> Mirtazapine has a half-life of approximately 20–40 hours.
>
> It has a transient sedation effect and has been used at nighttime.

An open-label study was conducted by Possey and colleagues (2001) on the efficacy and tolerability of mirtazapine in the treatment of associated symptoms of autism. The study included 26 subjects with a mean age of 10.1 +/– 4.8 years) diagnosed with ASD. Mirtazapine administered dose range was 7.5 to 45 mg daily. In all, 34.6% of the participants were judged responders ("much improved" or "very much improved" on the CGI) and had displayed an improvement in a variety of symptoms: aggression, self-injury, irritability, hyperactivity, anxiety, depression, and insomnia.

An open-label study was conducted by Coskun and colleagues (2009) to investigate the efficacy and safety of mirtazapine in the treatment of excessive masturbation and other inappropriate sexual behaviors (ISB) in children and adolescents with ASD. Mirtazapine was started at 7.5 to 15 mg per day and titrated up to 15 to 30 mg per day. Five subjects showed "very much," three showed "much," and one showed "moderate" improvement in excessive masturbation on CGI-Improvement scores.

Both studies reported that mirtazapine was well tolerated and that adverse effects were minimal, and included increased appetite and transient sedation.

Other antianxiety medication
Buspirone (Buspar)

> Buspirone works as a serotonin 5-HT1A receptor partial agonist; buspirone displays some affinity for DA2 autoreceptors and 5-HT2 receptors.
>
> After a single oral dose, the mean elimination half-life is 2.1 hours. Its active metabolite 1-(2-pyrimidinyl) piperazine (1-PP) has a mean elimination half-life of 6.1 hours.

Buitelaar and colleagues (1998) have conducted an open-label study of buspirone in the management of anxiety and irritability in children with ASD.

Twenty-two subjects, six to 17 years old, were treated with buspirone in dosages ranging from 15 to 45 mg per day for six to eight weeks. Nine subjects had a marked therapeutic response, and seven subjects a moderate response, on the Clinical Global Impressions scale after six to eight weeks of treatment.

During a three-week, double-blind, placebo-controlled crossover study on a child with ASD, McCormick and colleagues (1997) found that buspirone was safe and efficacious, without side effects, for decreasing hyperactivity and increasing performance completing tasks.

Realmuto and colleagues (1989) in open-blind four-week trial comparing buspirone to fenfluramine or methylphenidate and targeting hyperactivity have found out that two out of three treated children improved with buspirone.

Summary—Antidepressant medication use in ASD

Antidepressant medications have been used in the treatment of specific psychiatric comorbid disorders in individuals with ASD. They have also been used to target selected symptoms in ASD such as repetitive preoccupations, preseverative behaviors, and social anxiety. These reports have been anecdotal, small case studies, and small designed studies. Investigation has been limited by small sample size, broad age range, and being uncontrolled. The large double-blind, placebo-controlled study of citalopram in 149 children with ASD (Autism RUPP, and Hollander et al., 2009) found that there was no significant improvement on multiple measures.

Mood Stabilizers/Antiepileptic drugs (AEDs) in ASD

Antiepileptic medications are typically used for treatment of seizures, which may occur in approximately one third of children with ASD (often a two-peak distribution with a small peak before age five and a larger peak in adolescence (Tuchman & Rapin, 2002)). Mood-stabilizing antiepileptic drugs (AEDs) have also been used to treat mood instability, agitation and aggression in ASD. AEDs tend to be a second- or third-line option, behind atypical antipsychotics as well as alpha-2-adrenergic receptor agonists. None are specifically approved by the FDA for treatment of mood or behavior in children with ASD, and not all are approved for use in children. The use of this class of drugs is further complicated by the need for frequent blood draws for some AEDs to establish and maintain medication levels. There have been no controlled studies in the use of lithium in ASD. A few studies have also examined the possible efficacy of AEDs to treat repetitive behaviors and the core features of ASD.

Despite the availability of more than a handful of double-blind trials (most of which failed to support the use of AEDs), surveys of psycho-pharmacological use among children and adults with ASD suggest fairly frequent use. However, this may be due more to their role as anticonvulsant drugs than as medications prescribed to manage behavior. For example, 12.4% of Ohio families responding to a survey indicated that their family member with ASD was prescribed at least one AED (Aman et al., 2003).

A review of the ASD literature finds three double-blind, placebo-controlled trials of AEDs in this population. A 2005 study conducted by Hollander and colleagues used an eight-week, double-blind, placebo-controlled parallel groups trial of divalproex sodium (Depakote) to assess its safety and efficacy for treating repetitive behaviors in ASD. A total of 13 subjects (mean age 9.5 years) with research-reliable diagnoses of ASD were enrolled (mean dose of 823 +/– 326 mg/day; range = 500–1500 mg/day). Using the Children's Yale-Brown Obsessive Compulsive Scale, significant gains were noted on rates and severity of repetitive behavior while on active medication (p = 0.037), with an effect size of 1.6.

A second, larger well-controlled study was conducted by Hellings and colleagues (2005) to examine changes on measures of irritability/aggression (CGI and Irritability subscale of the Aberrant Behavior Checklist) with the use of valproate. The study involved a double-blind, placebo-controlled parallel groups trial of 30 children and adolescents with ASD. No significant group differences were found. In addition, increased serum ammonia levels were reported by two subjects, and a third subject withdrew after developing a skin rash.

Finally, Belsito and colleagues (2001) used a double-blind, placebo-controlled parallel group design to assess the possible impact of lamotrigine (Lamictal) on behavioral concerns as well as the core features of ASD. A total of 28 children, ranging from three to 11 years of age, were enrolled. However, no significant group differences were noted. All other studies of AEDs in ASD involved case reports or utilized open-label designs.

Given the limited amount of research in support of the use of AEDs for mood and behavior in children and adults with ASD, and the availability of other medications to treat aggression and irritability, the use of AEDs in this population should be reserved as an option only for individuals who consistently fail to respond to other treatment options.

Sleep Medications in ASD

A significant number of children with ASD experience sleep disturbances (see Chapter 9 on sleep). Treatment of a sleep disorder begins with a functional behavior assessment and the implementation of sleep hygiene techniques. Pharmacological interventions are typically reserved for use when children respond partially or fail to respond at all to psychosocial treatment. The available options are typically off-label and are used transiently.

Within the field of ASD, there is minimal empirical research examining the efficacy of pharmacotherapy to treat sleep disorders. The most well-researched option is melatonin, a herbal product sold over the counter. Melatonin (N-acetyl-5-methoxytryptamine) is a hormone derived from serotonin in the pineal gland that is involved in regulating the circadian rhythm (day/night, sleep/wake cycle). It has been suggested to be effective in reducing the time it takes to fall asleep but less so in reducing nighttime awakenings in children with neurodevelopmental disabilities (Phillips & Appleton, 2004).

Melatonin has been studied in a wide range of individuals and disorders, including populations who are visually impaired, individuals suffering from jet lag, geriatric populations, and disorders such as ADHD and depression. There have been a limited number of investigations in children with ASD, including both open-label studies as well as randomized, placebo-controlled trials (Garstang et al., 2006; Giannotti et al., 2006, 2008; Paavonen et al., 2003). All found melatonin to be effective in decreasing sleep latency and increasing sleep duration. A new prescription form of melatonin, ramelteon (Rozerem), has been marketed as a sleep-induction aid. A case report involving two children with ASD also showed effectiveness (Stigler et al., 2006).

Other options to address sleep concerns in ASD are available, but have minimal research support. The alpha-2-adrenergic agonist clonidine (Catapres—described above) has sedating effects and has been used for sleep induction. Duration is around three to four hours and sometimes results in the child's awakening in the middle of the night. Guanfacine (Tenex—described above) has slightly less sedating effect than clonidine. Diphenhydramine (Benadryl) has been used for sleep induction. However, it may have paradoxical, excitatory responses. If a child is being prescribed other medications that have some sedating effects, clinicians may arrange a dosing schedule that takes advantage of this. For example, if a child with ASD is prescribed risperidone or aripiprazole to address behavioral concerns, dosing in the evening may also help address sleep-related issues.

Polypharmacy in ASD

It is not uncommon for individuals with ASD to be prescribed more than one psychotropic medication. For example, in the 2005 ASD psychoactive medication survey conducted by Aman and colleagues, 9.8% of the sample were identified as taking two different drugs; 7.7% were taking three drugs (see Aman et al., 2005). In some cases, the medications are targeted to treat different psychiatric comorbidities. For example, an adolescent with ASD might be prescribed a stimulant to treat symptoms of hyperactivity and inattention as well as an SSRI to treat symptoms of anxiety. Other situations may find that an individual is only partially responsive to a first medication trial, resulting in the addition of a second medication to address the same disorder or symptoms.

To date, we are unaware of any randomized controlled trials involving the use of polypharmacy in ASD. As a result, the clinician needs to carefully consider the available information from studies involving the same disorder or symptoms (e.g., depression, anxiety, OCD) but with a different subject population. The clinician will also need to keep in mind the higher rate of side effects among individuals with ASD who are prescribed psychotropic agents. Consequently, the starting dose should be low and the dose titration should be slow.

Complementary Alternative Medicine (CAM) Treatments

Commonly used unconventional interventions are often defined in the literature as "complementary and alternative medicine" (CAM). Reports of the efficacy of CAM treatments are based predominantly on anecdotal reports from families and tend to lack scientific validation through large, randomized controlled trials. Parents of children with ASD often report that they selected CAM treatments for ASD because they believed the treatment was natural, safe, and had limited adverse side effects. Over 50% of parents surveyed used CAM because they hoped one or more alternative treatments would cure their child of ASD (Hanson et al., 2007; Wong & Smith, 2006; Levy, 2008). Even popular treatments, such as gluten-free/casein-free (GFCF) diets, have yet to be shown to be effective (Hyman, IMFAR Conference, 2010), and some treatments, such as facilitated communication and Secretin (see review in Sturmey, 2005) have been demonstrated to be ineffective. Consequently, psychiatrists, pediatricians, and other physicians need to have some knowledge of these treatments and how they might interact with other psychopharmacological agents.

Psychiatrists, pediatricians, and other physicians also need to regularly ask parents about the use of CAM treatments and be able to talk in a supportive manner with parents who have chosen to pursue these options. Simply stating that CAM interventions have not been shown to be effective will not help to build a working alliance with the family. The practitioner should not forget that the data on psychopharmacology and ASD are also limited. For many parents, the attraction of CAM treatments is based on a hope that such agents will address some of the core features of ASD, possibly even result in a cure. Traditional medicine and psychosocial/educational interventions cannot make such a claim.

An important caution regarding CAM treatments is that parents should not implement them to the exclusion of other, more evidence-based interventions. For example, it would be of concern if a parent chose to delay enrolling their child into an intensive preschool program so that the child could be placed in a CAM treatment. Most CAM treatments are unlikely to be harmful to a child. However, they often require considerable time, effort, and expense. In talking to parents about a CAM treatment, try to help them to think about how they will measure success with the new treatment and how long it will take for gains to be noted. Also, discuss the challenges of implementing a CAM treatment (such as the gluten-free/casein-free diet). For example, most proponents of the GFCF diet declare that any deviation from the diet will undo any positive effects. Consequently, how well will the parents be able to control the child's diet? See Table 6.1 in Chapter 6, which provides a list of some of the most commonly used CAM treatments in ASD, most of which are not covered in this book. None have been identified as "established" in the 2009 National Autism Center's National Standards Project and Maine's Department of Health and Human Services with the Maine Department of Education.

In summary, the clinician needs to be open to the idea of CAM treatments in order to maintain open communication with the parents of a child with ASD. The goals are to help guide the parents away from potentially harmful treatments (e.g., chelation), to insure that the treatment does not adversely interact with pharmacotherapy or remove the child from other, evidence-based treatments, and to help the parents critically assess the effectiveness of the selected CAM intervention.

Summary

In summary, there are no approved medications for the treatment of core features of ASD. Instead, pharmacotherapy in ASD is used to treat comorbid psychiatric disorders (e.g., depression, anxiety) and associated target symptoms, such as inattention/hyperactivity, aggression, or ritualistic behavior. Risperidone and aripiprazole remain the only FDA-approved drugs for the treatment of individual with ASD, having been approved specifically to treat irritability and agitation; all other pharmacological agents are considered to be off-label. There remain relatively few controlled trials available to guide the clinician. In general, children and adolescents with ASD tend to respond at somewhat lower rates than neurotypical individuals and also exhibit higher rates of side effects. Consequently, an approach of starting at a lower dose and titrating at a slower rate than would be typical is often recommended with this population. Finally, the use of pharmacotherapy among children and adolescents with ASD should always be done in collaboration with ongoing behavioral/psychosocial treatment and educational interventions.

Further Reading

1. Aman, M. G., Singh, N. N., Stewart, A.W., & Field, C. J. (1985). The Aberrant Behavior Checklist: A behavior rating scale for the assessment of treatment effects. *American Journal of Mental Deficiency*, 89, 485–491.

2. Aman, M. G., Lam, K. S., & Van Bourgondien, M. E.. (2005). Medication patterns in patients with autism: Temporal, regional, and demographic influences. *Journal of Child and Adolescent Psychopharmacology*, 15(1): 116–126.

3. American Psychiatric Association (2000). *Diagnostic and Statistical Manual of Mental Disorders* (5th ed.). Washington, DC: American Psychiatric Association.

4. Arnold, L. E., Aman, M. G., Cook, A., Witwer, A., Hall, K., Thompson, S., & Ramadan, Y. (2006). Atomoxetine for hyperactivity in autistic spectrum disorders: Placebo-controlled crossover trial. *Journal of the American Academy of Child and Adolescent Psychiatry*, 45, 1196–1205.

5. Belsito, K. M., Law, P. A., Kirk, K. S., Landa, R. J., & Zimmerman, A. W. (2001). Lamotrigine therapy for autistic disorder: A randomized, double-blind, placebo-controlled trial. *Journal of Autism & Developmental Disorders*, 31, 175–181.

6. Biederman, J., Melmed, R. D., Patel, A., McBurnett, K., Konow, J., Lyne, A., Scherer, N. (2008). A randomized, double-blind, placebo-controlled study of guanfacine extended release in children and adolescents with attention-deficit/hyperactivity disorder. *Pediatrics*, 121(1): e73–e84.

7. Carminati, G. G., Deriaz, N., & Bertschy, G. (2006). Low-dose venlafaxine in three adolescents and young adults with autistic disorder improves self-injurious behavior and attention deficit/hyperactivity disorders (ADHD)-like symptoms. *Progress in Neuro-Pschopharmacology and Biological Psychiatry*, 30, 312–315.

8. Correll, C. U., & Kane, J. M. (2007). One-Year Incidence Rates of Tardive Dyskinesia in Children and Adolescents Treated with Second-Generation Antipsychotics: A Systematic Review. *Journal of Child and Adolescent Psychopharmacology*, 17, 647–656.

9. Garnock-Jones, Karly, P., & Keating, Gillian, M. (2009). Atomoxetine: a review of its use in attention-deficit hyperactivity disorder in children and adolescents. *Paediatric Drugs*, 11, 203–226.

10. Garstang, J., Wallis, M. (2006). Randomized controlled trial of melatonin for children with autistic spectrum disorders and sleep problems. *Child Care Health Development*, 32, 585–589.

11. Giannotti, F., Cortesi, F., Cerquiglini, A., et al. (2006). An open-label study of controlled release melatonin in treatment of sleep disorders in children with autism. *Journal of Autism and Developmental Disorders*, 36, 741–752.

12. Giannotti, F., Cortesi, F., Cerquiglini, A., et al. (2008). The treatment of sleep disorders in childhood autism with melatonin or behavioral therapy: A randomized waiting list controlled study [abstract]. *Sleep*, 31, A58.

13. Greenhill, L. L., Swanson, J. M., Vitiello, B., Davies, M., Clevenger, W., Wu, M., Arnold, L. E., Abikoff, H. B., Bukstein, O. G., Conners, C. K., Elliott, G. R., Hechtman, L., Hinshaw, S. P., Hoza, B., Jensen, P. S., Kraemer, H. C., March, J. S., Newcorn, J. H., Severe, J. B., Wells, K., & Wigal, T. (2007). Impairment and deportment responses to different methylphenidate doses in children with, ADHD: The MTA titration trial. *Journal of the American Academy of Child and Adolescent Psychiatry*, 40,180–187.

14. Handen, B. L., Johnson, C. R., & Lubetsky, M. (2000). Efficacy of methylphenidate among children with autism and symptoms of attention-deficit hyperactivity disorder. *Journal of Autism and Developmental Disorders*, 30, 245–255.

15. Handen, B. L., Sahl, R., & Harden, A. Y. (2008). Guanfacine in children with autism and/or intellectual disabilities. *Journal of Developmental and Behavioral Pediatrics*, 29, 303–308.

16. Hellings, J. A., Weckbaugh, M., Nickel, E. J., Cain, S., Zarcone, J., Reese, R. M., Hall, S., Ermer, D., Tsai, L. Y., Schroeder, S. R., & Cook, E. H. ((2005).). A double-blind, placebo-controlled study of valproate for aggression in youth with pervasive developmental disorders. *Journal of Child and Adolescent Psychopharmacology*, 15, 682–692.

17. Hollander, E., Soorya, L., Wasserman, S., Esposito, K., Chaplin, W., & Anagnostou, E. (2006). Divalproex sodium vs. placebo in the treatment of repetitive behaviours in autism spectrum disorder. *International Journal of Neuropsychopharmacology*, 9, 209–213.

18. Jaselskis, C. A., Cook, E. H., Fletcher, K. E., & Leventhal, B. (1992). Clonidine treatment of hyperactivity and impulsive children with autistic disorder. *Journal of Clinical Psychopharmacology*, 12, 322–326.

19. Jou, R. J., Handen, B. L., & Hardan, A. Y. (2005). Retrospective assessment of atomoxetine in children and adolescents with pervasive developmental disorders. *Journal of Child and Adolescent Psychopharmacology*, 15, 325–330.

20. Lecavalier, L. (2006). Behavior and emotional problems in young people with pervasive developmental disorders: Relevant prevalence, effects of subject characteristics, and empirical classification. *Journal of Autism and Developmental Disorder, 36,* 1101–1114.

21. Marcus, R. N., Owen, R., Kamen, L., Manos, G, McQuade, R. D., Carson, W., & Aman, M. G. (2009). A placebo-controlled, fixed-dose study of aripiprazole in children and adolescents with irritability associated with autistic disorder. *Journal of the American Academy of Child and Adolescent Psychiatry, 48,* 1110–1119.

22. McCracken, J. T., McGough, J., Shah, B., Cronin, P., Hong, D., Aman, M. G., Arnold, L. E., Lindsay, R., Nash, P., Hollway, J., McDougle, C. J., Posey, D., Swiezy, N., Kohn, A., Scahill, L., Martin, A., Koenig, K., Volkmar, F., Carroll, D., Lancor, A., Tierney, E., Ghuman, J., Gonzalez, N. M., Grados, M., Vitiello, B., Ritz, L., Davies, M., Robinson, J., & McMahon, D. (2002). Research units on pediatric psychopharmacology autism network. Risperidone in children with autism and serious behavioral problems. *New England Journal of Medicine, 347,* 314–321.

23. Paavonen, E., von Wendt, T., Vanhala, N., et al. (2003). Effectiveness of melatonin in the treatment of sleep disturbances in children with Asperger's disorder. *Journal of Child and Adolescent Psychopharmacology, 13,* 83–95.

24. Pliszka, S. R. (2005). The neuropsychopharmacology of attention-deficit/hyperactivity disorder. *Biological Psychiatry, 57,* 1385–1390.

25. Poncin, Y., & Scahill, L. (2007). Stimulants and nonstimulants in the treatment of hyperactivity in autism. In E. Hollander and E. Anagnostou (Eds.), *Clinical manual for the treatment of autism* (pp. 131–152). Washington, DC: American Psychiatric Publishing Company.

26. Posey, D. J., Puntney, J. I., Sasher, T. M., Kem, D. L., & McDougle, C. J. (2004). Guanfacine treatment of hyperactivity and inattention in pervasive developmental disorders: A retrospective analysis of 80 cases. *Journal of Child and Adolescent Psychopharmacology, 14,* 233–241.

27. Posey, D. J., Wiegand, R. E., Wilkerson, J., Maynard, M., Stigler, K. A., & McDougles, C. J. (2006). Open-label atomoxetine for attention-deficit/hyperactivity disorder symptoms associated with high-functioning pervasive developmental disorders. *Journal of Child and Adolescent Psychopharmacology, 16,* 599–610.

28. Quintana, H., Birmaher, B., Stedge, D., Lennon, S., Freed, J., & Bridge, J. (1995). Use of methylphenidate in the treatment of children with autistic disorder. *Journal of Autism and Developmental Disorders, 25,* 283–294.

29. RUPP (2005). Randomized, controlled, crossover trial of methylphenidate in pervasive developmental disorders with hyperactivity. *Archives of General Psychiatry, 62,* 1266–1274.

30. Sallee, F. R,. Lyne, A. Wigal, T., & McGough, J. J. (2009). Long-term safety and efficacy of guanfacine extended release in children and adolescents with attention-deficit/hyperactivity disorder. *Journal of Child and Adolescent Psychopharmacology, 19,* 215–226.

31. Santosh, P. J., Baird, G., Pityaratstian, N., et al. (2006). Impact of comorbid Autism Spectrum Disorder on stimulant response in children with attention deficit hyperactivity disorder: A retrospective and prospective effectiveness study. *Child Care Health Development, 32,* 575–583.

32. Scahill, L., Aman, M. G., McDougle, C. J., McCracken, J. T., Tierney, E., Dziura, J., et al. (2006). A prospective open trial of guanfacine in children with pervasive developmental disorders. *Journal of Child and Adolescent Psychopharmacology, 16,* 589–598.

33. Shea, S., Turgay, A., Carrol, A., Schulz, M., Orlik, H., & Smith, I. (2004). Risperidone in the treatment of disruptive behavioral symptoms in children with autistic and other pervasive developmental disorders. *Pediatrics, 114,* e634Y–e641Y.

34. Stigler, K. A., Desmond, L. A., Posey, D. J., et al. (2004). A naturalistic retrospective analysis of psychostimulants in pervasive developmental disorders. *Journal of Child and Adolescent Psychopharmacology, 14,* 49–56.

35. Sturmey, P. (2005). Secretin is an ineffective treatment for pervasive developmental disabilities: A review of 15 double-blind randomized controlled trials. *Research in Developmental Disabilities, 26,* 87–97.

36. Tourette's Syndrome Study Group (2002). Treatment of ADHD in children with tics: A randomized controlled trial. *Neurology, 58,* 527–526.

37. Troost, P. W., Althaus, M., Lahuis, B. E., Buitelaar, J. K., Minderaa, R. B., & Hoekstra, P. J. (2006). Neuropsychological effects of risperidone in children with pervasive developmental disorders: A blinded discontinuation study. *Journal of Child and Adolescent Psychopharmacology, 16,* 561–573.

38. Troost, P.W., Steenhuis, M.P., Tuynman-Qua, H.G., Kalverdijk, L.J. Buitelaar, J.K., Minderaa, R.B, & Hoekstra, P.J. (2006). Atomoxetine for Attention-Deficit/Hyperactivity Disorder Symptoms in Children with Pervasive Developmental Disorders: A Pilot Study. *Journal of Child and Adolescent Psychopharmacology, 16,* 611–619.

39. Tsai, L. (2001). Taking the mystery out of medications in autism/Asperger syndromes. Arlington, TX: Future Horizons.
40. Werry, J. S., & Aman, M. G. (1999). Practitioner's guide to psychoactive drugs for children and adolescents (2nd ed.). New York: Plenum Medical Book Company.
41. Witwer, A., & Lecavalier, L. (2005). Treatment incidence and patterns in children and adolescents with Autism Spectrum Disorder. Journal of Child and Adolescent Psychopharmacology, 15, 671–681.

Questions

1. In general, studies of pharmacological treatment for symptoms of inattention, distractibility, hyperactivity, and impulsivity (ADHD) have found which of the following for children with ASD?
   a. Response rates tend to be lower than among typically developing children.
   b. Symptom improvement is often less robust.
   c. Side effects are more frequently reported.
   d. Significantly more children are unable to tolerate commonly prescribed medications.
   e. All of the above

2. Which of the following is not true about pharmacological treatment of inattention, distractibility, hyperactivity, and impulsivity (ADHD) for children with ASD?
   a. Autism RUPP 2005 study of methylphenidate showed 49% of study participants were labeled as responders, and 18% were discontinued from the trial due to adverse events.
   b. Studies have shown that atomoxetine (Strattera) efficacy does not match that of extended-release mixed amphetamine salts (Adderall, XR) or osmotically released MPH (Concerta).
   c. Clonidine and guanfacine use for the treatment of ADHD symptoms is off-label, and Guanfacine XR (GXR: Intuniv) recently received FDA approval as a monotherapy for treatment of ADHD in normally developing children ages 6–17 years.
   d. Atypical antipsychotics should be used as first-line therapy for children with ASD and ADHD symptoms.

3. All of the following are true about atypical antipsychotic use in individuals with ASD, except for which one?
   a. No atypical antipsychotic medications have been FDA-approved for use in children and adolescents with ASD.
   b. In the RUPP Autism Network double-blind placebo-controlled multicenter study in children with ASD, 69.4% of the children assigned to risperidone were noted to be "responders" with significant decrease in symptoms of irritability.
   c. Risperidone and aripiprazole received FDA approval for the treatment of irritability associated with autistic disorder, including symptoms of aggression towards others, deliberate self-injurious behavior, temper tantrums, and quickly changing moods in children and adolescents..

d. Though effective, antipsychotic medication must be used with caution in children, adolescents, and adults with ASD, due to the risk of increased appetite, weight gain, and metabolic changes that could impact glucose metabolism.

4. Which of the following is *true* about the use of antidepressants in individuals with ASD?
   a. In a double-blind, placebo-controlled study of citalopram in 149 children with ASD, there was no significant improvement on various measures, and the results did not support the use of citalopram for the treatment of repetitive behavior in children and adolescents with ASD.
   b. In a double-blind, placebo-controlled study of low-dose liquid fluoxetine in 45 children with ASD, it was superior to placebo in the treatment of repetitive behaviors, but only slightly but not significantly, superior to placebo on global improvement score.
   c. Antidepressants have been studied as a possible pharmacological intervention for depression and anxiety symptoms and obsessive-compulsive behaviors in individuals with ASD who are diagnosed with these DSM psychiatric disorders.
   d. The child, adolescent, or adult with ASD should be monitored for any increased risk of suicidal ideation (FDA Medication Guide, 2009).
   e. All of the above

5. Which of the following is *true* about mood stabilizers/antiepileptic drugs (AEDs) used in individuals with ASD?
   a. Anticonvulsant medications are typically used for treatment of seizures, which may occur in approximately one third of children with ASD.
   b. Mood stabilizing AEDs tend to be a second- or third-line option, behind atypical antipsychotics as well as alpha-2-adrenergic receptor agonists.
   c. None are specifically approved by the FDA for treatment of mood or behavior in children with ASD, and not all are approved for use in children.
   d. There have been no controlled studies in the use of lithium in ASD.
   e. All of the above

Answers

1. e. All of the above are true.
2. d. is Not true
3. a. is Not true
4. e. All of the above are true.
5. e. All of the above are true.

Future Directions

**Martin J. Lubetsky, Benjamin L. Handen,
John J. McGonigle, and co-authors**

Since the time of Kanner's early description of autism, there have
been advances in early identification, diagnostic classification,
assessment instruments, genetic and neurobiological mechanisms, educational models, behavioral therapies, pharmacological
interventions, and recognition of medical and psychiatric comorbidities. Autism (referred to as autism spectrum disorder) is now
viewed as a developmental neurobiological disorder. The increased
reported incidence of ASD over the past two decades has stimulated growth in research on etiology, diagnosis, and treatment, as
well as service provision. More recently, the expanded community
awareness of ASD has magnified the growing numbers and needs
of adults with ASD living in the community. Families and siblings
are increasingly asking for more services that involve them and
their family member with ASD. This book has provided a didactic
approach to understanding ASD across the lifespan and a range of
disciplines, assessments, and interventions.

As we look to the future, the study of ASD is progressing rapidly
in several ways.

With the upcoming proposed changes in DSM-5, the separate
diagnostic classifications under "pervasive developmental
disorder" (PDD) may be subsumed under one category of "ASD"
(www.dsm5.org). ASD would include autistic disorder (autism),
Asperger's disorder, childhood disintegrative disorder, and PDD
not otherwise specified. Rett's disorder will most likely be removed,
being reclassified as a genetic disorder. It is proposed that a single
diagnostic category be used, along with the inclusion of clinical
specifiers (e.g., severity, verbal abilities) and associated features
(e.g., known genetic disorders, epilepsy, intellectual disability).
Reorganization of subdomains increases clarity and continues to
provide adequate sensitivity while improving specificity through
provision of examples from different age ranges and language
levels. Unusual sensory behaviors are explicitly included within a
subdomain of stereotyped motor and verbal behaviors, expanding
the specification of different behaviors that can be coded within this
domain, with examples particularly relevant for younger children.

Considering that deficits in communication and social behaviors
are inseparable and more accurately considered as a single set
of symptoms with contextual and environmental specificities, the
DSM-IV-TR's three domains (communication deficits, social
deficits, stereotypic interests and behaviors) become two in
DSM-5: (a) social/communication deficits, and (b) fixated interests
and repetitive behaviors. The newly proposed diagnosis for ASD

requires that both criteria to be completely fulfilled. In addition, the current clinical and research consensus appears to be that Asperger's disorder is part of ASD. Research currently reflects that Asperger's disorder is not substantially different from other forms of "high-functioning" autism with good formal language skills and good (at least verbal) IQ.

Over the past 15 years, dramatic advances in the genetic and neurobiological characterization of ASD have resulted from the exponential growth in research technologies. These advances include a new understanding of the early and probably prenatal developmental neurobiological events that lead to subsequent brain developmental abnormalities, including alterations in forebrain connectivity. Fifteen to twenty percent of cases of ASD are now linked to genetic or chromosomal abnormalities. Recent genetic advances have identified a multitude of abnormal and mutated genes for ASD that all share a role in the development of neuronal connections. While the research is promising, the paucity of consistent results underscores the significant genetic variability involved as well as the need for even larger sample sizes in order to identify potential common risk alleles. In the near future, it is likely that ASD will be characterized, not by clinical nomenclature, but by the disturbance in developmental neurobiological mechanisms, and by genotype.

Current and future longitudinal research studies of "at risk" infant siblings are aimed at defining the earliest signs or symptoms of ASD, both to improve early diagnosis and to delve into implications regarding neurobiological mechanisms. Individuals with ASD display a broad but selective profile of deficits and intact or enhanced abilities. These findings could be characterized as reflecting a disorder of complex or integrative information processing, which results from altered development of cerebral cortical connectivity in ASD. Research has shown that ASD, as a whole, may be best characterized as having greatly heterogeneous brain-growth patterns relative to the non-affected population. Functional neuroimaging methods not only provide information on patterns of task-related activation abnormalities across networks, but also allow the assessment of the temporal synchronization of activation among regions, or *functional connectivity*, within these networks during a specific activity.

There have also been significant changes in the psychopharmacological treatment of individuals with ASD. Since the early studies of haloperidol for ASD in the 1970s, researchers have been examining a wide range of symptoms, including irritability, aggression, self-injury, and repetitive behaviors in ASD, which has led to two medications' being approved by the Food and Drug Administration, specifically to target these symptoms. While no medication has yet been identified that can treat the core features of ASD, future pharmacological trials will explore abnormalities in glutamatergic pathways that have been implicated in the pathophysiology of ASD, and the deficit in glutathione that has been linked to ASD.

The last 40 years have seen the growth of complementary and alternative treatments for ASD, in spite of limited scientific evidence and few studies. Most popular are the gluten-free/casein-free diet, nutritional supplements and vitamins; as well as omega-3 fatty acids, digestive enzymes, and melatonin for sleep. Future well-controlled scientific studies are needed to further test these interventions.

Finally, future advancements are also expected in educational approaches, from early childhood to adolescence, behavioral treatments, communication interventions, sensory therapies, social skills competency training, and adapted cognitive psychotherapies. There have been a number of recent national studies to categorize ASD treatments, based upon the quality and number of research studies supporting the scientific evidence for each treatment.

The ASD field has made impressive progress over the past few decades. It continues to be an area where our knowledge base will be rapidly changing and expanding as the results of numerous basic, translational, and clinical research studies become available.

Index

A

AAC. See augmentative and alternative communication
AAP. See American Academy of Pediatrics
ABA. See applied behavior analysis
ABAS-II. See Adaptive Behavior Assessment System
ABC. See Aberrant Behavior Checklist
ABC-CV. See Aberrant Behavior Checklist-Community Version
ABC data chart. See antecedent-behavior-consequence data chart
Aberrant Behavior Checklist (ABC) 61t
Aberrant Behavior Checklist-Community Version (ABC-CV) 312
ABLLS. See Assessment of Basic Language and Learning Skills
abstract concepts 281, 284
aCGH. See Array Comparative Genomic Hybridization
Achieving in Higher Education with Autism/Developmental Disabilities (AHEADD) 236
ACI. See Autism Comorbidity Interview
actigraphy 202
activities of daily living (ADL) skills 235, 243
acupuncture 141t
ADAMS. See Anxiety, Depression, and Mood Screen
Adams, Lynn 10
Adaptive Behavior Assessment System (ABAS-II) 290
adaptive behavior skills 29
ADD. See Assessment for Dual Diagnosis
adenylosuccinase deficit 53t
ADHD. See attention deficit hyperactivity disorder

ADI-R. See Autism Diagnostic Interview-Revised
ADL skills. See activities of daily living skills
adolescents
IEPs for 144
interventions for 254
school placements for 226–27
ADOS. See Autism Diagnostic Observation Schedule
adult living skills 234–35
adults 232
advocacy groups 142
AEDs. See antiepileptic drugs
aggressive episodes 259t
AGP. See Autism Genome Project
AGRE. See Autism Genetic Resource Exchange
AHEADD. See Achieving in Higher Education with Autism/Developmental Disabilities
allergies 247
alone condition 130
alpha-2-adrenergic receptor agonists 301–4, 318
alternative medicine. See complementary and alternative medicine
alternative strategies, in effective interventions 257
amenorrhea 308
American Academy of Pediatrics (AAP) 24, 35, 148–49
American Sign Language (ASL) 182
American Speech-Language-Hearing Association (ASHA) 175, 180
Angelman syndrome 49, 54t, 102t
anger 70t
anhedonia 70t
animal therapy 141t
antecedent-behavior-consequence (ABC) data chart 126–28, 129t
antecedents 119, 177, 258
changing 260–61, 266
in effective interventions 257
identifying 119, 125

antianxiety medication 315–16
antidepressants 310–16
antiepileptic drugs (AEDs) 316–17
antifungal treatment 141t
antipsychotics 306–9
atypical 302–3, 305
anxiety 45
in ASD 73t
diagnosing 72–75
disorders 99, 247
NLGN4X and 106
separation 72–73, 79
social motivation and 278
Anxiety, Depression, and Mood Screen (ADAMS) 61t
applied behavior analysis (ABA) 116–17, 130, 136, 148
efficacy of 255
for high-functioning autism 266
other intensive approaches 160–66
SCERTS model and 187
social skills teaching and 281
targeted behaviors of 255
applied verbal behavior (AVB) 148, 157–60, 188
curriculum and transition in 158–59
defining features of 157–58
empirical research base for 158
parental role in 159
prerequisites for 158
The Archives of Pediatric Adolescent Medicine, 24
aripiprazole 296, 303–4, 306–8
Array Comparative Genomic Hybridization (aCGH) 45
ASD. See autism spectrum disorder
ASD-CA. See Autism Spectrum Disorder-Comorbid for Adults
ASD-CC. See Autism Spectrum Disorder-Comorbid for Children
ASDS. See Asperger's Syndrome Diagnostic Scale

ASHA. See American Speech-Language-Hearing Association
ASL. See American Sign Language
Asperger, Hans 7, 11
 Kanner vs., 8–9, 8t
Asperger's disorder 7, 332
 in ASD diagnosis 20
 coping difficulties and 246–47
 diagnosis 33–34
 in DSM-IV-TR 13
 family history and 88
 poor jobs for 240
 stimulants and 299
"Asperger's Syndrome: A Clinical Account" (Wing) 7
Asperger's Syndrome Diagnostic Scale (ASDS) 28, 290
Assessment for Dual Diagnosis 64t
Assessment of Basic Language and Learning Skills (ABLLS) 158–59
assessments. See also functional behavioral assessment
 behavioral 116
 cognitive 29
 of comorbid disorders 56, 58
 diagnosis and 32–34
 domain 28–29
 ecological 128, 129t
 in effective interventions 257
 evaluation algorithms and 26–30
 evidence-based 20
 feeding disorder 196–97
 language 29, 176
 motivation 157
 of narrative discourse 189
 of psychiatric disorders 58–60
 rating scales 61t–63t
 related to challenging behaviors 177
 sleep disturbances 202
 social skills 290
 speech 29, 176
 systematic approach to 24
 toileting issues 206–7
 transition-age skills 234–35
associated symptoms, in early manifestations of autism 90
ASSQ. See Autism Spectrum Screening Questionnaire

atomoxetine (ATX) 300–301, 303–4
attention deficit hyperactivity disorder (ADHD) 45, 247
 brain-behavior correlations in 99
 diagnosing 75
 medications 298–304
 NLGN4X and 106
 primary differential diagnosis considerations for 79
ATX. See atomoxetine
auditory comprehension 174–75
auditory integration training 141t
augmentative and alternative communication (AAC) 181
autism 4. See also high-functioning autism
 atypical 34
 early manifestations of 90–91
 future directions for 331
 genetics of 100
 history of 12–13
 idiopathic 100
 neurobiology of 94–96
 at older ages 92–93
 origin of 5–6
 pathophysiology of 94–96
 psychogenic theory of 10–11
Autism: Explaining the Enigma (Frith) 5
Autism and Pervasive Developmental Disorders (Volkmar and Lord) 8
Autism Comorbidity Interview (ACI) 64t, 68–72
Autism Diagnostic Interview-Revised (ADI-R) 30, 88
Autism Diagnostic Observation Schedule (ADOS) 30, 35, 88
Autism Genetic Resource Exchange (AGRE) 104
Autism Genome Project (AGP) 104
Autism in History: The Case of Hugh Blair of Borgue (Frith) 5
Autism Partnership 156
autism spectrum disorder (ASD) 4
 anxiety in 73t
 in DSM-5, 14
 genetic etiology of 42
 increased prevalence of 35

 metabolic etiology of 42
 National Standards Project and 220
 neurobiology of 86
 non-syndromic 95–96, 100, 104, 109
 related syndromes 102t–103t
 subtypes 88–89
 syndromic 100, 102–3, 109
Autism Spectrum Disorder-Comorbid for Adults (ASD-CA) 61t
Autism Spectrum Disorder-Comorbid for Children (ASD-CC) 61t
Autism Spectrum Screening Questionnaire (ASSQ) 28
Autistic Disturbances of Affective Conduct (Kanner) 6, 11
automatic processing 99–100
AVB. See applied verbal behavior
avoidance 121
axonal pathfinding/positional information model 107–8

B

babbling, lack of 23
Baby and Infant Screen for Children with Autism Traits (BISCUIT) 64t
Baker, Lorian 10–11
Baron-Cohen, Simon 11
BASC. See Behavioral Assessment Scale for Children
Batelle Developmental Inventory (BDI) 29
Bayley Scales of Infant Development II 29
BCBA. See board certified behavior analyst
BDI. See Batelle Developmental Inventory
bedtime resistance 203–4
bedtime routines 203, 205t
Behavioral Assessment Scale for Children (BASC) 29, 128, 290
behavioral/emotional adjustment 29
behavioral psychology 152
behavioral support, in schools 219
behavioral syndrome 93
Behavior Problems Inventory (BPI-01) 62t

behaviors. *See also specific behaviors*
as compulsion 75
destructive 118
direct observation of 118–19, 126
disruptive 118
function of 121, 125, 258
identified for intervention 118
interfering 121–22
maintaining variable of 120
pivotal 187
prioritizing 125
problem 128–29
rating scale 127t
repetitive 14
replacement 266
targeted, by ABA 255
teaching alternative 262–63
visual cues for 188
best practices 145
Bettelheim, Bruno 10–11
biotinidase deficiency 53t
bipolar disorder 45, 69, 247
birth history 44
BISCUIT. *See Baby and Infant Screen for Children with Autism Traits*
Blair, Hugh 5
BMI. *See body mass index*
board certified behavior analyst (BCBA) 131
body mass index (BMI) 309
BPI-01. *See Behavior Problems Inventory*
brain-behavior correlations 99
brain development 90–91
brain growth 94–95, 332
brain malformation 48
brain volume (BV) 94–95
brain weight 95–96
bright light exposure 203
buspirone 314–15
BV. *See brain volume*

C

CAM. *See complementary and alternative medicine*
CAMs. *See cell adhesion molecules*
Cantwell, Dennis 10–11
CARE. *See Center for Autism and Related Disorders*
CARS 2. *See Childhood Autism Rating Scale 2*

Cases of Insane Children (Haslam) 5
catatonia 69
causal factors 86
CBT. *See cognitive-behavioral therapy*
CCC-SLP. *See Certificate of Clinical Competence in Speech-Language Pathology*
CDC. *See Centers for Disease Control*
cell adhesion molecules (CAMs) 106
Center for Autism and Related Disorders (CARE) 156
Centers for Disease Control (CDC) 20
  ASD prevalence 35
  early identification and 22–23
  median age of ASD diagnosis 22
central coherence deficit 276–77
cerebral palsy 91
Certificate of Clinical Competence in Speech-Language Pathology (CCC-SLP) 175
CGI Severity Scale. *See Clinical Global Impressions Severity Scale*
challenging behaviors
  assessments related to 177
  motivating factors for 121–22
  pediatric office visits and 52
character education 281
CHAT. *See Checklist for Autistic Toddlers*
CheapTalk 181
Checklist for Autistic Toddlers (CHAT) 27
chelation therapy 137, 141t
chewing skills 196
Child Behavior Checklist 59–60, 128
Child Find 222
Childhood Autism Rating Scale 2 (CARS 2) 28, 163
childhood disintegrative disorder 8–9, 13
childhood schizophrenic reaction 12
children
  IEPs for 144
  interventions for 254

Children's Sleep Habit Questionnaire 202
Children's Yale-Brown Obsessive Compulsive Scale modified for Pervasive Developmental Disorders (CYBOCS-PDD) 65t, 312, 316
Chinese medicine 141t
chlorpromazine 306
cholesterol biosynthesis, inborn errors of 53t
chromosomal/cytogenic microarray (CMA) 46
chromosomal deletions and duplications 103
chromosome analysis 45
Cincinnati Children's Hospital 239
citalopram 310, 312
classroom configuration 150
Clinical Global Impressions (CGI) Severity Scale 300
clomipramine 310, 313
clonidine 301–2, 317
clozapine 306, 308
CMA. *See chromosomal/ cytogenic microarray*
CNTN4 gene 107
CNTNAP2 gene 107
CNV. *See copy number variation*
coarse facies 48
cognitive-behavioral therapy (CBT) 263
cognitive deficits 121
cognitive disintegration 247
cognitive functioning, at older ages 92–93
cognitive skills 29
collaborative services, in natural settings 179
college preparation 236
colors 283
comic strip conversations 283, 283f
communication. *See also augmentative and alternative communication; social communication*
  of experiences 281
  functional 177, 262–63
  initiation of 284
  as motivating factor for challenging behaviors 121
  processes 157
  spontaneous 176
community
  experiences 234
  interventions in 144
  living 244

comorbid disorders 42, 78, 254
  assessments of 56, 58
  diagnostic clarification, identification and treatment of 246–47
  overdiagnosing 68
  pharmacological interventions for 296
complementary and alternative medicine (CAM) 137, 140, 296, 318–19
  IEPs and 144
  interventions 141t
compulsions 75
conduct disorder 45
connections 281
connectome 99
Conners Rating Scale-Revised 128, 300
consequences
  changing 265–66
  direct observation of 119
  in effective interventions 257
Consolidated Waiver 244
constipation 206
consultative services, speech-language therapy and 179
contingencies, for difficulty seating through meals 199
contingent attention condition 130
contingent escape condition 130
contracts 264, 264t
control condition 130
co-occurring disorders 247
coping difficulties 246–47
copy number variation (CNV) 103, 109, 109f
cortical dysplasia 107
cortical dysplasia-focal epilepsy syndrome 54t, 102t
cortical gyration 96
cortical neurons 96
Council on Children with Disabilities in Pediatrics 26–30
craniofacial therapy 141t
creatine deficiency syndromes 53t
crisis plans 245
criterion-referenced curriculum checklist 165
crying 198

CYBOCS-PDD. *See* Children's Yale-Brown Obsessive Compulsive Scale modified for Pervasive Developmental Disorders

D

daily living 235, 243
dangerous activities 71t
DAS. *See* Differential Abilities Scale
data analysis characteristics 124
Dawson, Geraldine 164
deafness, appearance of 22
deep pressure/squeeze machine 141t
dementia infantilis 8–9, 11
Denver Model 137, 165.
  See also Early Start Denver Model
Department of Public Welfare (DPW) 244
depressed mood 70t
depression 45, 247
  diagnosing 69
  NLGN4X and 106
descriptive sentences 282
developmental/academic skills 29
Developmental Behavior Checklist 62t
developmental differences 90
Developmental Individual Difference, Relationship-based model (DIR)/Floortime 167, 186–87
developmentally disabled populations
  assessment rating scales 61t–63t
  interviews 64t–66t
developmental psychology 150, 152
diagnosis 20, 32–33
  accuracy 35
  of ADHD 75, 79
  of anxiety 72–75
  of Asperger's disorder 33–34
  assessments and 32–34
  of bipolar disorder 69
  of catatonia 69
  confirmation of 29–30
  criteria 12–14
  of depression 69
  in early childhood 148–49
  gender and 35
  median age of 22
  of mood disorders 68–75

of OCD 74–75, 79
  of ODD 75–76
  of PDD 34
  primary differential 79
  proposed, in DSM-5, 331–32
Diagnostic and Statistical Manual of Mental Disorders-5 (DSM-5) 4, 14
  childhood disintegrative disorder and 9
  diagnostic criteria in 14
  PDD in 331
  proposed diagnosis in 331–32
  Proposed Draft Revisions to DSM Disorders and New Criteria 14
  subtypes in 88
  Task Force and Work Group 14
Diagnostic and Statistical Manual of Mental Disorders-I (DSM-I) 12
Diagnostic and Statistical Manual of Mental Disorders-II (DSM-II) 12
Diagnostic and Statistical Manual of Mental Disorders-III (DSM-III) 12
Diagnostic and Statistical Manual of Mental Disorders-III-R DSM-III-R) 12
Diagnostic and Statistical Manual of Mental Disorders-IV (DSM-IV) 13
Diagnostic and Statistical Manual of Mental Disorders-IV-TR (DSM-IV-TR) 4
  ADHD medications and 298
  ASD diagnosis 20
  childhood disintegrative disorder and 8–9
  diagnostic criteria 13, 32–34
  domains in 331–32
  Rett disorder and 9
Diagnostic Assessment for the Severely Handicapped-II 65t
diagnostic clarification 246–47
diagnostic evaluation 28–29
diaper rituals 208–11
diarrhea 206
Differential Abilities Scale (DAS) 29

diffusion imaging 99
dihydropyrimidine
    dehydrogenase
    deficiency 54t
diphenhydramine 317
directive sentences 282
direct observation 118–19,
    126, 129t
direct therapy 178–79
DIR/Floortime. *See*
    Developmental Individual
    Difference, Relationship-
    based model/Floortime
discrete trial training
    (DTT) 148, 151,
    154–57
    curriculum and transition
        in 156
    defining features
        of 154–55
    historical and empirical
        base of 155
    key facts 160
    parental role in 156–57
    prerequisites for 155–56
discriminative stimulus 154
disruptive behavior
    disorder 45
distractibility 70t
distractions, in mealtime
    routine 200
divalproex sodium 316–17
domain assessments 28–29
DPW. *See* Department of
    Public Welfare
DSM-5. *See* Diagnostic and
    Statistical Manual of
    Mental Disorders-5
DSM-I. *See* Diagnostic and
    Statistical Manual of
    Mental Disorders-I
DSM-II. *See* Diagnostic and
    Statistical Manual of
    Mental Disorders-II
DSM-III. *See* Diagnostic and
    Statistical Manual of
    Mental Disorders-III
DSM-III-R. *See* Diagnostic
    and Statistical Manual of
    Mental Disorders-III-R
DSM-IV. *See* Diagnostic
    and Statistical Manual of
    Mental Disorders-IV
DSM-IV-TR. *See* Diagnostic
    and Statistical Manual of
    Mental Disorders-IV-TR
DTT. *See* discrete trial
    training
dysgenic lesions 96
dysmorphic features
    46, 100
dysplasic lesions 96
dyssomnias 201, 211

E

early childhood
    interventions 148–49
    additional considerations
        for 153
    defining dimensions
        of 150–52
    degree of
        comprehensiveness
        of 150
    intensity of 150
    interventionists for 151
    location of 150–51
    parent education and
        training in 151
    structure of 151
    supportive materials
        for 151
    theoretical approaches
        to 150
early development 44
early identification 20,
    22–24
early intensive behavioral
    interventions (EIBI)
    154–60
Early Start Denver Model
    (ESDM) 164–66
    curriculum and transition
        in 165–66
    defining features of 164
    early childhood and 148
    empirical research base
        for 164–65
    key facts 166
    parental role in 166
    prerequisites for 165
eating too quickly 197, 199
echoic training 157
echolalia 6, 174
education 219. *See also*
    schools
    character 281
    future advances in 333
    goals 223
    placement options 226
    post-secondary 236
    regular 227t
educational law 218–20
EEG. *See*
    electroencephalography
EIBI. *See* early intensive
    behavioral interventions
Eisenberg, Leon 6
elated mood 71t
electroencephalography
    (EEG) 46–48
elimination record 210t
emotional regulation
    SCERTS model and 186
    techniques 281, 285
emotion dysregulation 99

empathy 23, 161
empirical evidence 153
employment 234, 238–42
    competitive 238
    models 239–42
    secured 238
    strategies 238
    supervision 241t
    supported 238
An Empty Fortress
    (Bettelheim) 10–11
epilepsy 45, 48, 107
EPS. *See* extra-pyramidal
    symptoms
ER. *See* Evaluation Report
ERK/PI3K pathway
    model 106
escape 121
escitalopram 310, 312
ESDM. *See* Early Start
    Denver Model
established evidence 255
established treatments
    255, 256t
etiology 42, 86
evaluation algorithms 26–30,
    26f, 27f
Evaluation Report (ER) 222
Evaluative Method for
    Determining Evidence
    Practice 138
evidence-based
    practice 138, 142–43,
    180–81
exam room 52
executive function
    deficits 11, 272, 277
experimental design 138
extinction 204, 265
extra-pyramidal symptoms
    (EPS) 306
eye contact, avoiding 22

F

facial responsiveness 22
facial weakness 48
faded bedtime
    procedure 203–4
family engagement, DTT
    and 157
family history 45
FAPE. *See* free and
    appropriate public
    education
FBA. *See* functional
    behavioral assessment
fc-MRI. *See* fMRI connectivity
FDA. *See* Food and Drug
    Administration
fear reactions 72
feeding disorders 194,
    196–200, 211

feelings, insights into 281
First Signs, Inc., 23
First Signs for Practitioners (CDC) 22–23
504 plan 216, 219
fixed interests 14
fluency training 160
fluoxetine 310–11
fluvoxamine 310–11
fMRI. See functional Magnetic Resonance Imaging
fMRI connectivity (fc-MRI) 98–100
FOAF. See Functional Observation Assessment Form
food, access to 199
Food and Drug Administration (FDA) 296, 300, 303, 307
food selectivity and/or texture problems 196–98
forebrain connectivity 332
foster care 244
Fragile X syndrome (FXS) 45–46, 48, 54t, 88–89
    ERK/PI3K pathway model and 106
    syndromic ASD and 100, 102
free and appropriate public education (FAPE) 218
Frith, Uta 5
functional analysis 260
Functional Assessment Interview 127t
functional behavioral assessment (FBA) 116
    completion of 121
    conducting 118–19
    core assumption of 120
    instruments 127t–128t
    interviews 118, 126
    necessity of 120–21
    purpose of 120–22
    qualifications for conducting 130–31
    rating scales 126
    setting for 124–29
    suitability of 130–31
    summary chart 125t
functional connectivity 98–99, 332
functional experimental analysis 130
functional Magnetic Resonance Imaging (fMRI) 46, 98–100
Functional Observation Assessment Form (FOAF) 128–29, 129t

G

galactorrhea 308
games, pretend 22
GARS-2. See Gilliam Autism Rating Scale, Second Edition
gastro-esophageal reflux disorder (GERD) 196
gastrointestinal (GI) symptoms 44, 247
gaze 7
gender 35
general health profile 30
generalized anxiety disorder 73–74, 79
genetics 86, 100
    advances in 332
    etiology 42
    factors 10
    models 106–8
    as motivating factor for challenging behaviors 121
    syndromes 45, 48–49, 55
GERD. See gastro-esophageal reflux disorder
gestalt processing 284
GFCF diet. See gluten-free/casein-free diet
Gilliam Asperger's Disorder Scale 290
Gilliam Autism Rating Scale, Second Edition (GARS-2) 28
GI symptoms. See gastrointestinal symptoms
gluten-free/casein-free (GFCF) diet 137, 141t, 318–19
GM. See gray matter
Go Talk 181
grammatical morphemes 187
Grandin, Temple 239
grandiosity 71t
Gray, Carol 282–83
gray matter (GM) 95
Greenspan, Stanley 167
group homes 244
group therapy 281
growth measurements 46
guanfacine 301–2, 317
guanfacine XR (GXR) 301–2
guilt 70t
Gutstein, Steven 167

GXR. See guanfacine XR
gynecomastia 308

H

haloperidol 137, 306
Hanen approach 186
Haslam, John 5
Hawk 181
HBOT. See hyperbaric oxygen treatment
HC. See head circumference
head circumference (HC) 94–95
Head Start 20
Heller, Theodore 8–9, 11
heterotopias 96
high-functioning autism 88
    ABA for 266
    poor jobs for 240
histidinemia 54t
holding therapy 141t
home-based programs
    early childhood 150–51
    education 226
    PRT and 161–62
housing options 244–45
human relatedness 284
humor 284
hyperactivity 298, 303–4
hyperbaric oxygen treatment (HBOT) 141t
hypersomnia 70t
hypothesis statement 124
hypothesis testing 130

I

ICD-10. See International Classification of Diseases-10
ID. See intellectual disability
IDEA. See Individuals with Disabilities Education Act
IEPs. See individual education plans
ignoring 265
ILAUGH model of social cognition 284
IMGSAC. See International Molecular Genetic Study of Autism Consortium
immunizations 50
immunoglobulin therapy 141t
impulsivity 298
inappropriate sexual behaviors (ISB) 314
inattention 298
incidental teaching 262
indecision 71t
independence skills 236, 243

individual education plans
(IEPs) 120, 144, 216
annual review 223–24
checklist 224t
document 223
IDEA and 218
meeting 223
process 222–25
referrals 222
social skills teaching in 280
transition planning 225
Individual Support Plan
(ISP) 244
Individuals with Disabilities
Education Act
(IDEA) 120, 136, 216,
218, 234, 248
*Infantile Autism: The
Syndrome and Its
Implications for a Neural
Theory of Behavior*
(Rimland) 11
infantile ceroid
lipofuscinosis 53t
infants
premature 91
at risk 90–91
informant
questionnaires 59–60
information-processing
demands 92
initiation, of
communication 284
insomnia 70t
intellectual disability (ID) 4,
42, 100, 107
intellectual distortion 247
interest, indication of 22
International Classification
of Diseases-10 (ICD-
10) 8–9
International Molecular
Genetic Study of
Autism Consortium
(IMGSAC) 104
interventions. *See also* early
childhood interventions
for adolescents 254
for bedtime
resistance 203–4
CAM 141t
category levels of 138
child 254
in communities 144
components of 257
development and
research 153
for difficulty seating
through meals 198–99
for eating too quickly 199
emerging 220
established 220
examples 257t

food selectivity and/or
texture problems 198
function of behavior in
determining 258
intensive behavioral 142
language 174–75,
180–83, 180t
National Standards Project
and 220
naturalistic
behavioral 160–67, 187
for nighttime
awakenings 204
overeating 199
overview of 136–37
pharmacological 137, 296
for sleep
disturbances 202–4
social cognition 284–85
social narrative 282–84
social skills 290–92
speech-language 180–83,
180t
toileting issues 207–11
unestablished 220
interviews 60, 64t–66t
employment 238
in FBA 118, 126
informant 60
intraverbal training 157
irritability 70t, 303, 307–8
ISB. *See* inappropriate sexual
behaviors
ischemic events 91
ISP. *See* Individual Support
Plan
Itard, Jean Marc Gaspard
5, 11

J

job-finding 238–42
joint-play routines 166
Joubert syndrome 54t, 102t

K

K-ABC. *See* Kaufman-
Assessment Battery for
Children
Kanner, Leo 5–6, 11
Asperger vs., 8–9, 8t
psychogenic theory
and 10
Kansas FBA Interview 127t
Kaufman-Assessment
Battery for Children
(K-ABC) 29
Kiddie Schedule for
Affective Disorder
and Schizophrenia
(K-SADS) 60

Klinger, Laura 10
Koegel Autism Center 162
K-SADS. *See* Kiddie
Schedule for Affective
Disorder and
Schizophrenia

L

laboratory workup 46–47
lamotrigine 316–17
Lancet 50
Landau-Kleffner
syndrome 44
language 29. *See also*
speech-language therapy;
spoken language
assessments 29, 176
AVB and 157–58
classification of 157
comprehension of 176
deficits 92
development 22–23
inferential 284
interventions 174–75,
180–83, 180t
natural 161
proficiency 174–75
therapy 144, 179
lead levels 45
LEAP. *See* Learning
Experiences: an
Alternative Program
for preschoolers and
parents
learning
observational 156
structured 262
Learning Experiences: an
Alternative Program
for preschoolers and
parents (LEAP) 136–37,
162–64, 166
curriculum and transition
in 163–64
defining features
of 162–63
empirical research base
for 163
parental role in 164
Learn the Signs - Act Early
(CDC) 22–23
least restrictive environment
(LRE) 218, 226
Leucine rich repeat (LRR)
family 107
LIFE. *See* Lovaas Institute for
Early Intervention
Lindsley, Ogden 160
listening 284
living arrangements 244
Lord, Catherine 8
Lovaas, Ivar 155

Lovaas Institute for Early Intervention (LIFE) 155–56
LRE. *See* least restrictive environment
LRR family. *See* Leucine rich repeat family

M

macrocephaly 6, 48
Magnetic Resonance Imaging (MRI) 46–47, 99
Mahler, Margaret 10
Mahoney, Gerald 167
Maine Department of Education 138
Maine Department of Health and Human Services (DHHS) 138, 140
    CAM treatments and 140, 318–19
    categories of 254
    established evidence 256t
    treatment recommendations 254–55
Maine DHHS. *See* Maine Department of Health and Human Services
maintaining variable, of behaviors 120
mands 157, 188
manners 235
manual signing 182
MAS. *See* Motivation Assessment Scale
MASS. *See* Mood and Anxiety Semi-Structured Interview for Patients with Intellectual Disabilities
massage therapy 141t
masturbation, excessive 314
Maudsley Henry 5
McCarthy Scales of Children's Ability (MSCA) 29
M-CHAT. *See* Modified Checklist for Autism in Toddlers
meals, difficulty sitting through 197–99
mealtime routines 198–200
MeCP2 gene 9
medical evaluations 30, 42
medical history 44–45, 48–49
medications. *See also* pharmacological interventions
    ADHD 298–305
    as antecedents 260–61

antianxiety 314–15
anticonvulsant 316–17
antidepressant 310–15
antipsychotic 306–9
atypical
    antipsychotic 302–3, 304
    common 296
    mood stabilizing antiepileptic 316–17
    multiple 318
    off-label 296
    overeating and 199
    side effects from 302
    sleep 317
    stimulant 299–300, 304
    timing of 198
mega-vitamin therapy 11
melatonin 317
meltdowns 258, 259t
memory 92
Mendelian mutations 104
menstruation 44–45
mental retardation 4
Mesibov, Gary 10
metabolic etiology 42
metabolic/mitochondrial workup 46–47
MET gene 106
methylphenidate (MPH) 299–300
microcephaly 48
mimetic training 157
mind blindness. *See* theory of mind deficit
mind types 239–40
minicolumns 96
mirtazapine 310, 314
MMR vaccine. *See* mumps, measles, rubella vaccine
MO. *See* motivative operation
Modified Checklist for Autism in Toddlers (M-CHAT) 27–28
Modified Simond & Parraga Sleep Questionnaire 202
molecular cascade 106, 108
Mood and Anxiety Semi-Structured Interview for Patients with Intellectual Disabilities (MASS) 65t
mood disorders 68–75, 70t–71t, 79
mood stabilizers 316–17
morphometric studies 94
motivating operations 257–58, 260–61
motivation
    assessment 157
    PRT and 161

social 278
Motivation Assessment Scale (MAS) 127t
motivative operation (MO) 154
motor apraxia 182
motor skills 29, 92
movement disorders 48, 247
MPH. *See* methylphenidate
MRI. *See* Magnetic Resonance Imaging
MSCA. *See* McCarthy Scales of Children's Ability
MSCS. *See* Multidimensional Self Concept Scale
Multidimensional Self Concept Scale (MSCS) 290
Multimodal Treatment Study for Children with ADHD 299
multiple cues, responsiveness to 161
mumps, measles, rubella (MMR) vaccine 50
music therapy 141t
mutations 104, 106–7, 110

N

NAC. *See* National Autism Center
narrative discourse 189
NaSSAs. *See* noradrenergic and specific serotonergic antidepressants
National Autism Center (NAC) 138
    CAM treatments and 140, 318–19
    established treatments 256t
    PRT and 161
    treatment recommendations 254–55
National Standards Project 138, 220, 254–55
natural language paradigm 161
neurexins 106–7
neurobiology 86, 94–96
neurodevelopmental disorders 90–91
neurofibromatosis type 1 (NF1) 106
neuroimaging 98
neuroligins 106
neurological exam 46
neurological functioning 92–93

neuro-metabolic
    disorders 53t–54t
neuronal migration 93, 110
neuronal organization 91,
    93, 110
*New England Journal of
    Medicine* 303
NF1. *See* neurofibromatosis
    type 1
nighttime awakenings 204
Nisonger Child Behavior
    Rating Form 290
NLGN3, 106
NLGN4X 106
No Child Left Behind 218
non-syndromic ASD 95–96,
    100, 104, 109
noradrenergic and
    specific serotonergic
    antidepressants
    (NaSSAs) 310
NOS. *See* not otherwise
    specified
not otherwise specified
    (NOS) 12
NRXN1, 106–7
nursing homes 244
nutritional supplements
    137, 141t

O

observational learning 156
obsessive-compulsive
    disorder (OCD) 45, 247
  brain-behavior correlations
    in 99
  CNTNAP2 gene and 107
  diagnosing 74–75
  primary differential
    diagnosis
    considerations for 79
occupational therapy
    (OT) 29, 144, 196
OCD. *See* obsessive-
    compulsive disorder
ODD. *See* oppositional
    defiant disorder
Office of Intellectual
    Disability (OID) 244
Office of Vocational
    Rehabilitation
    (OVR) 238
office visits. *See* pediatric
    office visits
OID. *See* Office of
    Intellectual Disability
Olanzapine 306, 308
operants 188
oppositional defiant disorder
    (ODD) 45, 75–76, 79
Options therapy 141t
organization skills 236

OT. *See* occupational
    therapy
overactivity, during
    mealtimes 198
overeating 197, 199
OVR. *See* Office of
    Vocational Rehabilitation

P

pain 47
panic disorder 73, 79
parasomnias 201, 211
parent questionnaires 59–60
parents
  AVB and 159
  DTT and 156–57
  education and training 151
  ESDM and 166
  evidence-based treatments
    and 142
  IEPs and 222–23
  interviews with 60
  LEAP and 164
  living with 244
  PRT and 162
  questions for 142–43
  telephone conferences
    with 52
PAS-ADD checklist. *See*
    Psychiatric Assessment
    Schedule for Adults
    with Developmental
    Disabilities checklist
The Pathology of Mind
    (Maudsley) 5
pathophysiology 86, 94–96,
    110
pattern thinkers 239
payment for services 153
PBS. *See* positive behavior
    support
PDD. *See* pervasive
    developmental disorder
PDDNOS. *See* pervasive
    developmental disorder-
    not otherwise specified
PDDST. *See* Pervasive
    Developmental Disorder
    Screening Test
PECS. *See* Picture Exchange
    Communication System
pediatric office visits 52
Pediatrics 50
peer-mediation, speech-
    language therapy
    and 179
peer mentoring 236
peer-to-peer support
    programs 243
Pennsylvania Autism
    Diagnostic
    Workgroup 26–30, 27f

performance deficits 262,
    290–91
perseverative
    utterances 174
personal care homes 244
personal hygiene 235, 243
personal space 52
Person/Family Directed
    Support (PFDS) 244
perspective sentences 282
perspective taking 284
pervasive developmental
    disorder (PDD) 4,
    12–13, 20, 34, 331
pervasive developmental
    disorder-not otherwise
    specified (PDDNOS) 88
Pervasive Developmental
    Disorder Screening Test
    (PDDST) 28
PET. *See* positron emission
    tomography
PFDS. *See* Person/Family
    Directed Support
pharmacological
    interventions 137, 296.
    See also medications
phenylketonuria 53t
physical exam 30, 46, 48–49
physical therapy (PT) 29,
    144
physiology 121
pica 45
Picture Exchange
    Communication System
    (PECS) 136, 182–83,
    184t, 255
pivotal response training
    (PRT) 160–62, 166, 187
  curriculum and transition
    in 161–62
  empirical research base
    for 161
  ESDM and 165
  parental role in 162
  prerequisites for 161
players, in transition
    planning 235
play skills 29
PMDD. *See* premenstrual
    dysphoric disorder
PMS. *See* pre-menstrual
    symptoms
point cards 264, 265t
polypharmacy 318
polysomnography
    (PSG) 202
positive behavior support
    (PBS) 117
positive behavior support
    plans 119, 124, 219
positron emission
    tomography (PET) 98

Potocki-Lupski
    syndrome 102t
Prader Willi syndrome 54t
pragmatics 174, 188
premenstrual dysphoric
    disorder (PMDD) 45
pre-menstrual symptoms
    (PMS) 45
prepositions 187
preschool programs 136–37
Prizant, Barry 167
Problem Behavior
    Questionnaire 127
Project SEARCH 239
PRT. See pivotal response
    training
PSG. See polysomnography
Psychiatric Assessment
    Schedule for Adults
    with Developmental
    Disabilities (PAS-ADD)
    checklist 62t, 65t
psychiatric disorders 58–60,
    68–74
psychogenic theory 10–11
psychomotor agitation 70t
psychosis, child 6
psychosocial masking 247
psychotherapy 281
PT. See physical therapy
Public Law 94-142, 136,
    216, 218
pull-out therapy 178–79
Purkinje neurons 95–96

Q

Quality Inclusion
    Curriculum 163–64
quetiapine 306, 308

R

race 22
racing thoughts 71t
rating scales
    for assessments 61t–63t
    behavior 127t
    FBA 126
    self 285, 287f
RDI. See Relationship
    Development
    Intervention
reading
    comprehension 174–75
referrals 47
    for IEPs 222
    to SLP 175
regurgitation 198
Rehabilitation Act of
    1973, 219
reinforcers 266
    changing 264

for difficulty seating
    through meals 199
motivating operations
    and 258
in PECS 183
Reiss Scales for Children's
    Dual Diagnosis 63t
Reiss Screen for Maladaptive
    Behavior 63t
related services 234
Relationship Development
    Intervention (RDI) 167,
    187
research, future 332
residential living 244
response cost 266
Responsive Teaching 167
Rett, Andreas 9
Rett disorder 8–9, 49,
    88–89, 102t
    in DSM-IV-TR 13
    ERK/PI3K pathway model
    and 106
    syndromic ASD and 100
"A Review of the
    State of Science for
    Pediatric Adolescent
    Medicine," 24
Rimland, Bernard 11
risperidone 296, 303–4, 306
Rogers, Sally 164
role play 283
RUPP Autism Network 307
Rutter, Michael 10–11

S

SAL. See System for
    Augmenting Language
sameness, insistence on 6,
    76, 241
Sanfilippo syndrome 53t
SAPPA. See Schedule for the
    Assessment of Psychiatric
    Problems Associated
    with Autism
SC. See Supports
    Coordinator
scaffolding proteins 107
scatter plots 128, 129t
SCERTS model. See Social
    Communication,
    Emotional Regulation and
    Transactional Support
    model
Schedule for Affective
    Disorder and
    Schizophrenia-Lifetime
    Version (SADS-LA) 60
Schedule for the Assessment
    of Psychiatric Problems
    Associated with Autism
    (SAPPA) 66t

schedules. See visual
    schedules
schizophrenia 5–6, 12, 247
schools
    classroom configuration
    in 150
    college preparation
    and 236
    IEPs and 144
    options 143
    placement in 226–27
    preschool programs
    136–37
    support services in 218–19
Scientific Merit Rating
    Scale 138
SCQ. See Social
    Communication
    Questionnaire
screenings 24, 27–28, 35.
    See also assessments
Screening Tool for Autism
    at Two-Year-Olds
    (STAT) 28
secretin 137, 141t
seizures 247
    nocturnal 201
    risk of 42
    syndromic ASD and 100
selective serotonin reuptake
    inhibitors (SSRIs) 310
self-advocacy 236, 245
self-initiated question-
    asking 187
self-management 161
self-rating scales 285, 287f
self-report
    questionnaires 58–59
sensory integration
    therapy 141t
sensory-motor skills 29
sensory perception 92, 242
sensory stimulation
    121–22
sentence types 282
separation anxiety 72–73, 79
serotonin-norepinephrine
    reuptake inhibitors
    (SNRIs) 310
sertraline 310, 312–13
setting events. See
    motivating operations
SHANK3, 106–7
shaping 198, 208
Shea, Victoria 10
side effects
    of antipsychotic
    medications 308–9
    to fluoxetine 311
    to fluvoxamine 311
    of GXR 302
    of haloperidol 306
    of risperidone 307

sitting
  for meals 197–99
  refusal to 208
situation options
  consequences choices
    strategy simulation
    (SOCCSS) 285, 287*f*
16p11 deletion 55*t*, 102*t*
skill-acquisition deficits
  262, 290
skills. *See also specific skills*
  break down of 155–56
  DTT and 154
  elementary 92, 110
  enhanced 92
  generalization of 156, 159
skin 46
Skinner, B. F. 150
sleep association
  problems 204
sleep diaries 202–3
sleep disorders 247
sleep disturbances 194,
  201–4, 211
  assessments 202
  common 202*t*
  interventions 202–3
  medications 317
  vulnerability for 201–2
sleep hygiene guidelines 203
sleep issues 44
sleep-wake cycle 201, 203
Slit proteins 108
SLP. *See* speech-language
  pathologist
Smith-Lemli-Optiz
  syndrome 102*t*
Smith-Magenis
  syndrome 100
snacks 200
SNAP-IV Hyperactivity-
  Impulsivity subscale 301
SNRIs. *See* serotonin-
  norepinephrine reuptake
  inhibitors
SOCCSS. *See* situation
  options consequences
  choices strategy
  simulation
social autopsy 285, 286*f*
social cognition
  interventions 284–85
social communication 189
  deficits 14
  impairment 174
  language difficulties 22
  PECS and 183
  SCERTS model and 186
Social Communication,
  Emotional Regulation and
  Transactional Support
  (SCERTS) model 167,
  186–87

Social Communication
  Questionnaire
  (SCQ) 27, 290
social competency
  training 243
social context 281
social development
  theories 276–77
social initiation 278
social interactions 29
  components of 280
  LEAP and 162
social motivation 278
social narrative
  strategies 281–84
social phobia 74, 79
social problem solving 281,
  284–85
social relatedness 274
Social Responsiveness Scale
  (SRS) 27, 290
social scripting 283–84
social skills
  assessments 290
  deficits 121
  IEPs and 144
  importance of 274
  programs 290–93
  teaching 280–81
  training 142, 272
Social Stories 187
social stories 188, 282
socioeconomic status 22
somatic therapy 141*t*
Son-Rise therapy 141*t*
specific phobia 74, 79
speech
  acquisition 6
  Asperger's disorder and 7
  assessments 29, 176
speech-language
  interventions 180–83, 180*t*
speech-language pathologist
  (SLP) 174–75
  ASHA guidelines for 180
  challenging behavior
    assessments and 177
  evidence-based practice
    and 180–81
speech-language
  therapy 144, 196
  models of service delivery
    for 178–79, 178*t*
  traditional 188–89
spoken language 174–75
  AAC and 181
  development 189
  PECS and 183
SRS. *See* Social
  Responsiveness Scale
SSRIs. *See* selective
  serotonin reuptake
  inhibitors

stakeholders, in transition
  planning 235
Stanford Binet Intelligence
  Scales, Fifth Edition 29
STAT. *See* Screening Tool
  for Autism at Two-
  Year-Olds
stem cell therapy 141*t*
stereotypy 6
stimulants 260–61,
  299–300, 304
stimulus fading
  strategies 204
Strain, Phillip 163
Strattera 300–301
strokes 91
structured learning 262
Student-Assisted
  Functional Assessment
  Interview 127*t*
subtypes, severity-based
  diagnostic 88
succinic semialdehyde
  dehydrogenase
  deficiency 54*t*
suicidal ideation/
  behavior 70*t*
support groups 142
supportive materials,
  for early childhood
  interventions 151
Supports Coordinator
  (SC) 244
susceptibility loci 104
swallowing skills 196
syndromic ASD 100,
  102–3, 109
systematic observation 126
System for Augmenting
  Language (SAL) 181–83

T

tact 157, 188
tantrums
  distinctions between
    meltdowns and 258,
    259*t*
  feeding problems and 198
  toileting issues and 207
tardive dyskinesia 308
TEACCH model.
  See Treatment and
  Education of Autistic and
  Communication-related
  handicapped Children
  model
teaching
  alternative behaviors
    262–63
  formats 156
  incidental 262
  precision 160

teaching (cont'd)
SAL 182
social skills 280–81
TechSpeak 181
TechTalk 181
telephone conferences 52
theory of mind deficit 11,
272, 276
thimerosal 50
thioridazine 306
thought bubbles 283
tic disorders 247
time management 236
time-outs 265
Timothy syndrome 54t, 102t
toileting issues 194,
206–11, 235
toilet training 209t
elimination record 210t
schedule and
independent 206–8
token economy 264
topographies 188
Total Communication 182
Tourette's syndrome 106
tractography 99
transactional support
(TS) 186
transition-age 232
training 234–35
transition planning 235, 248
across all age groups
241–42
social competency training
and 243
trauma 121
Treatment and Education
of Autistic and
Communication-related
handicapped Children
(TEACCH) model 136,
187, 239
treatments. See also
interventions
categorization of 333
established 255, 256t

teams 145
triggers. See antecedents
TS. See transactional support
TSC. See tuberous sclerosis
complex
tube-dependency 197
tuberous sclerosis complex
(TSC) 48–49, 54t, 88
ERK/PI3K pathway model
and 106
syndromic ASD and 100,
102, 103t
22q deletion syndrome
55t, 102t
2q37 deletion 55t

U

underconnectivity 98–99

V

VB MAPP. See Verbal
Behavior Milestones
Assessment and
Placement Program
venlafaxine 310, 314
verbal behavior 157
Verbal Behavior Milestones
Assessment and
Placement Program
(VB MAPP) 158–59
Victor, the wild boy of
Aveyron 5, 11
video modeling 188–89, 281
violence, unusual 71t
vision therapy 141t
visual cues 188
visual-graphic symbols 182
visual schedules
for bedtime routines 205t
for toilet training 208
transition planning
and 241
visual strategies 281

visual supports 285, 288f
visual thinkers 239
vitamins 11, 137, 141t
VOCA. See Voice Output
Communication Aid
vocational evaluation 235
vocational training 144
Voice Output
Communication Aid
(VOCA) 181
Volkmar, Fred 8
vomiting 198

W

Wakefield, Andrew 50
Walden Program 137
warning signs 20
Wechsler Intelligence Scale
for Children-IV 29
Wechsler Preschool and
Primary Scale
of Intelligence
(WPPSI) 29
weight gain 71t, 307–9
Wetherby, Amy 167
white matter (WM)
95, 99
Wieder, Serena 167
Wing, Lorna 7
WM. See white matter
Woodcock Johnson
Cognitive Abilities III 29
Wood's lamp 46
word bubbles 283
word fact thinkers 239
worrying 74
WPPSI. See Wechsler
Preschool and Primary
Scale of Intelligence
Wyatt vs. Stickney 136

Z

ziprasidone 306, 308